Emerging Respiratory Infections in the 21st Century

Guest Editors

ALIMUDDIN ZUMLA, FRCP, PhD(Lond), FRCPath
WING-WAI YEW, MBBS, FRCP (Edinb), FCCP
DAVID S.C. HUI, MD(UNSW), FRACP, FRCP

INFECTIOUS DISEASE CLINICS OF NORTH AMERICA

www.id.theclinics.com

Consulting Editor
ROBERT C. MOELLERING Jr, MD

September 2010 • Volume 24 • Number 3

SAUNDERS an imprint of ELSEVIER, Inc.

W.B. SAUNDERS COMPANY

A Division of Elsevier Inc.

1600 John F. Kennedy Blvd., Suite 1800, Philadelphia, PA 19103-2899.

http://www.theclinics.com

INFECTIOUS DISEASE CLINICS OF NORTH AMERICA Volume 24, Number 3
September 2010 ISSN 0891-5520, ISBN-13: 978-1-4377-2460-8

Editor: Barbara Cohen-Kligerman

Infectious Disease Clinics of North America (ISSN 0891-5520) is published in March, June, September, and December by Elsevier Inc., 360 Park Avenue South, New York, NY 10010-1710. Periodicals postage paid at New York, NY and additional mailing offices. Subscription prices are $235.00 per year for US individuals, $395.00 per year for US institutions, $118.00 per year for US students, $278.00 per year for Canadian individuals, $489.00 per year for Canadian institutions, $332.00 per year for international individuals, $489.00 per year for international institutions, and $163.00 per year for Canadian and international students. To receive student rate, orders must be accompanied by name of affiliated institution, date of term, and the *signature* of program/residency coordinator on institution letterhead. Orders will be billed at individual rate until proof of status is received. Foreign air speed delivery is included in all *Clinics* subscription prices. All prices are subject to change without notice. **POSTMASTER**: Send address changes to *Infectious Disease Clinics of North America*, Elsevier Health Sciences Division, Subcription Customer Service, 3251 Riverport Lane, Maryland Heights, MO 63043. **Customer Service: 1-800-654-2452 (US). From outside of the US and Canada, call 1-314-447-8871. Fax: 1-314-447-8029. E-mail: JournalsCustomerService-usa@elsevier.com (print support) or JournalsOnlineSupport-usa@elsevier.com (online support).**

Infectious Disease Clinics of North America is also published in Spanish by Editorial Inter-Médica, Junin 917, 1ᵉʳ A 1113, Buenos Aires, Argentina.

Reprints. For copies of 100 or more of articles in this publication, please contact the Commercial Reprints Department, Elsevier Inc., 360 Park Avenue South, New York, New York 10010-1710. Tel. (212) 633-3812, Fax: (212) 462-1935, E-mail: reprints@elsevier.com.

Infectious Disease Clinics of North America is covered in *MEDLINE/PubMed (Index Medicus), Current Contents/Clinical Medicine, Science Citation Alert, SCISEARCH,* and *Research Alert.*

Printed and bound by CPI Group (UK) Ltd, Croydon, CR0 4YY

Transferred to Digital Print 2011

Contributors

CONSULTING EDITOR

ROBERT C. MOELLERING JR, MD
Shields Warren-Mallinckrodt Professor of Medical Research, Harvard Medical School;
Department of Medicine, Beth Israel Deaconess Medical Center, Boston, Massachusetts

GUEST EDITORS

ALIMUDDIN ZUMLA, FRCP, PhD(Lond), FRCPath
Professor, Department of Infection, Centre for Infectious Diseases and International
Health, Windeyer Institute of Medical Sciences, University College London Medical
School, London, United Kingdom

WING-WAI YEW, MBBS, FRCP (Edinb), FCCP
Professor, Tuberculosis and Chest Unit, Grantham Hospital, Hong Kong, China

DAVID S.C. HUI, MD (UNSW), FRACP, FRCP
Professor and Head, Division of Respiratory Medicine; Director, Stanley Ho Center for
Emerging Infectious Diseases, The Chinese University of Hong Kong, Shatin,
New Territories, Hong Kong, China

AUTHORS

TREVOR P. ANDERSON, MSc
Microbiology Unit, Canterbury Health Laboratories, Christchurch, New Zealand

NIRANJAN BHAT, MD
Division of Infectious Diseases, Department of Pediatrics, Johns Hopkins School
of Medicine, Baltimore, Maryland

LAURENCE BRUNET, BSc
Department of Epidemiology, Biostatistics and Occupational Health, McGill University,
Montreal, Quebec, Canada

PAUL K.S. CHAN, MD, FRCPath
Professor, Department of Microbiology, The Chinese University of Hong Kong,
Shatin, New Territories, Hong Kong, China

DOO RYEON CHUNG, MD, PhD
Division of Infectious Diseases, Samsung Medical Center, Sungkyunkwan University
School of Medicine, Seoul, Korea

KEERTAN DHEDA, MBBcH, FCP(SA), FCCP, PhD(Lond), FRCP(Lond)
Lung Infection and Immunity Unit, Division of Pulmonology and Clinical Immunology
& UCT Lung Institute, Department of Medicine; Institute of Infectious Diseases and
Molecular Medicine, University of Cape Town, Cape Town, South Africa;

Centre for Infectious Diseases and International Health, Department of Infection, UCL Medical School, London, United Kingdom

STEVE DUNCAN, MD
Associate Professor, Division of Pulmonary, Allergy, and Critical Care Medicine, University of Pittsburgh, Pittsburgh, Pennsylvania

JEFF GLASSROTH, MD
Vice Dean and Chief Academic Officer, Professor of Medicine, Division of Pulmonary and Critical Care, Department of Medicine, Feinberg School of Medicine, Northwestern University, Chicago, Illinois

MARTIN P. GROBUSCH, MD, MSc, DTM&H, FRCP(Lond)
Infectious Diseases, Tropical Medicine and AIDS, Amsterdam Medical Centre, University of Amsterdam, The Netherlands; Medical Research Unit, Albert Schweitzer Hospital, Lambaréné, Gabon

K.L. ELLIS HON, MD, FAAP, FCCM
Professor, Department of Paediatrics, The Chinese University of Hong Kong, Shatin, Hong Kong Special Administrative Region, China

LI YANG HSU, MBBS, MRCP, MPH
Department of Medicine, National University Health System, Singapore

DAVID S.C. HUI, MD (UNSW), FRACP, FRCP
Professor and Head, Division of Respiratory Medicine; Director, Stanley Ho Center for Emerging Infectious Diseases, The Chinese University of Hong Kong, Shatin, New Territories, Hong Kong, China

LANCE C. JENNINGS, PhD, FRCPath
Department of Pathology, University of Otago Christchurch; Microbiology Unit, Canterbury Health Laboratories, Christchurch, New Zealand

TAREK KILANI, MD
Professor of Thoracic and Cardiovascular Surgery, Medical School, Tunis; Head, Department of Thoracic and Cardiovascular Surgery, Abderrahmane Mami Teaching Hospital, Ariana, Tunisia

LIANG PIU KOH, MBBS, MRCP
Department of Hematology/Oncology, National University Health System, Singapore, Singapore

TOMMY T.Y. LAM, PhD
Postgraduate Researcher, School of Biological Sciences, The University of Hong Kong, Hong Kong Special Administrative Region, China

CHI CHIU LEUNG, MBBS, FCCP
TB and Chest Service, Department of Health, Wanchai Chest Clinic, Wanchai, Hong Kong, China

DAPHNE LING, MPH
Respiratory Epidemiology and Clinical Research Unit, Montreal Chest Institute, McGill University, Montreal, Quebec, Canada

BEN J. MARAIS, MRCP (Paed UK), FCP (Paed SA), MMed (Paed), PhD
Professor, Department of Paediatrics and Child Health, Faculty of Health Sciences,
Tygerberg Children's Hospital, Stellenbosch University, Tygerberg, South Africa

DICK MENZIES, MD, MSc
Professor, Respiratory Epidemiology and Clinical Research Unit, Montreal Chest Institute,
McGill University, Montreal, Quebec, Canada

TORU MORI, MD, PhD
Director Emeritus, Research Institute of Tuberculosis, Japan Anti-Tuberculosis
Association, Kiyose, Tokyo, Japan

DAVID R. MURDOCH, MD, MSc, DTM&H, FRACP, FRCPA
Department of Pathology, University of Otago Christchurch; Microbiology Unit,
Canterbury Health Laboratories, Christchurch, New Zealand

ESTHER SHU-TING NG, MBBS
Department of Medicine, National University Health System, Singapore

SHAWN P.E. NISHI, MD
Fellow, Division of Pulmonary and Critical Care Medicine, University of Texas Medical
Branch, Galveston, Texas

MADHUKAR PAI, MD, PhD
Department of Epidemiology, Biostatistics and Occupational Health, McGill University,
Montreal, Quebec, Canada

H. SIMON SCHAAF, MMed (Paed), MD (Paed)
Professor, Department of Paediatrics and Child Health, Faculty of Health Sciences,
Tygerberg Children's Hospital, Stellenbosch University, Tygerberg, South Africa

NEIL W. SCHLUGER, MD
Chief, Division of Pulmonary, Allergy, and Critical Care Medicine, Professor of Medicine,
Epidemiology and Environmental Health Sciences, Columbia University College
of Physicians and Surgeons, New York, New York

NANDINI SHETTY, MSc, MD, FRCPath
Consultant Microbiologist, Department of Clinical Microbiology, University College
London Hospitals, Windeyer Institute of Medical Sciences, London, United Kingdom

JAE-HOON SONG, MD, PhD
Division of Infectious Diseases, Samsung Medical Center, Sungkyunkwan University
School of Medicine; Asian-Pacific Foundation for Infectious Diseases (APFID), Seoul,
Korea

BABAFEMI TAIWO, MBBS
Assistant Professor of Medicine, Division of Infectious Diseases, Department of Medicine,
Feinberg School of Medicine, Northwestern University, Chicago, Illinois

JULIAN W. TANG, PhD, MRCP, FRCPath
Consultant/Virologist, Divisions of Microbiology and Molecular Diagnosis Centre,
Department of Laboratory Medicine, National University Hospital, Singapore

VINCENT G. VALENTINE, MD
Professor, Internal Medicine; Director, Lung Transplantation; Medical Director, Division of Pulmonary and Critical Care Medicine, Texas Transplant Center, University of Texas Medical Branch, Galveston, Texas

RICHARD N. VAN ZYL-SMIT, MBChB, MRCP(UK)
Lung Infection and Immunity Unit, Division of Pulmonology and UCT Lung Institute, Department of Medicine, University of Cape Town, Cape Town, South Africa

VANNAN KANDI VIJAYAN, MD, PhD, DSc
Director, Vallabhbhai Patel Chest Institute; Head, Department of Respiratory Medicine, Vallabhbhai Patel Chest Institute, University of Delhi, Delhi, India

ROBERT S. WALLIS, MD, FIDSA
Senior Director, Pfizer, New London, Connecticut; Associate Professor, Department of Medicine, UMDNJ-New Jersey School of Medicine, Newark, New Jersey; Associate Professor, Department of Medicine, Case School of Medicine, Cleveland, Ohio

ROBIN M. WARREN, PhD
DST/NRF Centre of Excellence for Biomedical Tuberculosis Research/MRC Centre for Molecular and Cellular Biology, Division of Molecular Biology and Human Genetics, Faculty of Health Sciences, Stellenbosch University, Tygerberg, South Africa

WING-WAI YEW, MBBS, FRCP (Edinb), FCCP
Professor, Tuberculosis and Chest Unit, Grantham Hospital, Hong Kong, China

ALIMUDDIN ZUMLA, FRCP, PhD(Lond), FRCPath
Professor, Department of Infection, Centre for Infectious Diseases and International Health, Windeyer Institute of Medical Sciences, University College London Medical School, London, United Kingdom

Contents

> Kidney, liver, heart, pancreas, lung, and small intestine transplantations are viable therapeutic options for patients with end-stage organ failure. Ongoing advancements of surgical techniques, immunosuppressive regimens, and perioperative management have resulted in improved survival of allograft recipients. Despite these refinements, infections still contribute to substantial morbidity and mortality, limiting long-term success rates of these procedures. This article discusses the emerging bacterial, fungal, and viral respiratory infections in transplantation.

> Fungal pulmonary infections are becoming more prevalent as a consequence of the rising prevalence of immunocompromised patients. Besides ubiquitous opportunistic fungi such as *Aspergillus* spp and geographically delimited mycoses, fungi that were previously thought to be of uncertain pathogenicity, such as hyaline and dematiaceous molds, are increasingly being diagnosed as the causes of invasive disease in profoundly immunosuppressed hosts. Overall progress in the clinical management of fungal pulmonary infections has been slow compared with other areas of infectious diseases. However, recent encouraging advances in fungal diagnostics and therapeutics have resulted in improved clinical outcomes, particularly in vulnerable patient populations such as solid organ or allogeneic hematopoietic stem cell transplant recipients. This article provides an overview of endemic mycoses and other emerging fungal pulmonary infections. Recent developments in terms of the diagnosis and clinical management of these infections are also discussed.

> Many lung infestations from established and newly emerging parasites have been reported as a result of the emergence of HIV/AIDS, the increasing use of immunosuppressive drugs, increasing organ transplantations, the increase in global travel, and climate change. A renewed interest in parasitic lung infections has been observed recently because many protozoal and helminthic parasites cause clinically significant lung diseases. The diseases caused by these parasites may mimic common and complicated lung diseases ranging from asymptomatic disease to acute respiratory distress syndrome requiring critical care management. The availability of new molecular diagnostic methods and antiparasitic drugs enables early

diagnosis and prompt treatment to avoid the morbidity and mortality associated with these infestations. Good hygiene practices, improvement in socioeconomic conditions, vector control measures, and consumption of hygienically prepared and properly cooked food are essential to reduce the occurrence of parasitic infestations.

Influenza viruses continue to cause yearly epidemics and occasional pandemics in humans. In recent years, the threat of a possible influenza pandemic arising from the avian influenza A(H5N1) virus has prompted the development of comprehensive pandemic preparedness programs in many countries. The recent emergence of the pandemic influenza A(H1N1) 2009 virus from the Americas in early 2009, although surprising in its geographic and zoonotic origins, has tested these preparedness programs and revealed areas in which further work is necessary. Nevertheless, the plethora of epidemiologic, diagnostic, mathematical and phylogenetic modeling, and investigative methodologies developed since the severe acute respiratory syndrome outbreak of 2003 and the subsequent sporadic human cases of avian influenza have been applied effectively and rapidly to the emergence of this novel pandemic virus. This article summarizes some of the findings from such investigations, including recommendations for the management of patients infected with this newly emerged pathogen.

Severe acute respiratory syndrome (SARS) is a highly infectious disease with a significant morbidity and mortality. Respiratory failure is the major complication, and patients may progress to acute respiratory distress syndrome. Health care workers are particularly vulnerable to SARS. SARS has the potential of being converted from droplet to airborne transmission. There is currently no proven effective treatment of SARS, so early recognition, isolation, and stringent infection control are the key to controlling this highly contagious disease. Horseshoe bats are implicated in the emergence of novel coronavirus infection in humans. Further studies are needed to examine host genetic markers that may predict clinical outcome.

Pneumonia is the most common infection that is the leading cause of death. The increasing antimicrobial resistance in major respiratory pathogens such as *Streptococcus pneumoniae*, *Staphylococcus aureus* and gram-negative bacteria has severely restricted the treatment options. Respiratory infections caused by multidrug-resistant bacteria are associated with a greater likelihood of inappropriate antimicrobial therapy and poor clinical outcome. Especially, treatment of infections caused by pandrug-resistant gram-negative bacteria is a major challenge. Continuous efforts to control the global spread of drug-resistant bacteria are essential.

Occupational pulmonary infectious diseases include tuberculosis (TB) and many viral pathogens, including influenza, coronavirus (severe acute respiratory syndrome or SARS), varicella, respiratory syncytial virus, and hantavirus. This review focuses on TB, influenza, and SARS, because the published literature is extensive for these 3 infections. The lessons from these 3 are relevant for all nosocomial pulmonary infectious diseases.

The understanding of the infection risks posed by tumor necrosis factor (TNF) antagonists has continued to evolve in the 10 years since these drugs first were introduced. Recent prospective studies have confirmed the risk of tuberculosis (TB) reactivation posed by TNF antibodies to be several fold greater than soluble TNF receptor. Certolizumab pegol, a monovalent anti-TNF Fab' fragment, appears to share this risk, despite its lack of Fc and its inability to cross-link transmembrane TNF or activate complement. Two-step (boosted) tuberculin skin test screening and initiation of treatment for latent TB infection can greatly reduce the TB risk of anti-TNF treatment in western countries. Current recommendations for withdrawal of anti-TNF therapy when TB is diagnosed place patients at risk for paradoxical worsening due to recovery of TNF-dependent inflammation. Further research is needed to determine how best to prevent and manage their infectious complications and to determine their potential adjunctive therapeutic role in chronic infectious diseases.

At the beginning of the 21st century, we are facing the convergence of several epidemics. These include tobacco smoking, tuberculosis, HIV infection, influenza, and chronic obstructive pulmonary disease. These epidemics interact by way of increasing disease susceptibility and worsening outcomes. To control these interacting epidemics, we need to better understand each infection and how it influences the others. Multifaceted approaches will be necessary to reduce the impact on those in developing nations most likely to be affected by the convergence of all epidemics.

Widespread global use of rifampin for 2 decades preceded the emergence of clinically significant multidrug-resistant tuberculosis (MDR-TB) in the early 1990s. The prevalence of MDR-TB has gradually increased such that it accounts for ~5% of the global case burden of disease (approximately half a million cases in 2007). Eclipsing this worrying trend is the widespread emergence of extensively drug-resistant TB (XDR-TB). This article reviews the insights provided by clinical and molecular epidemiology regarding global trends and transmission dynamics of XDR-TB, and the challenges clinicians have to face in diagnosing and managing cases of XDR-TB. The ethical and management dilemmas posed by recurrent defaulters, XDR-TB treatment failures, and isolation of incurable patients are also discussed. Given the past global trends in MDR-TB, if aggressive preventive and management strategies are not implemented, XDR-TB has the potential to severely cripple global control efforts of TB.

Although awareness is growing, childhood tuberculosis (TB) remains a neglected disease in many resource-limited settings. In part this reflects operational difficulties, lack of visibility in official reports, as well as perceptions that children tend to develop mild disease, contribute little to disease transmission, and do not affect epidemic control. At an international level there is greater appreciation that children contribute significantly to the global TB disease burden and suffer severe TB-related morbidity and mortality, particularly in TB-endemic areas, where the disease often remains undiagnosed. However, this is not always the case at the national or local level and there remains an urgent need for feasible and implementable policies to guide clinical practice. Pediatric TB can be regarded as an emerging epidemic in areas where the adult epidemic remains out of control and *Mycobacterium tuberculosis* transmission is ongoing. This article reviews important concepts, challenges, and management principles related to childhood TB; it also summarizes the main priorities for future research.

Despite the decline in the overall incidence of tuberculosis (TB) in many developed countries, it remains an important problem among the older population. The control of TB in the elderly remains a major challenge because of the limitations of the existing tools for the diagnosis and treatment of latent TB infection and clinically active disease. This article examines the current and possible future status of TB in the elderly, focusing on epidemiology, risk factors, preventive treatment strategies, and clinical disease.

Nontuberculous mycobacteria (NTM) are generally hardy, ubiquitous environmental bacteria that vary in geographic distribution and pulmonary pathogenicity. Relatively few of the more than 115 species of NTM have been associated with lung disease. Diagnosis of disease due to NTM relies on a combination of clinical, imaging, and microbiologic data. Because

NTM may present as acid-fast bacilli in respiratory secretions of patients with clinical and radiologic features that mimic tuberculosis, laboratory discrimination of NTM from *Mycobacterium tuberculosis* is a priority. This discrimination is now often rapidly achievable using molecular techniques, although some tests have limited sensitivity. NTM species have different antibiotic response patterns, and success with medical treatment alone varies. Macrolides are an essential component of therapy for many species but must be combined with other drugs.

David R. Murdoch, Lance C. Jennings, Niranjan Bhat, and Trevor P. Anderson

Recent developments in rapid diagnostics for respiratory infections have mostly occurred in the areas of antigen and nucleic acid detection. Nucleic acid amplification tests have improved the ability to identify respiratory viruses in clinical specimens and have played pivotal roles in the rapid characterization of new viral pathogens. Antigen-detection assays in immunochromatographic or similar formats are most easily developed as near-patient tests, although they have been developed commercially only for a limited range of respiratory pathogens. New approaches for respiratory pathogen detection are needed, and breath analysis is an exciting area with enormous potential.

Lynne Strasfeld and Sunwen Chou

Erratum

Several typographical errors appeared in "Antiviral Drug Resistance: Mechanisms and Clinical Implications" by Lynne Strasfeld, MD, and Sunwen Chou, MD in the June 2010 issue, Volume 24, Number 2. The corrected article is reprinted in full in the current issue (September 2010, Volume 24, Number 3) beginning on page 809.

VISIT THE CLINICS ONLINE!

Access your subscription at:
www.theclinics.com

Preface

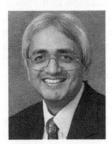 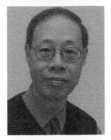 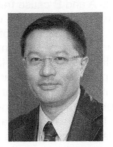

Alimuddin Zumla, FRCP,   Wing-Wai Yew, MBBS,   David S.C. Hui, MD
PhD(Lond), FRCPath   FRCP (Edinb), FCCP   (UNSW), FRACP, FRCP
                            Guest Editors

Respiratory infections are one of the most common causes of morbidity and mortality worldwide. As we enter the twenty-first century, several landmark events are unfolding in the area of respiratory infections. Some of these, by assuming the form of formidable disasters, have abruptly claimed lives and led to economic loss. Examples include severe acute respiratory syndrome (SARS) and bird and swine influenza. Viral and bacterial resistance to currently available antimicrobial drugs is thwarting efforts in the management of influenza and pulmonary sepsis. Newer and emerging viral lung infections are seen more frequently in clinical practice, including post-transplant viral infections other than cytomegalovirus and Epstein-Barr virus. The frequency and diversity of serious fungal infections are increasing. Persons who are severely immunocompromised are particularly vulnerable to infection from unusual molds and yeasts that are often found naturally in the environment. Other respiratory infections pose continuous health care challenges. Examples include the changing demography of tuberculosis (TB) and emerging deadly drug-resistant forms of TB worldwide. Pediatric TB and elderly TB are on the rise and the problem of coinfection with HIV is proving difficult to diagnose and manage. Anti–tumor necrosis factor (TNF)-α therapy for autoimmune conditions results in reactivation of TB. In addition, occupational lung diseases due to airborne microbes constitute another problematic issue. Protozoal and helminthic lung infestations continue to be important clinical problems in many parts of the world. This issue of *Infectious Diseases Clinics of North America* is aimed at giving an up-to-date and comprehensive overview of emerging respiratory infections in the twenty-first century through 14 articles written by authoritative experts from all around the globe.

David Hui and Paul Chan review SARS and coronavirus in detail, remind us of the enormous threat it posed to international health and the global economy, and state that at the end of the epidemic in July 2003, 8098 probable cases were reported in 29 countries and regions, with 774 deaths (9.6% mortality rate).

The recent panic over avian and swine influenza outbreaks has focused research-sequencing technologies and phylogenetic methods on how novel influenza viruses arise, usually from animal reservoirs. Julian Tang and colleagues describe how such knowledge allows more effective public health surveillance of seasonal human

---

Infect Dis Clin N Am 24 (2010) xiii–xvi
doi:10.1016/j.idc.2010.04.014
id.theclinics.com

influenza viruses as well as candidate pandemic viruses that may cross the species barrier from animal to man. Of the 3 known serotypes of influenza (A, B, and C), only influenza types A and B cause frequent and occasionally severe disease in humans. Although there is only one type of influenza B, influenza A has multiple subtypes, characterized by a combination of the 16 known hemagglutinin and 9 neuraminidase genes that code for these viral envelope or surface proteins. So far, only 3 subtypes of hemagglutinin (H1, H2, and H3) and 2 subtypes of neuraminidase (N1 and N2) have caused pandemics in humans. Influenza viruses will continue to pose a persistent and variable threat to human health for the foreseeable future.

Lower respiratory tract infections were ranked the third leading cause of death worldwide in 2004. The increasing prevalence of antimicrobial resistance in major respiratory pathogens has become a serious threat to clinical medicine with increased morbidity and mortality due to treatment failures. Antimicrobial resistance is a critical issue not only in community-acquired pneumonia due to resistance in *Streptococcus pneumoniae* but also in hospital-acquired pneumonia or ventilator-associated pneumonia due to methicillin-resistant *Staphylococcus aureus* (MRSA) or drug-resistant gram-negative bacilli. Jae-Hoon Song and Doo Ryeon Chung review current knowledge of respiratory infections caused by antibiotic-resistant pathogens and the treatment options available.

TB causes 1.8 million deaths annually, 5000 every day, and is one of the most common causes of death from an infectious disease. The emergence of multidrug-resistant TB and extensively drug-resistant TB (XDR-TB) in Eastern Europe, Asia, and South Africa now poses an ominous threat to global TB control. We review the insights provided by clinical and molecular epidemiology about global trends and transmission dynamics of XDR-TB and the challenges faced by clinicians in diagnosing and managing cases of XDR-TB. Keertan Dheda and colleagues review the clinical, management, and epidemiologic dilemmas posed by drug-resistant TB. Pediatric TB is now regarded as an emerging epidemic in areas where the adult epidemic remains out of control and *Mycobacterium tuberculosis* transmission is ongoing. Childhood TB remains a neglected disease in many resource-limited settings and the number of cases of pediatric TB is increasing. Ben Marais and Simon Schaaf emphasize in their article that children contribute significantly to the global TB disease burden and suffer severe TB-related morbidity and mortality. They describe current issues in the diagnosis, management, and prevention relevant to pediatric TB.

One third (over 2 billion people) of the world's population is latently infected with *M tuberculosis*. Although the risk of developing active TB disease is highest in the first two years after infection, considerable magnitude of risk persists in patients for the rest of their lives.

With waning immunity associated with advancing age and increasing use of immunosuppressants, there is an excess risk for the development of active clinical TB disease. Toru Mori and Chi Chiu Leung review TB in the ageing population, emphasizing that TB presents atypically among the elderly leading to delays in diagnosis and treatment.

Non-tuberculous mycobacteria (NTM) are environmental mycobacteria that are distinct from members of the Mycobacterium tuberculosis complex. Due to the advent of the HIV/AIDS epidemic and the increasing use of immunosuppressive drugs, infections due to NTM are increasingly being seen in clinical practice. Babafemi Taiwo and Jeff Glassroth describe the spectrum of NTM causing human disease. Lung involvement ranges from isolation of mycobacteria that may be benignly colonizing an individual, to benign nodules, disease in ostensibly healthy immune competent persons, disease in immune compromised hosts who may be infected with unusual or rarely encountered NTM, and hypersensitivity syndrome.

   Other risk factors for development of TB are discussed in two articles. TNF antagonists for treatment of rheumatoid disorders were first introduced 10 years ago. Robert Wallis and Neil Schluger review the risk of TB reactivation posed by TNF antibodies. Current recommendations for withdrawal of anti-TNF therapy when TB is diagnosed place patients at risk for paradoxic worsening due to recovery of TNF-dependent inflammation. Further research is needed to determine how best to prevent and manage their infectious complications. Richard N. van Zyl-Smit and coworkers attempt to link the interactions between smoking, TB, HIV infection, and chronic obstructive pulmonary disease (COPD), suggesting these epidemics interact by means of increased susceptibility or worsening outcomes. For example, tobacco smoking increases the risk of TB, and this in turn increases the risk of subsequent COPD. They warn of the possibility that new global influenza pandemics are more likely to occur in those with predisposing factors, such as smoking, COPD, or HIV infection.

   With increasing use of immunosuppressive therapy and the advent of the HIV epidemic, fungal pulmonary infections are increasingly seen in clinical practice. Li Yang Hsu and colleagues give a succinct overview of the diagnosis, treatment, and prevention of common and emerging new fungal infections causing respiratory illness.

   Occupational pulmonary infectious diseases are also important causes of morbidity worldwide and these include TB and many viral pathogens, including influenza, varicella, respiratory syncytial virus, and hantavirus. Daphne Ling and Dick Menzies focus on TB, influenza, and SARS. The lessons from these three are relevant for all nosocomial pulmonary infectious diseases. TB is the most important occupational infectious disease worldwide. Rates of infection are 5- to 10-fold higher in health care workers than in the general population whereas rates of disease are 2- to 5-fold higher. Risk is increased among occupations associated with performance of aerosol-producing procedures, such as sputum induction, bronchoscopy, or autopsy. SARS was unusual because of the severity of illness and high rate of nosocomial transmission via the droplet (and perhaps also airborne) route, so that health care workers accounted for 21% of all known cases. Hence, infection control measures are of primary importance. This means identification of patients (or workers) with these illnesses and their immediate separation from other patients. Personal protective equipment recommended for influenza and SARS include gown, gloves, and masks with eye-shields, whereas for TB, only masks (personal respirators) are recommended.

   Kidney, liver, heart, pancreas, lung, and small intestine transplantations are now viable therapeutic options for patients with end-stage organ failure. Infections still contribute to substantial morbidity and mortality, limiting long-term success rates of these procedures. Immunosuppressive regimens are necessary to limit allograft rejection and also weaken host immune responses to exogenously acquired pathogens and enable endogenous reactivation of latent infection. Frequent medical care of newly transplanted patients exposes recipients to potentially drug-resistant pathogens. To help prevent the occurrence of common opportunistic infections in transplant recipients, prophylactic strategies have been used; despite these efforts, emerging pathogens continue to pose unique challenges for clinicians to recognize, diagnose, and treat. Shawn Nishi and colleagues describe some of these organisms responsible for emerging respiratory infections in transplantation recipients.

   A decline in parasitic infestations was observed in the past century, especially in developed countries, due to improved socioeconomic conditions, good vector control, and excellent hygiene practices. Vannan Kandi Vijayan and Tarek Kilani review the emerging problems of respiratory parasitic infections, particularly due to protozoa and helminths. The increasing occurrence of immunosuppression in individuals due to HIV infection, organ transplantations, and use of immunosuppressive drugs has made these individuals prone to the development of parasitic pulmonary infestations de novo from the environment or recrudescence from dormant infestations.

Rapid and accurate diagnosis of respiratory pathogens can lead to effective and specific treatment resulting in low morbidity and mortality rates. David Murdoch and colleagues review recent developments in rapid diagnostics for respiratory infections, particularly in the areas of antigen and nucleic acid detection. They conclude that new approaches for respiratory pathogen detection are needed, and breath analysis is an exciting new area with enormous potential. Their review provides encouragement that recent developments in technology will eventually yield point-of-care, rapid diagnostic tests for screening of multiple pathogens in resource-poor developing countries where current technologic equipment could be run on solar-powered computers.

ACKNOWLEDGMENTS

We are extremely grateful to all the contributors for their comprehensive contributions to this excellent volume on emerging respiratory diseases of the twenty-first century. Our sincere thanks Barbara Cohen-Kligerman, Senior Elsevier Editor, and her staff for their kind assistance and diligence throughout the development of this issue. It was a pleasure to work with them. Dr Robert Moellering, Consulting Editor for *Infectious Disease Clinics of North America*, gave his unflinching support to this project. Adam Zumla provided administrative support to Professor Zumla. We thank our families for their support and patience during the many long hours spent on this project.

Alimuddin Zumla, FRCP, PhD(Lond), FRCPath
Department of Infection
Centre for Infectious Diseases and International Health
Windeyer Institute of Medical Sciences
University College London Medical School
46 Cleveland Street
London W1T 4JF, UK

Wing-Wai Yew, MBBS, FRCP (Edinb), FCCP
Tuberculosis and Chest Unit, Grantham Hospital
125 Wong Chuk Hang Road
Hong Kong, China

David S.C. Hui, MD(UNSW), FRACP, FRCP
Division of Respiratory Medicine
Stanley Ho Center for Emerging Infectious Diseases
Prince of Wales Hospital
The Chinese University of Hong Kong
30-32 Ngan Shing Street, Shatin, NT
Hong Kong, China

E-mail addresses:
a.zumla@ucl.ac.uk (A. Zumla)
yewww@ha.org.hk (W.-W. Yew)
dschui@cuhk.edu.hk (D.S.C. Hui)

Emerging Bacterial, Fungal, and Viral Respiratory Infections in Transplantation

Shawn P.E. Nishi, MD[a], Vincent G. Valentine, MD[b,*],
Steve Duncan, MD[c]

KEYWORDS

• Emerging • Transplant • Respiratory infections

Kidney, liver, heart, pancreas, lung, and small intestine transplantations are viable therapeutic options for patients with end-stage organ failure. Ongoing advancements of surgical techniques, immunosuppressive regimens, and perioperative management have resulted in improved survival of allograft recipients. Despite these refinements, infections still contribute to substantial morbidity and mortality, limiting long-term success rates of these procedures.

Infections are particularly problematic among transplant recipients for several reasons. Immunosuppressive regimens are necessary to limit allograft rejection but weaken host immune responses to exogenously acquired pathogens and enable endogenous reactivation of latent infection. Frequent medical care of newly transplanted patients exposes them to potentially drug-resistant pathogens. Infections of the respiratory tract are common and could herald the development of more severe diseases. This is largely because of constant contact with the environment, which uniquely predisposes the respiratory system to direct microbial inoculation. Moreover, lung recipients specifically suffer from mucociliary dyskinesia, with reduced mechanical clearance of respiratory pathogens, as a result of airway anastomoses and a denervated allograft.

[a] Division of Pulmonary and Critical Care Medicine, University of Texas Medical Branch, 301 University Boulevard, Galveston, TX 77555, USA
[b] Division of Pulmonary and Critical Care Medicine, Texas Transplant Center, University of Texas Medical Branch, 301 University Boulevard, Galveston, TX 77555, USA
[c] Division of Pulmonary, Allergy, and Critical Care Medicine, University of Pittsburgh, 628 NW MUH, 3459 Fifth Avenue, Pittsburgh, PA 15213, USA
* Corresponding author.
E-mail address: vgvalent@utmb.edu

Infect Dis Clin N Am 24 (2010) 541–555
doi:10.1016/j.idc.2010.04.005
0891-5520/10/$ – see front matter © 2010 Elsevier Inc. All rights reserved.

id.theclinics.com

To help prevent the occurrence of common opportunistic infections in transplant recipients, prophylactic strategies have been used, but despite these efforts, emerging pathogens continue to pose unique challenges for clinicians to recognize, diagnose, and treat. One useful paradigm relevant to emerging infections in recipients of transplants stratifies these microbes into 3 categories.[1] The first category consists of known microbes causing infection with previously unrecognized pathogenicity causing human disease. Category 2 includes known microbes with already appreciated pathogenicity but cause more frequent or severe disease. The third category comprises newly discovered pathogens. This last category is growing apace in large part from technological advances that result in diagnosis or differentiation of new microbial pathogens. This article describes some of the organisms responsible for emerging respiratory infections in transplantation (**Box 1**).

EMERGING BACTERIAL RESPIRATORY INFECTIONS IN TRANSPLANTATION
Nocardia

Nocardia is a gram-positive filamentous aerobic actinomycete with variable acid-fast staining characteristics. Among more commonly reported opportunists in transplantation, pulmonary nocardiosis infection rates range from 0.7% to 3.5%.[2–7] The largest case series in transplantation describes these infections to be more common among lung recipients (3.5%), followed by recipients of heart (2.5%), intestine (1.3%), kidney (0.2%), and liver (0.1%).[7] However, literature reviews are difficult to systematically assess. With more than 50 species in existence, taxonomic classification is fraught with confusion and controversy. Until recently, most isolates causing human disease were labeled "*Nocardia asteroides*" and included organisms with considerable differences in antimicrobial susceptibility patterns.[8] With technological advances in molecular genotyping, isolates previously described as *N asteroides* have been subspeciated.[8] *N asteroides* is now denoted as *N asteroides* complex and includes *Nocardia nova* complex, *Nocardia farcinica*, *Nocardia transvalensis* complex, *Nocardia*

Box 1
Selected emerging pathogens in solid organ transplantation

Emerging bacterial respiratory tract infections

    Nocardia spp

    Mycobacterium abscessus

    Rhodococcus equi

Emerging fungal respiratory tract infections

    Aspergillus ustus

    Aspergillus terreus

    Fusarium spp

    Scedosporium apiospermum

    Scedosporium prolificans

Emerging viral respiratory tract infections

    Human metapneumovirus

    Lymphocytic choriomeningitis virus

    Severe acute respiratory syndrome virus

abscessus, and, newly, *Nocardia cyriacigeorgica.*[8,9] Moreover, additional species will emerge with continued advances in genotyping methods.

Clinically and radiographically, most nocardial infections are nonspecific and often confined to the lungs, which usually have a favorable prognosis.[10,11] These pathogens hematogenously disseminate in 20% to 25% of cases to the central nervous system, skin, and other organs, and, although much less frequently reported, extrapulmonary extension of infection is almost always fatal.[3,5,7,10,12,13] Therefore, early recognition and prompt therapy is crucial.

With ill-defined clinicoradiographic features, diagnosis is frequently delayed. *Nocardia* is a slow growing organism, with a mean duration of 2 weeks before a diagnosis is established. Concurrent infection or contamination by other microbes can overwhelm the growth of *Nocardia* species in laboratory culture media and further impede diagnosis.[6] Several studies suggest that *Nocardia* as the sole pathogen is uncommon in comparison with nocardial infections with other coisolates of cytomegalovirus, *Aspergillus*, or opportunistic fungi.[14–16] Given the delays in diagnosis, the clinician should have a low threshold to institute therapy early while awaiting culture results.

Trimethoprim-sulfamethoxazole (TMP-SMX) prophylaxis for *Pneumocystis jiroveci* pneumonitis is widely thought to afford protection against *Nocardia* infections.[13] However, more than 60% of nocardiosis have occurred in patients receiving TMP-SMX prophylaxis. Conversion to high-dose therapy has been curative, suggesting that prophylaxis dosages are ineffective for nocardiosis prevention but does not indicate a reduced susceptibility once infection is established.[3,6,7,10,17] Most therapeutic regimens use TMP-SMX combined with imipenem, amikacin, third-generation cephalosporins, minocycline, moxifloxacin, or linezolid from concerns about resistance.[6,18] To avoid recidivism, a protracted course of at least 6 to 12 months in immunocompromised patients is recommended.[5]

Mycobacterium abscessus

M abscessus is a gram-positive rod classified as rapid-growing nontuberculous mycobacteria. It is ubiquitously present in sewage, drinking water, decaying vegetation and the normal skin flora. Genotyping by polymerase chain reaction (PCR) methods have enabled distinction and subspeciation of this pathogen from *Mycobacterium chelonae* in 1992.[19]

M abscessus is identified frequently in patients with cystic fibrosis (CF), less often in others with structural lung abnormalities caused by chronic respiratory disease, and occasionally among immunocompromised hosts. In a prevalence study of nontuberculous mycobacterium isolated from sputum cultures of patients with CF, *M abscessus* was second to *Mycobacterium avium* complex (72%). The sensitivity of sputum culture to detect disease due to *M abscessus* is low and increases little with serial sputum samples from 7% to 13%.[20] Clinicoradiological findings are nonspecific and complicated by underlying structural lung disease, making the diagnosis elusive.[21,22] Infection is confined to the lungs in patients with CF, but dissemination is not uncommon among immunocompromised patients, including transplant recipients, which usually portends a poor prognosis.[20,23–27]

Whether *M abscessus* colonization before lung transplantation should be a contraindication is unknown.[24–26] Current guidelines urge caution in the face of virulent or resistant mycobacteria, especially with positive results for sputum smears before transplant, reflecting high airway mycobacterial loads.[25] The allograft can be secondarily colonized by microbes that persist proximally to the anastomoses and predisposes the recipient to infection of the newly transplanted lung. Treatment to establish and maintain serial smear negativity before transplantation and extension of treatment intraoperatively and postoperatively have had some success.[25]

Treatment of *M abscessus* is complex and difficult for patients and clinicians. *M abscessus* isolates are resistant to most antimycobacterial agents, including tetracyclines, fluoroquinolones, and sulfonamides.[28] Initial therapy should include a combination of clarithromycin, amikacin, and cefoxitin or a carbapenem, pending sensitivity studies. Directed combination therapy should continue a minimum of 12 months after negative results of sputum cultures to avoid relapse.[20,29] Maintenance suppressive therapy with clarithromycin and aerosolized amikacin has also been suggested, as relapse after extended therapy has occurred.[29] The toxic effects of therapy and interactions with transplant medications limit adequate treatment.

Rhodococcus equi

R equi is an asporogenous, nonmotile, pleomorphic gram-positive coccobacilli and an obligate aerobe belonging to the family Nocardioform, order Actinomycetes.[30] The organism is present in soil, thrives in freshwater and marine habitats, and can live in the intestines of bloodsucking arthropods. It can be acquired by inhalation from the soil, direct inoculation, ingestion, colonization, and person-to-person transmission.[30]

R equi was first isolated as a causative agent of equine bronchopneumonia in 1923. The first human infection of *R equi* was reported in 1967 as cavitary pneumonia in a patient with autoimmune hepatitis receiving immunosuppressive therapy. Only 13 other cases have been reported up to 1983.[30] Subsequently, a marked increase in reported cases has occurred commensurate with human immunodeficiency virus, advances in cancer therapies, and transplantation.[30] More than 100 cases have now been reported, with 29 involving organ recipients, of which 23 involved the lungs.[31]

Establishing a diagnosis of *R equi* is difficult. Imaging is nonspecific and occasionally normal.[32–34] Identification of *R equi* from culture has proven difficult because of variable acid-fast staining and pleomorphic appearance in laboratory media.[30] Two studies have reported *R equi* lung infections in heart recipients initially misdiagnosed when laboratory cultures grew "diptheroids" mistaken for contaminants. Two other cases involving the kidney and pancreas and a pancreas recipient were misdiagnosed as tuberculosis, based on acid-fast staining and radiographs showing an upper lobe cavity, small satellite nodules, perihilar mass, and nonspecific infiltrate.[35,36] Final diagnosis was confirmed by bronchoalveolar lavage cultures prompted by worsening respiratory symptoms.

Given the limited number of cases, heterogeneous patient populations, and diverse clinical manifestations, standard treatments for *R equi* infection do not exist. However, success has been reported with dual antibiotic therapy for a minimum of 6 months and surgical drainage of complicated cases.[30,37,38] Combinations using vancomycin, imipenem, aminoglycosides, and fluoroquinolones are suggested empiric regimens until antimicrobial susceptibilities of the isolate are known.[30,34,39]

EMERGING FUNGAL RESPIRATORY INFECTIONS IN TRANSPLANTATION
Aspergillus species: Aspergillus ustus and Aspergillus terreus

Aside from *Candida* species, *Aspergillus* species are the most common fungal pathogens causing infection in transplant patients. This genus comprises more than 175 species, and although only a few are human pathogens, mortality of invasive aspergillosis varies from 74% to 92%.[40] *Aspergillus fumigatus* is the most common cause of disease, followed by *Aspergillus flavus* and rarely *A terreus*, *Aspergillus niger*, or

Aspergillus nidulans.[41] Recently, *A ustus* and *A terreus* have gained attention as rare, mycelial fungi responsible for fatalities with posttransplant respiratory infection.[40,42–50] Primary modes of acquisition are inhalation of environmental microconidia, similar to other mycelial fungi, or direct inoculation through the skin.[51] Predisposing factors include prolonged and severe neutropenia, high-dose steroid treatment, nosocomial exposure in hospitals undergoing construction, and prophylactic use of amphotericin B aerosols.[42,49,50,52] Once a primary respiratory infection is established, the organism has a proclivity to disseminate.

Most cases of *A terreus* and *A ustus* infections were described in the last 15 years.[45] This increase is attributed to the growing population of severely immunosuppressed patients and better diagnostic methods. Among cases reviewing these pathogens in transplant recipients, infection involved the lungs in all but one case noted with *A ustus*.[51,53–63] More than half disseminated and a third involved the central nervous system or skin.[62] *A terreus* is emerging as the next most common invasive pulmonary aspergillosis after *A fumigatus* and *A flavus*.[42–50]

Clinicians must possess an index of suspicion and a low threshold for aggressive and often invasive diagnostic procedures necessary for sampling. In many instances, *Aspergillus* species have unique histomorphologic characteristics from culture isolates facilitating identification. However, rarely encountered *Aspergillus* species such as *A ustus* and *A terreus* are not readily identified. Diagnoses by growth in culture may also be hindered by concurrent infecting organisms, most frequently other *Aspergillus* species, in nearly half of patients.[44] PCR analysis has advantages for rapid diagnosis because definitive speciation by culture takes weeks.[43,51,56,58,60,63] Early antifungal therapy is routinely initiated once a fungal pathogen is suspected or presumptively identified. However, this strategy is tempered by highly variable susceptibilities of *A terreus* and *A ustus*.[42,43,45,47,49]

Growing recognition of *A ustus* and *A terreus* is clinically important, as these species are resistant to amphotericin B, which has been standard therapy for most invasive *Aspergillus* infections.[42,45,47] Reports involving a series of 17 patients noted that 3 of 4 patients with *A ustus* who survived received voriconazole combined with caspofungin, although other reports using the same antifungal regimen as prophylaxis or as empiric therapy have not proven successful.[51,54,56,62,63] Unfortunately, *A terreus* infections are difficult to treat, with few reported successes. Only isolated respiratory infection has been amenable to amphotericin B with itraconazole after surgical lobectomy in a nonneutropenic transplant recipient.[43] Firm data for treating *A ustus* and *A terreus* infections are not available, as reflected by the multitude of antifungal regimens used. Other nonpharmacologic methods such as reduction in immunosuppression and local surgical debridement have had some success as adjunctive therapy.[42,47,49,52,57,64] Overall, however, treatment results are disappointing.

Fusarium

Fusarium solani is a colorless, septated mycelial fungus found in the soil, with increased frequency among transplant recipients.[65] The portal of entry is unclear, but inhalation, ingestion, and direct inoculation are suspected. Infection disseminates by vascular invasion with formation of yeast-like structures in the blood (adventitious sporulation), which are easily cultured.[65] Other than the characteristic fusiform or canoe-shaped macroconidia, *Fusarium* species are indistinguishable from *Aspergillus* species by routine histology.[65] Diagnosis ultimately requires speciation from culture.[66]

Among transplant recipients, reported infections have mostly occurred in hematopoietic stem cell transplantation (HSCT) recipients with prolonged neutropenia and are rarely seen in solid organ recipients. Notable differences exist between HSCT and organ recipients. First, fusariosis in HSCT recipients occurs in a trimodal distribution: early posttransplant during extreme neutropenia, a median of 70 days after transplant associated with acute graft versus host disease (GvHD) (while receiving corticosteroid therapy), and more than 1 year posttransplant in association with extensive GvHD; however, in solid organ recipients, fusariosis occurs after the first year of transplantation.[67,68] Next, HSCT recipients typically have fungemia with disseminated fusariosis, whereas organ recipients develop isolated infection. Only 6 cases have been reported up to 2001 in solid organ recipients, with only 1 disseminated and others isolated to lung (n = 1) or skin (n = 4).[68–70] Localized infection in HSCT recipients, although much less reported, includes septic arthritis, endophthalmitis, osteomyelitis, cystitis, brain abscess, and cutaneous necrotizing lesions.[66] Lung (pneumonia, nonspecific alveolar or interstitial infiltrates, nodules, cavities) is the most commonly involved site of infection, accounting for 39% of HSCT recipients who develop invasive disease.[67] Last, especially in the setting of prolonged neutropenia, fusariosis mortality rates are up to 70% to 100% in HSCT recipients. No deaths due to fusariosis have been seen in organ recipients.[68]

Effective treatment regimens for fusariosis in transplantation are unknown but invariably require correction of neutropenia.[66,67] Response rates of disseminated fusariosis to antifungal therapy are disappointing, as most organisms are resistant to currently available antifungals.[66,71] Surgical resection of localized disease combined with topical antifungal therapy has been successful in most patients,[66] whereas treatment with amphotericin B alone has only a 32% response rate.[72] Response rates up to 45% are reported with voriconazole and posaconazole salvage treatment after amphotericin B failure.[48,73] Adjunctive therapy with granulocyte transfusions and granulocyte colony-stimulating factor has shown some benefit but has not been extensively studied.[65]

Scedosporium apiospermum and Scedosporium prolificans

The genus Scedosporium includes two important human pathogens, S apiospermum and S prolificans. Historically, Scedosporium species are found in patients with hematologic malignancy or destructive chronic lung disease such as CF. Scedosporium species are the second most common mold (after Aspergillus species) colonizing airways of patients with CF.[74–77] These organisms are found ubiquitously in soil, sewage, and polluted waters and are histologically indistinct from Aspergillus, Fusarium, and other mycelial fungi.[78] Infection occurs via inhalation of spores or direct tissue inoculation and most commonly involves the respiratory tract.[78,79]

Before 2000, there were only 4 cases of disseminated infection in organ transplant recipients.[80] Recently, Scedosporium has emerged as a pathogen among the growing immunocompromised population, particularly transplant recipients. PCR methods are being developed to facilitate early identification of this pathogen.[75] The spectrum of disease for both Scedosporium species resembles aspergillosis. However, there are notable clinical differences between these 2 pathogens. S apiospermum, the asexual anamorph of Pseudallescheria boydii, is found throughout the world, whereas S prolificans is geographically concentrated in Spain, Australia, and the southern United States.[76–78,81] Rates of invasive infection are reported in 6% of cases with S apiospermum and in more than half of patients with S prolificans.[76] In addition, mortality rates of S apiospermum and S prolificans infection range from 47% to 68% and from 50% to 100%, respectively, with respiratory involvement associated with higher mortality.[74,76,77,79,82,83]

Scedosporium infections have been reported since 1985 in bone marrow transplant recipients but only recently in solid organ transplantation with prominent differences in manifestations of infection within these 2 populations.[77] In a comparison between 23 HSCT and 57 solid organ recipients with *Scedosporium* species infection, the former were more likely to have infection by *S prolificans* and have early infections (within 90 days compared with >1 year) given that solid organ recipients rarely become neutropenic. HSCT recipients were also more likely to develop fungemia and had the poorest response to therapy (40%–45% compared with 63%).[77,80,81,84] Reported rates of fungemia (70%) and dissemination (44%) with *S prolificans* are notably greater than with *Aspergillus* species and is attributed to the organism's ability to undergo adventitious sporulation.[83,84]

Unfortunately, effective antifungal therapy for *Scedosporium* infection is lacking. *S apiospermum* and *S prolificans* are resistant to amphotericin B and most antifungals. *S apiospermum* may have some susceptibility to the newer triazoles, and anecdotal regimens based on prior successfully treated cases are reported using voriconazole as monotherapy or in combination with terbinafine or an echinocandin.[74,81,82,85,86] *S prolificans*, however, remains resistant to all antifungals, as no therapy was shown to reduce mortality.[83,85] Only surgical excision and recovery from neutropenia were independently associated with survival from *S prolificans*.[83] Long-term itraconazole treatment in combination with fluconazole among patients with structurally abnormal airways who were colonized with *Scedosporium* species have lower rates of dissemination, suggesting a possible role of maintenance therapy to prevent disease progression.[84]

EMERGING VIRAL RESPIRATORY INFECTIONS IN TRANSPLANTATION
Human Metapneumovirus

Human metapneumovirus (hMPV) is a nonsegmented, single-stranded RNA virus belonging to the Paramyxoviridae family. First described in 2001 in the Netherlands among children with acute respiratory viral symptoms, hMPV has since been increasingly noted to have worldwide distribution among children and immunocompromised adults, including transplant recipients.[87–91]

Infection with hMPV mimics the course of respiratory syncytial virus (RSV), with a spectrum from mild respiratory symptoms and wheezing to severe bronchiolitis and pneumonia. Symptomatic infection occurs in less than 5% of the general population and up to about 5% to 10% of the immunocompromised population.[87,89,92] In temperate climates, seasonal variation occurs predominantly in late winter (January to April).[87–89] The clinical and radiographic courses of the disease closely resemble that of RSV infection, and this diagnosis should be considered after RSV infection is ruled out.[87]

The first case of hMPV in transplantation involved an HSCT recipient who died within a week because of pneumonia and respiratory failure.[93] Since then, multiple series among HSCT, lung, and a liver recipient have been published.[88–90,93–101] One study involving lung transplantation recipients showed an association between detection of replicating hMPV in bronchoalveolar lavage specimens and allograft rejection.[96] Despite intensifying immunosuppression to treat acute rejection, viral clearance and reduced viral replication to lower than detectable levels was still achievable in contrast to other respiratory viral data, particularly cytomegalovirus infection data, which show increased viral replication with intensification of immunosuppression.[96] This observation suggests differing mechanisms of viral clearance between these 2 pathogens, which has not been elucidated.

Diagnosis of hMPV disease is confounded by several factors. First, persistent detection of the virus in nasopharyngeal aspirates is reported in up to 85% of asymptomatic HSCT and lung recipients.[96,98] No long-term respiratory sequelae in persistently infected patients have been noted.[98] Second, primary infection is nearly universal by age 5 years, necessitating a 4-fold increase in antibody titer or seroconversion to establish a diagnosis in adults.[87] Third, although isolation of hMPV with standard cell culture techniques is the definitive method of detection, it is technically difficult, as the virus does not grow efficiently in traditional cell lines used for viral isolation.[87] PCR is the most widely used method of detection of hMPV but largely limited to research investigation.[87] Fourth, although nasopharyngeal aspirates are easily obtainable, detection is less sensitive than in bronchoalveolar lavage specimens.[95]

No agent has been approved to treat hMPV in immunocompromised hosts, but because of the close clinical correlation to RSV, similar therapies have been used.[99] A combination of intravenous ribavirin and immunoglobulin has been successful in the treatment of an HSCT recipient.[88,99] Intravenous ribavirin treatment has been used in a lung transplant recipient after isolated respiratory symptoms progressed to systemic disease and shock despite inhalational treatment. After repeat bronchoalveolar lavage specimens tested negative by PCR, therapy was discontinued.[88]

With increasing reports in the transplant literature of hMPV causing disease, it would be prudent to include hMPV in the differential diagnosis of respiratory infections, especially in winter months. Early diagnosis of hMPV infection may reduce injudicious use of antibiotics and invasive diagnostic investigations and promote appropriate infection control practices to prevent nosocomial spread.[94]

Lymphocytic Choriomeningitis Virus

Lymphocytic choriomeningitis virus (LCM) is an RNA arenavirus. Serologic surveys estimate that 5% of the US population has been infected but remained asymptomatic or had only mild self-limited infection.[102,103] LCM in immunocompromised individuals, however, can cause an acute febrile illness with fatal dissemination.[102–104] Posttransplant infections present as an acute, nonspecific febrile illness, often with abdominal symptoms that frequently progress to severe illness. Diagnosis is made by serologic testing for anti-LCM IgG or IgM antibodies, isolation of the virus from blood or cerebral spinal fluid, and immunohistochemical staining of tissue specimens or PCR.[102,103]

Infection occurs from either direct or indirect exposure to aerosolized rat urine or excrement of the common house mouse, the natural host for the virus.[102,103] Human-to-human transmission has also been documented from mother to fetus and via donor organs to recipients.[102–104] Among the clusters of LCM transmission by donor organs, 12 of 13 recipients died of multisystem organ failure, and the lone surviving patient responded to ribavirin therapy and reduction of immunosuppression.[102–104] Interestingly, none of the donors responsible for transmission had clinical signs of infection, none had IgG or IgM antibodies to LCM, and only one had an identified rodent exposure. No known treatment trials have been reported. Ribavirin use is based on in vitro viral susceptibility, but the effectiveness of this therapy and need to reduce immunosuppression remains unclear.

Diagnosis of lymphocytic choriomeningitis is difficult. Current assays to detect LCM are notably insensitive, with frequent false-negative test results during donor screening.[102,103] Lack of accurate and sensitive diagnostics for LCM necessitate rapid 2-way communication between organ procurement organizations and transplantation centers to help identify clustering of patient infections stemming from a common donor.

Severe Acute Respiratory Syndrome

A corona virus causes the severe acute respiratory syndrome (SARS) associated with an outbreak in the Toronto area linked to an index case of a traveler from Hong Kong.

Several SARS cases diagnosed by PCR of bronchoalveolar lavage samples occurred in 2003 among solid-organ and HSCT recipients. In 2 cases, despite treatment with ribavirin and reduction of immunosuppression, rapid, fatal progression to respiratory failure ensued.[1,105] One allogeneic bone marrow recipient survivor was treated with oral prednisolone and ribavirin.[106]

Subsequently, a risk stratification tool initially used for donor screening of SARS based on hospital exposure, clinical symptoms, imaging studies, and contact history was developed.[1,105] A modified version was later implemented for potential recipients. This screening protocol highlights the need for high clinical suspicion and early initiation of specific diagnostic testing with existing serologic tests or PCR methods, if available.

SUMMARY

Respiratory infections in transplantation medicine will continue to pose significant obstacles with associated detrimental effects on morbidity and mortality. The high morbidity and mortality observed from emerging infections stem from protean manifestations of disease, which delay diagnosis as well as appropriate diagnostic and therapeutic interventions. Early institution and maintenance of antimicrobial therapy is often restricted by toxicity and interactions with necessary immunosuppressive drugs. Also, limited data on effective antimicrobial regimens exist, with most therapeutic strategies based on anecdotal experiences.

Despite the introduction of newer antimicrobials, infections continue to emerge, especially among transplantation recipients. The interaction of several additional factors including transplant type, surgical technique, underlying metabolic defects, epidemiologic exposures, extent and nature of immunosuppression, and prior antimicrobial use contribute to development of infection. Technological advances have improved diagnostic techniques and modalities to define few new, previously uncharacterized pathogens. Innovations have also enabled definitive genotypic distinctions of pathogens formerly characterized exclusively by phenotypic differences. Finally, the transplant population has experienced increasing numbers, intensification of immunosuppressive regimens, and prolonged survival. Clinicians should focus on prevention of infections if at all possible, consider a broad but rational range of causes of infections in patients presenting with respiratory symptoms and perform early interventional procedures such as bronchoscopy with bronchoalveolar lavage and/or transbronchial biopsy or surgical biopsy as clinically indicated for adequate diagnostic sampling while maintaining awareness of the potential for multidrug resistance.

REFERENCES

1. Kumar D, Humar A. Emerging viral infections in transplant recipients. Curr Opin Infect Dis 2005;18(4):337–41.
2. Roberts SA, Franklin JC, Mijch A, et al. Nocardia infection in heart-lung transplant recipients at Alfred Hospital, Melbourne, Australia, 1989–1998. Clin Infect Dis 2000;31(4):968–72.
3. Husain S, McCurry K, Dauber J, et al. Nocardia infection in lung transplant recipients. J Heart Lung Transplant 2002;21(3):354–9.
4. Wiesmayr S, Stelzmueller I, Tabarelli W, et al. Nocardiosis following solid organ transplantation: a single-centre experience. Transpl Int 2005;18(9):1048–53.
5. Peraira JR, Segovia J, Fuentes R, et al. Pulmonary nocardiosis in heart transplant recipients: treatment and outcome. Transplant Proc 2003;35(5):2006–8.

6. Poonyagariyagorn HK, Gershman A, Avery R, et al. Challenges in the diagnosis and management of Nocardia infections in lung transplant recipients. Transpl Infect Dis 2008;10(6):403–8.

7. Peleg AY, Husain S, Qureshi ZA, et al. Risk factors, clinical characteristics, and outcome of Nocardia infection in organ transplant recipients: a matched case-control study. Clin Infect Dis 2007;44(10):1307–14.

8. Brown-Elliott BA, Brown JM, Conville PS, et al. Clinical and laboratory features of the Nocardia spp. based on current molecular taxonomy. Clin Microbiol Rev 2006;19(2):259–82.

9. Wallace RJ, Brown BA, Brown JM, et al. Taxonomy of Nocardia species. Clin Infect Dis 1994;18(3):476–7.

10. Khan BA, Duncan M, Reynolds J, et al. Nocardia infection in lung transplant recipients. Clin Transplant 2008;22(5):562–6.

11. Oszoyoglu AA, Kirsch J, Mohammed TL. Pulmonary nocardiosis after lung transplantation: CT findings in 7 patients and review of the literature. J Thorac Imaging 2007;22(2):143–8.

12. Simpson GL, Stinson EB, Egger MJ, et al. Nocardial infections in the immuno-compromised host: A detailed study in a defined population. Rev Infect Dis 1981;3(3):492–507.

13. Montoya JG, Giraldo LF, Efron B, et al. Infectious complications among 620 consecutive heart transplant patients at Stanford University Medical Center. Clin Infect Dis 2001;33(5):629–40.

14. Lopez FA, Johnson F, Novosad DM, et al. Successful management of disseminated Nocardia transvalensis infection in a heart transplant recipient after development of sulfonamide resistance: case report and review. J Heart Lung Transplant 2003;22(4):492–7.

15. McNeil MM, Brown JM, Magruder CH, et al. Disseminated Nocardia transvalensis infection: an unusual opportunistic pathogen in severely immunocompromised patients. J Infect Dis 1992;165(1):175–8.

16. McNeil MM, Brown JM, Georghiou PR, et al. Infections due to Nocardia transvalensis: clinical spectrum and antimicrobial therapy. Clin Infect Dis 1992;15(3):453–63.

17. Weinberger M, Eid A, Schreiber L, et al. Disseminated Nocardia transvalensis infection resembling pulmonary infarction in a liver transplant recipient. Eur J Clin Microbiol Infect Dis 1995;14(4):337–41.

18. Threlkeld SC, Hooper DC. Update on management of patients with Nocardia infection. Curr Clin Top Infect Dis 1997;17:1–23.

19. Ezaki T. [Rapid genetic identification system of mycobacteria]. Kekkaku 1992;67(12):803–8 [in Japanese].

20. Olivier KN, Weber DJ, Wallace RJ Jr, et al. Nontuberculous mycobacteria. I: Multicenter prevalence study in cystic fibrosis. Am J Respir Crit Care Med 2003;167(6):828–34.

21. Chernenko SM, Humar A, Hutcheon M, et al. Mycobacterium abscessus infections in lung transplant recipients: the international experience. J Heart Lung Transplant 2006;25(12):1447–55.

22. Fairhurst RM, Kubak BM, Shpiner RB, et al. Mycobacterium abscessus empyema in a lung transplant recipient. J Heart Lung Transplant 2002;21(3):391–4.

23. Sanguinetti M, Ardito F, Fiscarelli E, et al. Fatal pulmonary infection due to multidrug-resistant Mycobacterium abscessus in a patient with cystic fibrosis. J Clin Microbiol 2001;39(2):816–9.

24. Chalermskulrat W, Sood N, Neuringer IP, et al. Non-tuberculous mycobacteria in end stage cystic fibrosis: implications for lung transplantation. Thorax 2006; 61(6):507–13.
25. Zaidi S, Elidemir O, Heinle JS, et al. *Mycobacterium abscessus* in cystic fibrosis lung transplant recipients: report of 2 cases and risk for recurrence. Transpl Infect Dis 2009;11(3):243–8.
26. Taylor JL, Palmer SM. *Mycobacterium abscessus* chest wall and pulmonary infection in a cystic fibrosis lung transplant recipient. J Heart Lung Transplant 2006;25(8):985–8.
27. Morales P, Ros JA, Blanes M, et al. Successful recovery after disseminated infection due to *Mycobacterium abscessus* in a lung transplant patient: subcutaneous nodule as first manifestation–a case report. Transplant Proc 2007;39(7):2413–5.
28. Petrini B. *Mycobacterium abscessus*: an emerging rapid-growing potential pathogen. APMIS 2006;114(5):319–28.
29. Wallace RJ Jr. Recent changes in taxonomy and disease manifestations of the rapidly growing mycobacteria. Eur J Clin Microbiol Infect Dis 1994;13(11): 953–60.
30. Weinstock DM, Brown AE. *Rhodococcus equi*: an emerging pathogen. Clin Infect Dis 2002;34(10):1379–85.
31. Arya B, Hussian S, Hariharan S. *Rhodococcus equi* pneumonia in a renal transplant patient: a case report and review of literature. Clin Transplant 2004;18(6): 748–52.
32. Tse KC, Tang SC, Chan TM, et al. Rhodococcus lung abscess complicating kidney transplantation: successful management by combination antibiotic therapy. Transpl Infect Dis 2008;10(1):44–7.
33. Sabater L, Andreu H, Garcia-Valdecasas JC, et al. *Rhodococcus equi* infection after liver transplantation. Transplantation 1996;61(6):980–2.
34. Simsir A, Oldach D, Forest G, et al. *Rhodococcus equi* and cytomegalovirus pneumonia in a renal transplant patient: diagnosis by fine-needle aspiration biopsy. Diagn Cytopathol 2001;24(2):129–31.
35. La Rocca E, Gesu G, Caldara R, et al. Pulmonary infection caused by *Rhodococcus equi* in a kidney and pancreas transplant recipient: a case report. Transplantation 1998;65(11):1524–5.
36. Lo A, Stratta RJ, Trofe J, et al. *Rhodococcus equi* pulmonary infection in a pancreas-alone transplant recipient: consequence of intense immunosuppression. Transpl Infect Dis 2002;4(1):46–51.
37. Schilz RJ, Kavuru MS, Hall G, et al. Spontaneous resolution of rhodococcal pulmonary infection in a liver transplant recipient. South Med J 1997;90(8): 851–4.
38. Stiles BM, Isaacs RB, Daniel TM, et al. Role of surgery in *Rhodococcus equi* pulmonary infections. J Infect 2002;45(1):59–61.
39. Munoz P, Burillo A, Palomo J, et al. *Rhodococcus equi* infection in transplant recipients: case report and review of the literature. Transplantation 1998;65(3): 449–53.
40. Singh N, Paterson DL. Aspergillus infections in transplant recipients. Clin Microbiol Rev 2005;18(1):44–69.
41. Richardson M, Lass-Florl C. Changing epidemiology of systemic fungal infections. Clin Microbiol Infect 2008;14(Suppl 4):5–24.
42. Hachem RY, Kontoyiannis DP, Boktour MR, et al. *Aspergillus terreus*: an emerging amphotericin B-resistant opportunistic mold in patients with hematologic malignancies. Cancer 2004;101(7):1594–600.

43. Iwen PC, Rupp ME, Langnas AN, et al. Invasive pulmonary aspergillosis due to *Aspergillus terreus*: 12-year experience and review of the literature. Clin Infect Dis 1998;26(5):1092–7.

44. Steinbach WJ, Benjamin DK Jr, Kontoyiannis DP, et al. Infections due to *Aspergillus terreus*: a multicenter retrospective analysis of 83 cases. Clin Infect Dis 2004;39(2):192–8.

45. Steinbach WJ, Perfect JR, Schell WA, et al. In vitro analyses, animal models, and 60 clinical cases of invasive *Aspergillus terreus* infection. Antimicrob Agents Chemother 2004;48(9):3217–25.

46. Tokimatsu I, Kushima H, Iwata A, et al. Invasive pulmonary aspergillosis with hematological malignancy caused by *Aspergillus terreus* and in vitro susceptibility of *A. terreus* isolate to micafungin. Intern Med 2007;46(11):775–9.

47. Walsh TJ, Petraitis V, Petraitiene R, et al. Experimental pulmonary aspergillosis due to *Aspergillus terreus*: pathogenesis and treatment of an emerging fungal pathogen resistant to amphotericin B. J Infect Dis 2003;188(2):305–19.

48. Perfect JR, Marr KA, Walsh TJ, et al. Voriconazole treatment for less-common, emerging, or refractory fungal infections. Clin Infect Dis 2003;36(9):1122–31.

49. Lass-Florl C, Griff K, Mayr A, et al. Epidemiology and outcome of infections due to *Aspergillus terreus*: 10-year single centre experience. Br J Haematol 2005; 131(2):201–7.

50. Caston JJ, Linares MJ, Gallego C, et al. Risk factors for pulmonary *Aspergillus terreus* infection in patients with positive culture for filamentous fungi. Chest 2007;131(1):230–6.

51. Panackal AA, Imhof A, Hanley EW, et al. *Aspergillus ustus* infections among transplant recipients. Emerg Infect Dis 2006;12(3):403–8.

52. Cooke FJ, Terpos E, Boyle J, et al. Disseminated *Aspergillus terreus* infection arising from cutaneous inoculation treated with caspofungin. Clin Microbiol Infect 2003;9(12):1238–41.

53. Stiller MJ, Teperman L, Rosenthal SA, et al. Primary cutaneous infection by *Aspergillus ustus* in a 62-year-old liver transplant recipient. J Am Acad Dermatol 1994;31(2 Pt 2):344–7.

54. Pavie J, Lacroix C, Hermoso DG, et al. Breakthrough disseminated *Aspergillus ustus* infection in allogeneic hematopoietic stem cell transplant recipients receiving voriconazole or caspofungin prophylaxis. J Clin Microbiol 2005; 43(9):4902–4.

55. Baddley JW, Stroud TP, Salzman D, et al. Invasive mold infections in allogeneic bone marrow transplant recipients. Clin Infect Dis 2001;32(9):1319–24.

56. Nakai K, Kanda Y, Mineishi S, et al. Primary cutaneous aspergillosis caused by *Aspergillus ustus* following reduced-intensity stem cell transplantation. Ann Hematol 2002;81(10):593–6.

57. Azzola A, Passweg JR, Habicht JM, et al. Use of lung resection and voriconazole for successful treatment of invasive pulmonary *Aspergillus ustus* infection. J Clin Microbiol 2004;42(10):4805–8.

58. Verweij PE, van den Bergh MF, Rath PM, et al. Invasive aspergillosis caused by *Aspergillus ustus*: case report and review. J Clin Microbiol 1999;37(5):1606–9.

59. Iwen PC, Rupp ME, Bishop MR, et al. Disseminated aspergillosis caused by *Aspergillus ustus* in a patient following allogeneic peripheral stem cell transplantation. J Clin Microbiol 1998;36(12):3713–7.

60. Bretagne S, Marmorat-Khuong A, Kuentz M, et al. Serum *Aspergillus galactomannan* antigen testing by sandwich ELISA: practical use in neutropenic patients. J Infect 1997;35(1):7–15.

61. Vagefi PA, Cosimi AB, Ginns LC, et al. Cutaneous *Aspergillus ustus* in a lung transplant recipient: emergence of a new opportunistic fungal pathogen. J Heart Lung Transplant 2008;27(1):131–4.

62. Olorunnipa O, Zhang AY, Curtin CM. Invasive aspergillosis of the hand caused by *Aspergillus ustus*: a case report. Hand (N Y) 2010;(5):102–5.

63. Florescu DF, Iwen PC, Hill LA, et al. Cerebral aspergillosis caused by *Aspergillus ustus* following orthotopic heart transplantation: case report and review of the literature. Clin Transplant 2009;23(1):116–20.

64. Goldberg SL, Geha DJ, Marshall WF, et al. Successful treatment of simultaneous pulmonary *Pseudallescheria boydii* and *Aspergillus terreus* infection with oral itraconazole. Clin Infect Dis 1993;16(6):803–5.

65. Merz WG, Karp JE, Hoagland M, et al. Diagnosis and successful treatment of fusariosis in the compromised host. J Infect Dis 1988;158(5):1046–55.

66. Gupta AK, Baran R, Summerbell RC. Fusarium infections of the skin. Curr Opin Infect Dis 2000;13(2):121–8.

67. Nucci M, Marr KA, Queiroz-Telles F, et al. Fusarium infection in hematopoietic stem cell transplant recipients. Clin Infect Dis 2004;38(9):1237–42.

68. Sampathkumar P, Paya CV. Fusarium infection after solid-organ transplantation. Clin Infect Dis 2001;32(8):1237–40.

69. Arney KL, Tiernan R, Judson MA. Primary pulmonary involvement of *Fusarium solani* in a lung transplant recipient. Chest 1997;112(4):1128–30.

70. Guinvarc'h A, Guilbert L, Marmorat-Khuong A, et al. Disseminated *Fusarium solani* infection with endocarditis in a lung transplant recipient. Mycoses 1998;41(1–2):59–61.

71. Pfaller MA, Marco F, Messer SA, et al. In vitro activity of two echinocandin derivatives, LY303366 and MK-0991 (L-743,792), against clinical isolates of *Aspergillus, Fusarium, Rhizopus*, and other filamentous fungi. Diagn Microbiol Infect Dis 1998;30(4):251–5.

72. Nucci M, Anaissie E. *Fusarium* infections in immunocompromised patients. Clin Microbiol Rev 2007;20(4):695–704.

73. Raad II, Hachem RY, Herbrecht R, et al. Posaconazole as salvage treatment for invasive fusariosis in patients with underlying hematologic malignancy and other conditions. Clin Infect Dis 2006;42(10):1398–403.

74. Castiglioni B, Sutton DA, Rinaldi MG, et al. *Pseudallescheria boydii* (anamorph *Scedosporium apiospermum*). Infection in solid organ transplant recipients in a tertiary medical center and review of the literature. Medicine (Baltimore) 2002;81(5):333–48.

75. Cimon B, Carrere J, Vinatier JF, et al. Clinical significance of *Scedosporium apiospermum* in patients with cystic fibrosis. Eur J Clin Microbiol Infect Dis 2000;19(1):53–6.

76. Cooley L, Spelman D, Thursky K, et al. Infection with *Scedosporium apiospermum* and *S. prolificans*, Australia. Emerg Infect Dis 2007;13(8):1170–7.

77. Husain S, Munoz P, Forrest G, et al. Infections due to *Scedosporium apiospermum* and *Scedosporium prolificans* in transplant recipients: clinical characteristics and impact of antifungal agent therapy on outcome. Clin Infect Dis 2005;40(1):89–99.

78. Tadros TS, Workowski KA, Siegel RJ, et al. Pathology of hyalohyphomycosis caused by *Scedosporium apiospermum* (*Pseudallescheria boydii*): an emerging mycosis. Hum Pathol 1998;29(11):1266–72.

79. Panackal AA, Marr KA. *Scedosporium/Pseudallescheria* infections. Semin Respir Crit Care Med 2004;25(2):171–81.

80. Raj R, Frost AE. *Scedosporium apiospermum* fungemia in a lung transplant recipient. Chest 2002;121(5):1714–6.

81. Troke P, Aguirrebengoa K, Arteaga C, et al. Treatment of scedosporiosis with voriconazole: clinical experience with 107 patients. Antimicrob Agents Chemother 2008;52(5):1743–50.

82. Sahi H, Avery RK, Minai OA, et al. *Scedosporium apiospermum* (*Pseudoallescheria boydii*) infection in lung transplant recipients. J Heart Lung Transplant 2007;26(4):350–6.

83. Rodriguez-Tudela JL, Berenguer J, Guarro J, et al. Epidemiology and outcome of *Scedosporium prolificans* infection, a review of 162 cases. Med Mycol 2009; 47(4):359–70.

84. Tamm M, Malouf M, Glanville A. Pulmonary scedosporium infection following lung transplantation. Transpl Infect Dis 2001;3(4):189–94.

85. Meletiadis J, Mouton JW, Meis JF, et al. In vitro drug interaction modeling of combinations of azoles with terbinafine against clinical *Scedosporium prolificans* isolates. Antimicrob Agents Chemother 2003;47(1):106–17.

86. Rogasi PG, Zanazzi M, Nocentini J, et al. Disseminated *Scedosporium apiospermum* infection in renal transplant recipient: long-term successful treatment with voriconazole: a case report. Transplant Proc 2007;39(6):2033–5.

87. Falsey AR. Human metapneumovirus infection in adults. Pediatr Infect Dis J 2008;27(10 Suppl):S80–3.

88. Raza K, Ismailjee SB, Crespo M, et al. Successful outcome of human metapneumovirus (hMPV) pneumonia in a lung transplant recipient treated with intravenous ribavirin. J Heart Lung Transplant 2007;26(8):862–4.

89. Dare R, Sanghavi S, Bullotta A, et al. Diagnosis of human metapneumovirus infection in immunosuppressed lung transplant recipients and children evaluated for pertussis. J Clin Microbiol 2007;45(2):548–52.

90. Hopkins P, McNeil K, Kermeen F, et al. Human metapneumovirus in lung transplant recipients and comparison to respiratory syncytial virus. Am J Respir Crit Care Med 2008;178(8):876–81.

91. van den Hoogen BG, de Jong JC, Groen J, et al. A newly discovered human pneumovirus isolated from young children with respiratory tract disease. Nat Med 2001;7(6):719–24.

92. Williams JV, Martino R, Rabella N, et al. A prospective study comparing human metapneumovirus with other respiratory viruses in adults with hematologic malignancies and respiratory tract infections. J Infect Dis 2005;192(6):1061–5.

93. Cane PA, van den Hoogen BG, Chakrabarti S, et al. Human metapneumovirus in a haematopoietic stem cell transplant recipient with fatal lower respiratory tract disease. Bone Marrow Transplant 2003;31(4):309–10.

94. Evashuk KM, Forgie SE, Gilmour S, et al. Respiratory failure associated with human metapneumovirus infection in an infant posthepatic transplant. Am J Transplant 2008;8(7):1567–9.

95. Gerna G, Vitulo P, Rovida F, et al. Impact of human metapneumovirus and human cytomegalovirus versus other respiratory viruses on the lower respiratory tract infections of lung transplant recipients. J Med Virol 2006;78(3):408–16.

96. Larcher C, Geltner C, Fischer H, et al. Human metapneumovirus infection in lung transplant recipients: clinical presentation and epidemiology. J Heart Lung Transplant 2005;24(11):1891–901.

97. Oliveira R, Machado A, Tateno A, et al. Frequency of human metapneumovirus infection in hematopoietic SCT recipients during 3 consecutive years. Bone Marrow Transplant 2008;42(4):265–9.

98. Debiaggi M, Canducci F, Terulla C, et al. Long-term study on symptomless human metapneumovirus infection in hematopoietic stem cell transplant recipients. New Microbiol 2007;30(3):255–8.
99. Kamble RT, Bollard C, Demmler G, et al. Human metapneumovirus infection in a hematopoietic transplant recipient. Bone Marrow Transplant 2007;40(7): 699–700.
100. Huck B, Egger M, Bertz H, et al. Human metapneumovirus infection in a hematopoietic stem cell transplant recipient with relapsed multiple myeloma and rapidly progressing lung cancer. J Clin Microbiol 2006;44(6):2300–3.
101. Englund JA, Boeckh M, Kuypers J, et al. Brief communication: fatal human metapneumovirus infection in stem-cell transplant recipients. Ann Intern Med 2006;144(5):344–9.
102. Centers for Disease Control and Prevention (CDC). Brief report: Lymphocytic choriomeningitis virus transmitted through solid organ transplantation–Massachusetts, 2008. MMWR Morb Mortal Wkly Rep 2008;57(29):799–801.
103. Fischer SA, Graham MB, Kuehnert MJ, et al. Transmission of lymphocytic choriomeningitis virus by organ transplantation. N Engl J Med 2006;354(21): 2235–49.
104. Palacios G, Druce J, Du L, et al. A new arenavirus in a cluster of fatal transplant-associated diseases. N Engl J Med 2008;358(10):991–8.
105. Kumar D, Tellier R, Draker R, et al. Severe acute respiratory syndrome (SARS) in a liver transplant recipient and guidelines for donor SARS screening. Am J Transplant 2003;3(8):977–81.
106. Lam MF, Ooi GC, Lam B, et al. An indolent case of severe acute respiratory syndrome. Am J Respir Crit Care Med 2004;169(1):125–8.

Common and Emerging Fungal Pulmonary Infections

Li Yang Hsu, MBBS, MRCP, MPH[a],*, Esther Shu-Ting Ng, MBBS[a],
Liang Piu Koh, MBBS, MRCP[b]

KEYWORDS

- Pulmonary fungal infections • Epidemiology
- Diagnostic tests • Antifungal agents
- Antifungal drug resistance • Prevention and control

The epidemiology of human fungal infections has evolved considerably over the past 3 decades, mainly due to the rising prevalence of immunocompromised patients worldwide consequent to the spread of human immunodeficiency virus (HIV) as well as increasing iatrogenic immunosuppression from chemotherapy for malignancies, solid organ/stem cell transplantation, and the use of biologic agents such as tumor necrosis factor (TNF) inhibitors. These factors have resulted in an expanding subpopulation at risk for opportunistic fungal infections, including fungi that were heretofore considered poorly virulent, such as the hyaline and dematiaceous molds.[1–3]

Secondary epidemiologic shifts in pathogenic fungi within the immunocompromised host population have resulted from steps taken to prevent more common fungal infections. As an example, the relatively recent use of fluconazole prophylaxis in patients undergoing chemotherapy or hematopoietic stem cell transplantation (HSCT) has resulted in a reduction in the incidence of invasive candidiasis, but with relative increase in proportion of fluconazole-resistant non-*albicans Candida* spp, as well as a corresponding increase in invasive mold diseases.[2,4–6] An increase in azole-resistant *Candida* spp colonization but not infection has been documented in the case of posaconazole use,[7] while early data suggest a possible association between voriconazole prophylaxis and zygomycosis.[8]

Funding: No specific funding was utilized in the writing of this article.
Disclosures: L.P.K. is currently the site principal investigator for a multicenter study funded by Pfizer Inc. L.Y.H. has received research funding from Pfizer Inc, and Merck, Sharpe & Dohme, as well as paid consultancy from Pfizer Inc. E.S.N. has no competing interests to declare.
[a] Department of Medicine, National University Health System, 5 Lower Kent Ridge Road, Singapore 119074, Singapore
[b] Department of Hematology/Oncology, National University Health System, 5 Lower Kent Ridge Road, Singapore 119074, Singapore
* Corresponding author.
E-mail address: liyang_hsu@yahoo.com

Infect Dis Clin N Am 24 (2010) 557–577
doi:10.1016/j.idc.2010.04.003
0891-5520/10/$ – see front matter © 2010 Elsevier Inc. All rights reserved.

The influence of climate change on the distribution of pathogenic fungi, particularly endemic mycoses, is another area that has not been well studied.[9] The sudden emergence of *Cryptococcus gattii* as a cause of disease in British Columbia and the Pacific Northwest of North America in the past decade may have been due to the materialization of a favorable ecological niche in these regions as a consequence of climate change, although conclusive proof remains elusive.[10]

An overview of the epidemiologic trends has thus led to the recognition that invasive fungal infections are now more prevalent and clinically important than ever before, with a progressively growing list of fungi that may cause disease in humans. This review centers on pulmonary infections caused by emerging dimorphic and opportunistic fungi (**Table 1**), and summarizes the microbiology, clinical presentation, diagnosis, and management of each of these organisms. In particular, emphasis is placed on the discussion of recent developments in terms of diagnostics, therapeutics, and prophylaxis where applicable. Because intensive care–related and transplant-related infections are dealt with in other related articles in this issue, the fungal pathogens common in such scenarios, namely *Candida* spp and *Aspergillus* spp, are not discussed herein.

ENDEMIC MYCOSES

The term "endemic mycoses" is applied to a heterogeneous group of fungi sharing similar characteristics:[11]

- They may cause disease in both immunocompetent and immunocompromised hosts. In particular, the advent of AIDS, organ transplantation, and more recently biologics such as TNF-α inhibitors have resulted in an increase in the incidence of disease caused by endemic mycoses.
- They occupy defined ecological niches in the environment.
- They display temperature dimorphism, existing as yeasts (or spherules in the case of *Coccidioides* spp) at body temperatures and as molds at environmental temperatures. Thus human-to-human transmission, except via organ transplantation, is extremely rare.

For the latter reason, *Cryptococcus gattii* is not considered an endemic mycosis, although it has a circumscribed geographic distribution and is dimorphic under certain environmental conditions.[12]

The major endemic areas for histoplasmosis, coccidioidomycosis, blastomycosis, paracoccidioidomycosis, and penicilliosis are shown in **Fig. 1**. Sporotrichosis has a worldwide distribution, although it is most common in tropical and subtropical areas, especially South America.

Histoplasmosis

Histoplasmosis is the most common endemic mycosis reported worldwide. Two varieties of *Histoplasma* are responsible for human histoplasmosis: *H capsulatum* var. *capsulatum* (*H capsulatum*) and *H capsulatum* var. *duboisii* (*H duboisii*). *H capsulatum*, the more common cause of human disease, is distributed worldwide although it is most frequently reported from the Ohio and Mississippi River valleys (see **Fig. 1**), growing abundantly in soil that is rich with bird or bat droppings.[13] *H duboisii*, the cause of African histoplasmosis, coexists with *H capsulatum* in central and western sub-Saharan Africa. Far less is known about the pathogenesis of this fungus, although it exhibits tropism for cutaneous and skeletal structures with negligible pulmonary involvement, unlike *H capsulatum*.[13] Treatment options for African histoplasmosis are extrapolated from guidelines for the treatment of H capsulatum.[14] The rest of this section pertains to infection caused by H capsulatum.

Infection occurs when aerosolized microconidia formed in the mold stage of the fungus are inhaled and phagocytized by alveolar macrophages, wherein these microconidia convert to the yeast stage and are spread to hilar and mediastinal lymph nodes with subsequent hematogenous dissemination.[11] The clinical presentation and severity of disease is dependent on the number of inhaled microconidia and the immune status of the host.[11] Infection is asymptomatic or presents as a mild nonspecific respiratory illness in the great majority of immunocompetent individuals. When specific cell-mediated immunity develops, T-cell–activated macrophages are able to destroy the majority of intracellular yeasts, although some survive in tissue in a latent state for years, reactivating and causing disease when cell-mediated immunity wanes,[11] or very rarely when infected organs are transplanted.[15] This situation may create a diagnostic dilemma if the infected patient has moved away from the endemic area.

Immunocompromised patients or healthy individuals who have inhaled a large inoculum of microconidia may develop more severe, even life-threatening, acute pneumonia. Symptoms include high fever, dyspnea, nonproductive cough, and chest pain. Patients often appear toxic, with acute respiratory distress developing rapidly, while diffuse reticulonodular infiltrates and hilar lymphadenopathy are present on chest imaging.[11]

Although the vast majority of patients with acute pulmonary histoplasmosis have self-limited disease or respond well to antifungal therapy, fewer than 1% will develop one of several delayed complications: pericarditis, granulomatous mediastinitis, histoplasmoma, broncholithiasis, and the very rare fibrosing mediastinitis. These complications represent different inflammatory responses to the organism, with the first 2 generally resolving after several months, whereas the last—which may occur years to decades after the initial infection—is progressive and poorly responsive to pharmacologic and surgical therapy.[11] Symptoms of fibrosing mediastinitis are related to the vessel(s) or airway(s) entrapped by the fibrous tissue, and bilateral involvement may be life-threatening.[16] Histoplasmomas are slowly enlarging pulmonary nodules that seldom cause clinical problems but may be mistaken for bronchogenic carcinoma. Broncholithiasis occurs when peribronchial calcific nodal disease causes bronchial obstruction via direct obstruction or airway distortion via inflammation.[17]

Chronic cavitary pulmonary histoplasmosis occurs almost invariably in older patients with underlying chronic obstructive pulmonary disease (COPD), with clinical and radiologic manifestations that are indistinguishable from pulmonary tuberculosis. Whether this is due to reactivation or new infection is unclear, but it is progressive and life-threatening if untreated.[11]

Acute and chronic progressive disseminated histoplasmosis is beyond the scope of this article, but pulmonary involvement is not uncommon, with diffuse infiltrates on chest imaging occasionally mimicking miliary tuberculosis.[18]

The wide variety of diagnostic tests available for histoplasmosis is summarized in **Table 2**: the choice of diagnostic tests should be based on both type of disease and laboratory capabilities. In general, culture remains the definitive method although time to recovery of the fungus is slow (4–6 weeks on average).[11] Antibody assays are most useful in relatively immunocompetent patients with chronic pulmonary or disseminated histoplasmosis. However, they may be falsely negative in immunosuppressed patients or those with delayed mediastinal complications, and treatment outcomes have little correlation with antibody levels.[19] Antigen detection in urine is increasingly being used, with several commercial assays now available on the market.

Table 1
Common and emerging fungi associated with invasive pulmonary disease

Fungus	Host	Pulmonary Presentation
Endemic mycoses		
Histoplasma capsulatum	Immunocompetent	1. Nonspecific respiratory illness to acute fulminant pneumonia depending on inhaled microconidia load 2. Chronic cavitary pulmonary histoplasmosis in older patients with chronic obstructive lung disease (COPD); resembles tuberculosis 3. Histoplasmoma and other complications post acute infection
	Immunocompromised	1. Acute pneumonia (as in immunocompetent host above) 2. Acute or chronic progressive disseminated disease (variety of pulmonary findings)
Coccidioides imitis	Immunocompetent & immuno compromised (clinical syndromes more common with immunocompromised hosts)	1. Asymptomatic or subclinical infection 2. Primary pulmonary coccidioidomycosis (may be fulminant in immunocompromised host or post-inhalation of large arthroconidia load) 3. Pulmonary nodules ± thin-walled cavitary disease 4. Chronic progressive coccidioidal pneumonia (resembles tuberculosis)
Blastomyces dermatitidis	Immunocompetent & immunocompromised (morbidity/mortality higher with immunocompromised)	1. Acute pulmonary blastomycosis (indistinguishable clinically from other acute pulmonary infections) 2. Chronic pulmonary blastomycosis (variety of chest findings ranging from nodules to military disease and pleural effusion) 3. Disseminated disease with pulmonary involvement (lung involvement as per chronic blastomycosis above)
Paracoccidioides brasiliensis	Immunocompetent & immunocompromised	1. Pulmonary involvement rare in children 2. Chronic pulmonary paracoccidioidomycosis (infiltrates and nodules over central and lower portion of the lung fields) 3. Disseminated disease especially with mucosal and cutaneous features in addition to pulmonary involvement is common
Penicillium marneffei	Immunocompetent	1. Asymptomatic or subclinical disease (clinical disease very rare in immunocompetent hosts)
	Immunocompromised (especially AIDS patients)	1. Chronic disseminated disease in most cases (variety of pulmonary findings ranging from diffuse alveolar lesions to cavitary disease)

Sporothrix schenckii	Immunocompetent (alcoholics or patients with COPD)	1. Chronic fibronodular cavitary disease
	Immunocompromised	1. Pulmonary involvement as part of disseminated disease (variety of pulmonary findings)
Molds		
Zygomycetes	Immunocompromised (diabetes mellitus, AIDS, stem cell or solid organ transplantation, corticosteroids, and so forth)	1. Infection extremely rare in immunocompetent host 2. Pulmonary infection commonly in combination with sinus involvement, otherwise indistinguishable from invasive pulmonary aspergillosis (IPA)
Hyalohyphomycosis	Immunocompetent (mainly *Scedosporium apiospermum*)	1. Allergic bronchopulmonary disease (ABPD) similar to allergic bronchopulmonary aspergillosis 2. Pulmonary mycetoma 3. Sinopulmonary infection ± brain abscess in near-drowning victims
	Immunocompromised	1. Disseminated disease with pulmonary findings resembling invasive pulmonary aspergillosis. Cutaneous lesions mimicking ecthyma gangrenosum characteristic for fusariosis
Phaehyphomycosis	Immunocompetent (patients with asthma)	1. ABPD
	Immunocompromised	1. Variety of pulmonary manifestations including solitary nodules, endobronchial lesions and pneumonia
Yeasts		
Cryptococcus gattii	Immunocompetent & immunocompromised	1. Pulmonary cryptococcosis (variety of findings from pulmonary nodules to ground-glass opacities and adenopathy) 2. Pulmonary involvement as part of disseminated disease (prominently meningitis)

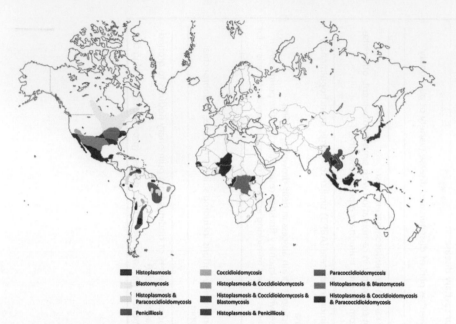

Fig. 1. Geographic distribution of major endemic mycoses: histoplasmosis,[86–92] coccidioidomycosis,[87,93] paracoccidioidomycosis,[87] blastomycosis,[94,95] penicilliosis.[44]

Of importance is that there may be differences in sensitivity and specificity among these assays, and false-positive reactions may occur with a variety of other endemic mycoses.[19] Lower sensitivity of urine antigen testing for most forms of pulmonary histoplasmosis has led to investigators using the assays on bronchoalveolar lavage fluid, with promising initial results.[20]

The Infectious Diseases Society of America (IDSA) revised the guidelines for the management of histoplasmosis in 2007.[14] In general, itraconazole was recommended for mild to moderate disease while amphotericin B (including lipid formulations) was reserved for severe disease. Concomitant methylprednisolone was recommended for the first 1 to 2 weeks for patients with severe acute pulmonary histoplasmosis with respiratory complications. Antifungal treatment was generally not recommended for patients with delayed complications, unless corticosteroids were prescribed.[14] The newer azoles (voriconazole and posaconazole) are also active against *H capsulatum*, but clinical experience remains limited at present.

Prevention of exposure to *H capsulatum* is difficult given the omnipresent nature of the fungus. The National Institute for Occupational Safety and Health recommends the wearing of well-fitting particulate respirators for workers involved in high-risk activities. Water sprays or other dust suppression techniques should also be used during demolition work to minimize the risk of aerosolizing microconidia.[21] Pharmacologic prophylaxis with itraconazole or posaconazole may be considered in high-risk immunocompromised patients living in highly endemic areas.

In conclusion, the armamentarium of tests used to diagnose histoplasmosis is constantly evolving, and clinicians need to be aware of the pitfalls associated with each investigation. More studies are required to define the role of prophylaxis and the patient population that will benefit from this.

Table 2
Diagnostic modalities for endemic mycoses

Mycoses	Direct Microscopy/ Histopathology	Culture	Serology	Antigen Testing	Molecular Testing
Histoplasmosis[19]	Good sensitivity (70%) for chronic pulmonary histoplasmosis. Poor for other forms of disease	Good sensitivity for various types of histoplasmosis	Multiple kits available. CF test best currently Useful for all forms of histoplasmosis	Urine/serum antigen (ELISA) test available. High sensitivity (>90%) in immunosuppressed patients	Various primers and publications; no commercial kit available
Coccidioi-domycosis[19]	Variable sensitivity (15%–64%)	Low sensitivity in acute coccidioidal pneumonia. One week to culture on average	High sensitivity (up to 82%) for various serologic assays	ELISA seroassay available: good sensitivity (71%) and specificity (98%)	Various primers and publications; no commercial kit available
Blastomycosis[19]	High sensitivity (90%) from tissue specimens	Good sensitivity (66%). Long time to positivity (4–6 wk)	Not recommended. Current tests have low sensitivity/ specificity	Highly sensitive (93%) for chronic pneumonia. Cross-reacts with histoplasmosis	No commercial kit available
Paracoccidioi-domycosis[37–42]	High sensitivity/ specificity	High sensitivity. Long time to positivity (5 wk)	Multiple kits available. Immunodiffusion the current test of choice	Multiple kits available	No commercial kit available
Penicilliosis[45,46]	Good sensitivity/ specificity	High sensitivity from blood (76%), skin (90%), bone marrow (100%)	ELISA and other kits available. Varying sensitivities/ specificities	Platelia *Aspergillus* seroassay may cross-react Urinary antigen testing available	Experimental only. No commercial kit available
Sporotrichosis[11,54,55]	Poor sensitivity/ specificity	Tissue cultures: high sensitivity/ specificity Growth in 7 days	ELISA: high sensitivity (~90%)	Not available	Experimental only. No commercial kit available

Abbreviations: CF, complement fixation; ELISA, enzyme-linked immunosorbent assay.

Coccidioidomycosis

Coccidioidomycosis is endemic to the Americas between latitudes 40°N and 40°S, particularly within south Arizona, Utah, California (San Joaquin Valley), Nevada, west Texas, south New Mexico, and northwestern Mexico (see **Fig. 1**).[22,23] Infection is caused by inhalation of arthroconidia of either *Coccidioides imitis* (geographically limited to San Joaquin Valley) or *Coccidioides posadasii* (located in all other endemic regions).[22] Arthroconidia develop into spherules filled with endospores within tissue, and each endospore will develop into a new spherule on release, thus resulting in extension of disease.[22] Over the past decade, there has been a resurgence in the incidence of coccidioidomycosis in the United States.[22]

Up to two-thirds of individuals infected by *Coccidioides* spp are asymptomatic or have subclinical disease for which no medical attention is sought.[24] In the rest, 3 main pulmonary clinical syndromes have been described besides disseminated disease, which may or may not involve the meninges and is more likely to develop in immunocompromised patients or those from certain ethnic groups such as Filipinos and African Americans.[25]

Primary pulmonary coccidioidomycosis the most common presentation, manifesting between 7 and 21 days post exposure.[26] This condition is underdiagnosed because the symptoms are indistinguishable from other respiratory illnesses. Cutaneous manifestations such as erythema nodosum or erythema multiforme may also be seen, and appear to predict a favorable outcome. Chest radiography demonstrates a variety of findings ranging from pulmonary infiltrates and consolidation to hilar adenopathy and pleural effusion.[26] Similar to histoplasmosis, a fulminant process with diffuse lung infiltrates and acute respiratory failure may rarely develop as a consequence of host immunosuppression or inhalation of large arthroconidia loads.[26]

Up to 5% of patients with primary coccidioidal pneumonia will develop pulmonary nodules or thin-walled cavities. The former are typically asymptomatic but are indistinguishable from lung tumors without the benefit of histology. The latter generally close within 2 years, although complications, such as mycetoma or rupture into a pleural space resulting in pyopneumothorax, may rarely occur.[26]

Chronic progressive coccidioidal pneumonia is uncommon and appears to be associated with diabetes mellitus or preexisting pulmonary fibrosis. Symptoms persist beyond 3 months and include weight loss, low-grade fever, and chronic cough. Radiologic findings may resemble pulmonary tuberculosis.[26]

Currently available diagnostic tests for coccidioidomycosis are listed in **Table 2**. Cultures are more likely to be positive in chronic pneumonia and disseminated disease,[19] but it is imperative that microbiology laboratories, especially in nonendemic areas, be warned about the possibility of coccidioidomycosis for biosafety reasons.[27] Serologic testing is the most common means of diagnosing coccidioidomycosis, with many antibody-testing methods available commercially. Results may, however, be false-negative in immunocompromised patients, or for the first few months after infection.[19] Antigen detection is a relatively new modality with high sensitivity (up to 71%) and specificity (up to 98%) in limited studies, but cross-reactivity with other endemic mycoses may occur.[19]

Treatment guidelines were established in 2005 by IDSA, and are due to be revised next year.[28] Initiating antifungal therapy in acute coccidioidal pneumonia remains controversial, although oral azoles are recommended for severe disease and/or infected immunocompromised patients. Patients with chronic fibrocavitary coccidioidomycosis will benefit from long-term oral azole therapy or even from surgery for refractory disease, while evidence is lacking that antifungal therapy is useful for patients with pulmonary nodules or cavities.[28] Amphotericin B formulations and the newer azoles are also active against *Coccidioides* spp.[28]

Prophylaxis has been attempted in 2 at-risk populations living in endemic areas, with mixed results. Primary prophylaxis was not effective for the majority of HIV-positive patients.[29] On the other hand, a targeted approach wherein fluconazole was prescribed to solid organ transplant recipients with either positive history or serologic results for coccidioidomycosis has been more successful.[30]

Blastomycosis

Blastomyces dermatitidis, the etiologic agent of blastomycosis, has traditionally been restricted to the midwestern, southeastern, and south central states of the United States, as well as the Canadian provinces bordering the Great Lakes at St Lawrence Seaway (see **Fig. 1**).[31] Autochthonous cases have also been reported from parts of Africa and the Middle East.[11] As with most of the other endemic mycoses, infection occurs most commonly following inhalation of conidia, with the transformation of mold into yeast stage occurring within macrophages. Immunity is also T-cell mediated.[32]

Blastomycosis is a systemic disease with protean pulmonary and extrapulmonary manifestations, with severity ranging from asymptomatic to rapidly fatal. The majority of acute pulmonary infections are nonspecific in terms of symptomatology and radiologic findings, which typically show segmental or lobar consolidation.[33] Outside of the outbreak setting, acute pulmonary blastomycosis is rarely identified. Chronic pulmonary blastomycosis is more commonly diagnosed, presenting with low-grade fever, weight loss, fatigue, and productive cough. Masslike lesions (mimicking lung cancer), multiple nodules, lobar infiltrates, and cavitary lesions are frequently seen on chest imaging, whereas hilar adenopathy, miliary disease, and pleural effusions are comparatively rare.[33]

A wide variety of cutaneous and subcutaneous manifestations are seen in blastomycosis, and skin involvement may occur in up to 60% of patients. These and other extrapulmonary manifestations are outside the scope of this article, but they may heighten clinical suspicion for blastomycosis in a patient from an endemic region.

In contrast to the other endemic mycoses, immunocompromised patients, including transplant patients and those with HIV infection, appear not to be at higher risk of developing blastomycosis, although morbidity and mortality rates are higher once infection has occurred.[34] Early findings are backed by more recent reports suggesting higher rates of acute respiratory distress syndrome and miliary disease in infected solid organ transplant recipients (15%),[35] patients with AIDS (20%),[36] and HSCT recipients (40%),[34] with high rates of disease-associated mortality in these vulnerable populations.

Diagnostic testing for blastomycosis is comparatively problematic compared with the other endemic mycoses (see **Table 2**). Cultures can be positive in up to two-thirds of cases after 4 to 6 weeks of incubation—a delay that may impact on the management of acute and disseminated infections.[19] Antigen detection appears to be highly sensitive (93%), especially for chronic pneumonia, but cross-reactions occur with histoplasmosis. Currently available serologic tests are not recommended by experts.[19]

Treatment guidelines for blastomycosis were recently updated by IDSA in 2008.[31] In summary, although it was acknowledged that acute pulmonary blastomycosis in immunocompetent patients could be mild and self limited, it was recommended that all infected patients should receive antifungal therapy to prevent extrapulmonary dissemination.[31] Antifungal therapy was also recommended for all other forms of blastomycosis, including mild acute pneumonia in immunocompromised patients, and generally comprised an initial 1 to 2 weeks of amphotericin B followed by oral itraconazole. The newer azoles did not appear to confer any advantage over itraconazole.[31] The exception was in infected pregnant women, in whom azoles (but not amphotericin B) were not recommended because they may be teratogenic.[31]

There are currently no viable strategies for preventing blastomycosis in individuals living in endemic areas.

Paracoccidioidomycosis

Paracoccidioidomycosis is the most prevalent endemic mycosis in Latin America. The causative agent has a restricted geographic distribution ranging from Mexico to Argentina (latitudes 23°N to 34°S), although not all countries within these latitudes are affected and Brazil accounts for a disproportionate (80%) number of cases.[37,38] Molecular phylogenetic analysis has shown that *Paracoccidioides brasiliensis* is not a single species, but rather a species complex that includes at least 3 cryptic species: phylogenetic species (PS) 1 (Brazil, Argentina, Paraguay, Peru, and Venezuela), PS2 (Brazil and Venezuela), and PS3 (Colombia).[39]

Paracoccidioidomycosis is rare in children (3%), occurring mostly in men aged 30 to 50 years who are involved in agricultural work.[38] Primary infection is usually transient and subclinical, with the yeast stage capable of remaining dormant in tissue for years until reactivated by immunosuppression. Two patterns of disease are commonly seen: a subacute (juvenile) form seen in children and adolescents (3%–5% of cases) where reticuloendothelial system involvement is predominant with minimal lung involvement, and a chronic (adult) form (>90% of all cases) in which the lungs are predominantly affected.[37,38] In AIDS patients, the disease occurs at a younger age especially in those with CD4 count of <200 cells/µL, and progresses more rapidly, with more extrapulmonary involvement. However, mortality is similar to the chronic form if antifungal therapy is initiated.[40]

Patients with chronic pulmonary paracoccidioidomycosis generally present with chronic cough and constitutional symptoms such as night sweats, fever, and weight loss. Where multifocal disease exists, symptoms from mucosal and cutaneous involvement tend to predominate over pulmonary symptoms despite significant lung involvement.[37,38] Chest radiography frequently reveals bilateral patchy or nodular infiltrates over the central and lower portion of the lungs, with cavities but not hilar adenopathy. Fibrosis and bullae formation are common long-term sequelae.[37,38]

The diagnosis of paracoccidioidomycosis is usually made by the detection of characteristic budding yeasts ("steering wheels" or "Mickey Mouse" appearance) from sputum, in a tissue biopsy or scrapings of skin/mucosal lesions.[37,38] Cultures are recommended, although time to positivity may be up to 6 weeks.[37,38] Serologic tests are useful both for diagnosis and follow-up. Various commercial kits are available, although immunodiffusion is the current test of choice while the utility of complement fixation and enzyme-linked immunosorbent assay (ELISA) are limited due to cross-reactivity with other fungi.[41] In unifocal disease or where serologic titers may be low, antigen detection (gp48 and gp70) using an immunoenzymatic assay may be helpful.[42]

P brasiliensis is sensitive to amphotericin B, azoles, terbinafine, and sulfonamides. Brazilian guidelines for the management of paracoccidioidomycosis were published in 2006.[43] For mild to moderate disease, oral itraconazole is the drug of choice. For severe disease, intravenous amphotericin B or trimethoprim-sulfamethoxazole is recommended.[37,38,43] Relapses tend to occur only in patients with disseminated disease, with higher rates in AIDS patients.[40]

There are no commercially available vaccines or any tested strategies for the primary prevention of paracoccidioidomycosis in individuals living in endemic areas.

Penicilliosis

Penicillium marneffei, the only thermally dimorphic *Penicillium* sp, is an emerging endemic mycosis geographically limited to tropical Asia, especially Thailand, southern China, northwestern India, Taiwan, and Vietnam.[44] Rare as a cause of human disease before 1988, the advent of the HIV epidemic has resulted in an explosive increase in the prevalence of penicilliosis in Asia.[44,45] In northern Thailand, it remains the third most common opportunistic infection in AIDS patients.[45] Although no association was found between human disease and exposure to bamboo rats—from which *P marneffei* was originally isolated[46]—molecular studies have shown that human and rat isolates are genetically identical.[47]

Asymptomatic or subclinical infection likely occurs via inhalation of airborne conidia, with conversion to yeast stage within lung macrophages. Cell-mediated immunity in immunocompetent hosts results in clearance of the fungus within weeks. Clinical disease develops mainly in immunocompromised patients, more commonly in AIDS patients and less so in transplant or corticosteroid recipients.[44] Chronic disseminated disease is the norm, with cutaneous lesions resembling molluscum contagiosum and generalized lymphadenopathy reported in the majority of cases.[48] Chest imaging in cases where lung involvement has occurred demonstrates a variety of findings including reticulonodular and diffuse alveolar infiltrates, with cavitary lesions seen less commonly.[48] Unless treated, penicilliosis is progressive and often fatal.

Diagnostic tests for penicilliosis are summarized in **Table 2**. In contrast to other endemic mycoses, cultures, even from blood samples (76% sensitivity), are often positive, although diagnosis is most commonly made from direct microscopy of infected samples.[45] Several serologic and antigen detection kits are available commercially, with varying sensitivities and specificities.[44] Of note, the Platelia *Aspergillus* seroassay cross-reacts with *P marneffei* and may be considered as a diagnostic modality for penicilliosis.[49] Various promising polymerase chain reaction–based methods have been developed, although none are commercially available as yet.[44]

P marneffei is sensitive to amphotericin B and most azoles except for fluconazole.[50] Current treatment with amphotericin B for 2 weeks initially followed by oral itraconazole for 10 weeks has yielded an excellent response (97.3%).[51] AIDS patients should be maintained on secondary itraconazole prophylaxis until CD4 counts exceed 100 cells/μL for 6 months.[52]

Sporotrichosis

Sporothrix schenckii can be found in tropical and temperate zones worldwide in decaying material, hay, soil, and sphagnum moss. Unlike other endemic mycoses, infection occurs primarily by cutaneous inoculation, and is more common among gardeners and landscapers.[11] Infection can also be caused by zoonotic spread via scratches from digging animals or infected cats.[53] Unsurprisingly, cutaneous or lymphocutaneous presentations of sporotrichosis are the most common. Rarely, involvement of the lungs can occur via inhalation of the *S schenckii* conidia or when systemic dissemination occurs in immunocompromised patients, typically those with advanced HIV disease.[11]

Pulmonary sporotrichosis typically presents as chronic fibronodular cavitary disease mimicking tuberculosis in middle-aged alcoholic men or those with underlying COPD. Presenting symptoms include fever, night sweats, cough with purulent sputum, and other constitutional symptoms.[53] Outcomes are often poor because of diagnostic delay and severe underlying pulmonary disease.[53,54]

In terms of diagnostic approaches, culture of infected material offers the best yield, with positive growth documented within 7 days on average.[11] An ELISA serologic test appears to offer excellent sensitivity (90%), although false-positive results may occur with leishmaniasis.[55] Direct microscopic examination of infected samples is of low yield, as the organism is rare in tissue and small in size.[5] There are no antigen or molecular tests that are of clinical utility at present.

Guidelines for the treatment of sporotrichosis were updated by IDSA in 2007.[53] In patients with severe or life-threatening pulmonary disease, amphotericin B formulations are the drugs of choice, followed by itraconazole for up to 12 weeks if a favorable initial outcome is demonstrated. Oral itraconazole may be used first-line for less severe disease, while surgery combined with an antifungal agent is recommended in some cases. Overall, the pharmacologic management of disseminated disease is essentially similar to the management of pulmonary disease.[53] There are no viable strategies for primary prophylaxis against sporotrichosis, although AIDS patients with sporotrichosis may benefit from secondary prophylaxis using itraconazole.[53]

EMERGING PULMONARY MOLD INFECTIONS

Recent medical advances, particularly aggressive interventions for patients with malignancies and/or HSCT, have resulted in progressively lengthening periods of profound immunosuppression and improved survival for these individuals. Coupled with changes in terms of prophylaxis and therapy against common invasive mycoses such as *Candida* spp initially and *Aspergillus* spp more recently, rare and previously nonpathogenic molds are now emerging as a cause of infection in these vulnerable patients. The 3 main groups of emerging medically important molds are the Zygomycetes, hyaline septated molds, and dematiaceous molds. In specific host populations, namely HSCT, guidelines have been published to minimize the risk of exposure and disease during especially vulnerable periods.[56]

Zygomycosis

Zygomycosis is a term used to collectively describe fungal infections caused by molds belonging to the class Zygomycetes of the phylum Zygomycota. The most common species causing angioinvasive zygomycosis are *Rhizopus arrhizus* (*Rhizopus oryzae*), followed by *Rhizopus microsporus* var. *rhizopodiformis* and *Rhizomucor pusillus*.[57]

These fungi are commonly found in decaying vegetation and soil, releasing large numbers of airborne spores. Distribution is worldwide. Risk factors include diabetes mellitus, corticosteroid therapy, HSCT, solid organ transplantation, treatment with desferrioxamine, iron overload, AIDS, and metabolic acidosis.[58] It has recently been shown that the use of voriconazole in immunocompromised patients may be associated with zygomycosis.[8]

Zygomycosis commonly presents as rhino-orbital-cerebral, pulmonary, gastrointestinal, cutaneous, renal, or isolated central nervous system (CNS) infection.[57,58] Clinical manifestations of pulmonary zygomycosis mimic those of invasive pulmonary aspergillosis. Patients may present with fever and cough, pleuritic chest pain, and pleural effusion. Rarely, invasion of the adjacent organs of the chest wall (such as mediastinum, pericardium, or hilar vessels) resulting in massive and potentially fatal hemoptysis have been reported.[59] Chest imaging is nonspecific, encompassing infiltrates, consolidation, nodules, cavitation, atelectasis, effusion, and hilar lymphadenopathy.[60]

The major diagnostic issue lies in differentiating zygomycosis from invasive aspergillosis, as optimal therapy for each differs. An observational study highlighted the presence of multiple nodules and pleural effusions as the differentiating features of zygomycosis on computed tomography imaging.[61] The presence on microscopic examination of broad, ribbonlike, wide-angled branching, pauciseptate hyphae accompanying tissue necrosis, and angioinvasion can be helpful, as *Aspergillus* spp hyphae are narrower and septated. Galactomannan and β-D-glucan antigen testing are also negative in zygomycosis.[62] The correlation between clinical response and minimum inhibitory concentration values of antifungal agents are uncertain, hence there is a limited role for routine antifungal susceptibility testing in zygomycosis.

Lipid formulations of amphotericin B are considered the drugs of choice for this disease.[63] There is increasing evidence for posaconazole as an option for oral step-down therapy in those who have responded to amphotericin or salvage therapy in those who have not, with the largest retrospective study showing 60% complete/partial response in 91 compassionate-use subjects.[64] The oral iron-chelating agent deferasirox showed a possible benefit when used in combination with antifungal agents to treat zygomycosis.[65] Correction of metabolic disturbances such as diabetic ketoacidosis and reversal of immunosuppression is essential, along with debridement of necrotic/infected tissue where possible. The role of adjunctive measures for improving immunity, such as granulocyte colony stimulating factor (G-CSF) and interferon-γ, is still unclear.[66]

Posaconazole appears to be an effective antifungal prophylaxis in high-risk patients such as HSCT recipients, although several cases of breakthrough zygomycosis have been reported.[67]

Hyalohyphomycosis

Hyalohyphomycosis collectively refers to infections caused by colorless (hyaline) septate molds (see **Tables 1** and **2**). *Fusarium* and *Scedosporium* infections, the most common hyalohyphomycoses, are summarized here. Naggie and Perfect[68] have recently published an excellent review of these and other medically important hyaline molds.

Fusariosis, caused by *Fusarium* spp (in particular *F solani*, *F oxysporum*, and *F moniliforme*), is the most common of these infections. Localized disease occurs in immunocompetent hosts, the most devastating of which is keratitis, with a recent multi-country outbreak occurring in 2005 to 2006 associated with Bausch & Lomb's ReNu contact lens solution.[69] In immunocompromised patients, particularly HSCT recipients and those with prolonged neutropenia or graft-versus-host disease (GVHD), disseminated disease with pulmonary involvement occurs, with 90-day mortality exceeding 80%.[70] This condition is difficult to differentiate clinically from other invasive fungal diseases in such patients, although the presence of characteristic "bull's eye" skin lesions (mimicking ecthyma gangrenosum in some cases) may help.[71] Chest radiographic features range from nonspecific alveolar infiltrates to nodules and cavitary disease.[70,71] Diagnosis is made by histopathologic examination of affected tissue and/or culture, with positive blood cultures occurring in up to 75% of patients with disseminated disease.[71] In disseminated disease, immune reconstitution is a critical part of therapy, as variable species-dependant resistance to amphotericin B and the azoles may occur.[72] Optimal antifungal therapy is dependent on susceptibility testing—both lipid amphotericin B and the newer azoles such as voriconazole or posaconazole have been used with success.[72] Topical antifungals, with or without a systemic agent such as voriconazole, are used for localized infections.[72]

Scedosporium apiospermum (with *Pseudoallescheria boydii* as its teleomorph state) is probably the next most common cause of hyalohyphomycosis after the various *Fusarium* spp. Exposure occurs via inhalation or cutaneous inoculation following trauma. *S apiospermum* can cause 3 distinctive clinical syndromes in relatively immunocompetent hosts: allergic bronchopulmonary disease (ABPD) similar to that caused by *Aspergillus* spp,[73] pulmonary or cutaneous mycetoma,[73] and sinopulmonary infection with concomitant brain abscesses in near-drowning victims.[74] The mortality rate of the last is about 70%.[74] Disease in immunocompromised patients resembles fusariosis, with similar rates of fungemia and mortality.[68] Diagnosis is made via microscopy or culture of the fungus from infected tissue or blood; there are no commercially available molecular tests at present. Voriconazole is the drug of choice, while posaconazole or combinations of antifungals have been studied.[68] Outcomes have generally been poor in disseminated disease (<50% survival), and immune reconstitution is critical.

Phaeohyphomycosis

Phaeohyphomycosis refers to infections caused by more than 100 species of ubiquitous dematiaceous (black) molds. The characteristic brown-black color of the cells is caused by melanin, which is believed to confer a protective advantage by scavenging free radicals and hypochlorite that are produced by phagocytic cells in their oxidative burst.[75] In addition, melanin may bind to hydrolytic enzymes, preventing their action on the plasma membrane.[75]

Exposure occurs via inhalation or cutaneous inoculation (trauma). These molds may infect both immunocompetent and immunocompromised hosts. In the former, it presents as skin or CNS infections whereas in the latter, sinusitis, pulmonary involvement, CNS infection, and disseminated disease occurs.[68] Both allergic and nonallergic pulmonary manifestations have been described.

ABPD is typically seen in patients who have asthma. All cases caused by dematiaceous molds were related to *Bipolaris* spp or *Curvularia* spp and were associated with eosinophilia or elevated IgE levels.[76] Systemic steroids prescribed over 2 to 3 months have been the primary therapy. Itraconazole has been used as a steroid-sparing agent, but its efficacy is not clear.[77]

Non-ABPD is rare, seen only in immunocompromised patients or those with underlying lung disease. Non-ABPD may be caused by a wide variety of species including *Ochronosis gallopava*, *Cladophialophora* spp, *Wangiella dermatitidis*. and *Curvularia* spp[68] Clinical manifestations include pneumonia, asymptomatic solitary pulmonary nodules, and endobronchial lesions that may cause hemoptysis. Obtaining histologic confirmation is critical because dematiaceous molds are common airway colonizers. It can be difficult to distinguish tissue-invasive phaeohyphomycosis from invasive aspergillosis on radiography or histology (**Fig. 2**), although fortunately antifungal susceptibility profiles are similar. Therapy consists of systemic antifungal agents, usually amphotericin B or itraconazole initially, followed by itraconazole for a more prolonged period.[78]

EMERGING PULMONARY YEAST INFECTION: *CRYPTOCOCCUS GATTII*

As with the filamentous and dimorphic fungi, an increasing number of less common yeast infections have been reported over the past two decades. This trend coincides with the advent of the HIV pandemic, medical advances especially in terms of iatrogenic immunosuppression, and perhaps even climate change and human ecological activities.[1,4–6,9] The majority of these yeasts are not associated with any specific

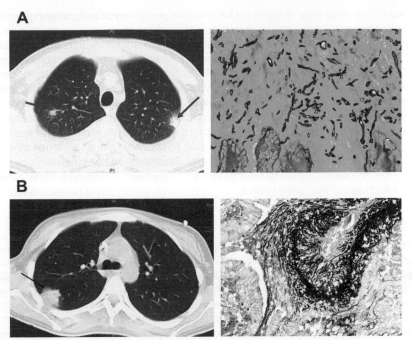

Fig. 2. Dematiaceous mold infections. (*A, left*) Computed tomography (CT) thorax image. *Exserohilum* spp invasive pulmonary disease in an allogeneic stem cell transplant recipient. (*A, right*) Grocott methenamine silver (GMS) stain of tissue (sinus) biopsy demonstrating *Exserohilum* spp hyphae from the same patient. (Original magnification ×100). (*B, left*) CT thorax image. *Rhinocladiella* spp invasive pulmonary disease in a neutropenic patient post auto stem cell transplantation for acute lymphoblastic leukemia. (*B, right*) GMS stain of tissue (lung) biopsy demonstrating *Rhinocladiella* spp hyphae from the same patient. (Original magnification ×100).

pulmonary syndrome except as part of disseminated disease, and a review of these is beyond the scope of this article.

Cryptococcus gattii

Cryptococcus gattii is one of two major pathogenic cryptococcal species, with a comparatively narrower geographic distribution because its environmental reservoir is mainly eucalyptus trees, although it may occasionally be associated with other species of trees.[79] Cases have mainly been reported from Australia, Papua New Guinea, and Vancouver (Canada). As with the endemic mycoses, infection occurs almost invariably from environmental exposure (inhalation). Unlike *Cryptococcus neoformans*, *C gattii* is far more likely to infect immunocompetent hosts, although clinical features are indistinguishable between the two *Cryptococcus* spp.[80]

Although the primary clinical findings are largely caused by pulmonary and neurologic disease, *C gattii*, like *C neoformans*, is capable of systemic dissemination. Underlying risk factors significantly influence the disease manifestations—symptomatic pulmonary cryptococcosis was proportionately about 7 times more common in patients with chronic lung disease in one study.[81] The signs and symptoms of pulmonary cryptococcosis are nonspecific, and chest imaging findings run the gamut from pulmonary nodules (most commonly seen) to ground-glass opacities and adenopathy.[82] Acute respiratory failure secondary to severe pulmonary disease has been reported.[83] The diagnosis is clinched on positive serum cryptococcal antigen titers, and less commonly via positive cultures or histopathology.

Guidelines for the management of cryptococcosis were last published by IDSA in 2000, with an update due in 2010.[84] These guidelines do not distinguish C gattii from C neoformans. In general, fluconazole is recommended for mild to moderate pulmonary disease if there is no concomitant meningitis, while an initial course of amphotericin B combined with flucytosine is recommended for severe disease.[84] The newer azoles are effective against cryptococcosis, but experience with these agents is limited. In asymptomatic immunocompetent patients in whom the diagnosis of cryptococcosis was made after removal of a pulmonary nodule, an initial period of observation before initiating antifungal therapy is considered reasonable.[85]

There are no viable strategies for the primary prevention of C gattii or other cryptococcal infections at this point in time.

SUMMARY

The incidence of fungal infection, and by extension fungal pulmonary disease, has risen over the past few decades, with previously rare fungi being isolated at increasing frequencies even as newer prophylactic strategies reduce but do not completely abrogate the risk of infection by more common fungi such as Candida spp. Even with improved diagnostic capabilities and new antifungal agents, outcomes remain poor for many types of fungal infections. Better diagnostic tests are required, in particular for the filamentous fungi that cause disease in severely immunocompromised patients, while cost-effective and affordable prophylactic strategies are urgently required for patients who are at risk for these diverse fungal infections. More research is required to understand the ecology of the endemic mycoses, as well as how to limit their widening geographic reach.

REFERENCES

1. Lass-Flörl C. The changing face of epidemiology of invasive fungal disease in Europe. Mycoses 2009;52(3):197–205.
2. Erjavec Z, Kluin-Nelemans H, Verweij PE. Trends in invasive fungal infections, with emphasis on invasive aspergillosis. Clin Microbiol Infect 2009;15(7):625–33.
3. Malani AN, Kauffman CA. Changing epidemiology of rare mould infections: implications for therapy. Drugs 2007;67:1803–12.
4. Richardson M, Lass-Flörl C. Changing epidemiology of systemic fungal infections. Clin Microbiol Infect 2008;14(Suppl 4):5–24.
5. Marr KA. Fungal infections in oncology patients: update on epidemiology, prevention, and treatment. Curr Opin Oncol 2010;22(2):138–42.
6. Lewis RE. Overview of the changing epidemiology of candidemia. Curr Med Res Opin 2009;25(7):1732–40.
7. Mann PA, McNicholas PM, Chau AS, et al. Impact of antifungal prophylaxis on colonization and azole susceptibility of Candida species. Antimicrob Agents Chemother 2009;53(12):5026–34.
8. Pongas GN, Lewis RE, Samonis G, et al. Voriconazole-associated zygomycosis: a significant consequence of evolving antifungal prophylaxis and immunosuppression practices? Clin Microbiol Infect 2009;15(Suppl 5):93–7.
9. Greer A, Ng V, Fisman D. Climate change and infectious diseases in North America: the road ahead. CMAJ 2008;178(6):715–22.

10. Datta K, Bartlett KH, Marr KA. *Cryptococcus gattii*: emergence in western North America: exploitation of a novel ecological niche. Interdiscip Perspect Infect Dis 2009;2009:176532.

11. Kauffman CA. Endemic mycoses: blastomycosis, histoplasmosis, and sporotrichosis. Infect Dis Clin North Am 2006;20(3):645–62, vii.

12. Wickes BL, Mayorga ME, Edman U, et al. Dimorphism and haploid fruiting in *Cryptococcus neoformans*: association with the α-mating type. Proc Natl Acad Sci U S A 1996;93(14):7327–31.

13. Loulergue P, Bastides F, Baudouin V, et al. Literature review and case histories of *Histoplasma capsulatum* var. *duboisii* infections in HIV-infected patients. Emerg Infect Dis 2007;13(11):1647–52.

14. Wheat LJ, Freifeld AG, Kleiman MB, et al. Clinical practice guidelines for the management of patients with histoplasmosis: 2007 update by the Infectious Diseases Society of America. Clin Infect Dis 2007;45(7):807–25.

15. Cuellar-Rodriguez J, Avery RK, Lard M, et al. Histoplasmosis in solid organ transplant recipients: 10 years of experience at a large transplant center in an endemic area. Clin Infect Dis 2009;49(5):710–6.

16. Wheat LJ, Conces D, Allen SD, et al. Pulmonary histoplasmosis syndromes: recognition, diagnosis and management. Semin Respir Crit Care Med 2004; 25(2):129–44.

17. Gurney JW, Conces DJ Jr. Pulmonary histoplasmosis. Radiology 1996;199(2): 297–306.

18. Sathapatayavongs B, Batteiger BE, Wheat J, et al. Clinical and laboratory features of disseminated histoplasmosis during two large urban outbreaks. Medicine (Baltimore) 1983;62(5):263–70.

19. Wheat LJ. Approach to the diagnosis of endemic mycoses. Clin Chest Med 2009; 30(2):379–89, viii.

20. Hage CA, Davis TE, Fuller D, et al. Diagnosis of histoplasmosis by antigen detection in bronchoalveolar fluid. Chest 2010;137(3):623–8.

21. Lenhart SW, Schafer MP, Singal M, et al. NIOSH: histoplasmosis: protecting workers at risk - revised edition. 2004. Available at: http://www.elcosh.org/en/document/718/d000679/niosh%253A-histoplasmosis%253A-protecting-workers-at-risk-revised-edition.html. Accessed May 22, 2010.

22. Laniado-Laborin R. Expanding understanding of epidemiology of coccidioidomycosis in the Western hemisphere. Ann N Y Acad Sci 2007;1111:19–34.

23. Centers for Disease Control and Prevention (CDC). Increase in coccidioidomycosis—California, 2000–2007. MMWR Morb Mortal Wkly Rep 2009;58(5):105–9.

24. Smith CE, Beard RR, Whiting EG, et al. Varieties of coccidioidal infection in relation to the epidemiology and control of the disease. Am J Public Health 1946;36: 1394–402.

25. Kirkland TN, Fierer J. Coccidioidomycosis: a reemerging infectious disease. Emerg Infect Dis 1996;2(3):192–9.

26. Galgiani J. Coccidioides immitis. In: Mandell GL, Bennett JE, Dolin R, editors. Principles and practice of infectious diseases. 5th edition. Philadelphia: Churchill Livingstone; 2000. p. 2746–57.

27. Sutton DA. Diagnosis of coccidioidomycosis by culture: safety considerations, traditional methods, and susceptibility testing. Ann N Y Acad Sci 2007;1111: 315–25.

28. Galgiani JN, Ampel NM, Blair JE, et al. Coccidioidomycosis. Clin Infect Dis 2005; 41(9):1217–23.

29. Woods CW, McRill C, Plikaytis BD, et al. Coccidioidomycosis during human immunodeficiency virus infection: results of a prospective study in a coccidioidal endemic area. Am J Med 1993;94(3):235–40.
30. Blair JE. Approach to the solid organ transplant patient with latent infection and disease caused by *Coccidioides* spp. Curr Opin Infect Dis 2008;21(4):415–20.
31. Chapman SW, Dismukes WE, Proia LA, et al. Clinical practice guidelines for the management of blastomycosis: 2008 update by the Infectious Diseases Society of America. Clin Infect Dis 2008;46(12):1801–12.
32. Chang WL, Audet RG, Aizenstein BD, et al. T-cell epitopes and human leukocyte antigen restriction elements of an immunodominant antigen of *Blastomyces dermatitidis*. Infect Immun 2000;68(2):502–10.
33. Brown LR, Sweasen SJ, VanScoy RE, et al. Roentgenologic features of pulmonary blastomycosis. Mayo Clin Proc 1991;66:29–38.
34. Pappas PG, Threlkeld MG, Bedsole GD, et al. Blastomycosis in immunocompromised patients. Medicine (Baltimore) 1993;72(5):311–25.
35. Gauthier GM, Safdar N, Klein BS, et al. Blastomycosis in solid organ transplant recipients. Transpl Infect Dis 2007;9:310–7.
36. Pappas PG, Pottage JC, Powderly WG, et al. Blastomycosis in patients with the acquired immunodeficiency syndrome. Ann Intern Med 1992;116:847–53.
37. Restrepo A, Benard G, de Castro CC, et al. Pulmonary paracoccidioidomycosis. Semin Respir Crit Care Med 2008;29(2):182–97.
38. Laniado-Laborin R. Coccidioidomycosis and other endemic mycoses in Mexico. Rev Iberoam Micol 2007;24(4):249–58.
39. Theodoro RC, Bagagli E, Oliveira C. Phylogenetic analysis of PRP8 intein in *Paracoccidioides brasiliensis* species complex. Fungal Genet Biol 2008;45(9):1284–91.
40. Morejón KM, Machado AA, Martinez R. Paracoccidioidomycosis in patients infected with and not infected with human immunodeficiency virus: a case-control study. Am J Trop Med Hyg 2009;80(3):359–66.
41. de Camargo ZP. Serology of paracoccidioidomycosis. Mycopathologia 2008;165(4–5):289–302.
42. Marques da Silva SH, Colombo AL, Blotta MH, et al. Detection of circulating gp43 antigen in serum, cerebrospinal fluid, and bronchoalveolar lavage fluid of patients with paracoccidioidomycosis. J Clin Microbiol 2003;41(8):3675–80.
43. Shikanai-Yasuda MA, Telles Filho Fde Q, Mendes RP, et al. [Guidelines in paracoccidioidomycosis]. Rev Soc Bras Med Trop 2006;39(3):297–310 [in Portuguese].
44. Vanittanakom N, Cooper CR Jr, Fisher MC, et al. *Penicillium marneffei* infection and recent advances in the epidemiology and molecular biology aspects [Review]. Clin Microbiol Rev 2006;19(1):95–110.
45. Supparatpinyo K, Khamwan C, Baosoung V, et al. Disseminated *Penicillium marneffei* infection in Southeast Asia. Lancet 1994;344(8915):110–3.
46. Capponi M, Sureau P, Segretain G. [Penicillosis from *Rhizomys sinensis*]. Bull Soc Pathol Exot 1956;49(3):418–21 [in French].
47. Fisher M, Aanensen CD, de Hoog S, et al. Multilocus microsatellite typing system for *Penicillium marneffei* reveals spatially structured populations. J Clin Microbiol 2004;42(11):5065–9.
48. Duong TA. Infection due to *Penicillium marneffei*, an emerging pathogen: review of 155 reported cases. Clin Infect Dis 1996;23(1):125–30.
49. Huang YT, Hung CC, Liao CH, et al. Detection of circulating galactomannan in serum samples for diagnosis of *Penicillium marneffei* infection and

cryptococcosis among patients infected with human immunodeficiency virus. J Clin Microbiol 2007;45(9):2858–62.

50. Supparatpinyo K, Nelson KE, Merz WG, et al. Response to antifungal therapy by human immunodeficiency virus-infected patients with disseminated *Penicillium marneffei* infections and in vitro susceptibilities of isolates from clinical specimens. Antimicrob Agents Chemother 1993;37(11):2407–11.

51. Sirisanthana T, Supparatpinyo K, Perriens J, et al. Amphotericin B and itraconazole for treatment of disseminated *Penicillium marneffei* infections and human immunodeficiency virus-infected patients. Clin Infect Dis 1998;26(5):1107–10.

52. Chalwarith R, Charoenyos N, Sirisanthana T, et al. Discontinuation of secondary prophylaxis against penicilliosis marneffei in AIDS patients after HAART. AIDS 2007;21(3):365–7.

53. Kauffman CA, Bustamante B, Chapman SW, et al. Clinical practice guidelines for the management of sporotrichosis: 2007 updated by the Infectious Diseases Society of America. Clin Infect Dis 2007;45(10):1255–65.

54. Pluss JL, Opal SM. Pulmonary sporotrichosis: review of treatment and outcome. Medicine (Baltimore) 1986;65(3):143–53.

55. Bernardes-Engemann AR, Costa RC, Miguens BR, et al. Development of an enzyme-linked immunosorbent assay for the serodiagnosis of several clinical forms of sporotrichosis. Med Mycol 2005;43(6):487–93.

56. Tomblyn M, Chiller T, Einsele H, et al. Guidelines for preventing infectious complications among hematopoietic cell transplantation recipients: a global perspective. Biol Blood Marrow Transplant 2009;15(10):1143–238.

57. Sugar AM. Agents of mucormycosis and related species. In: Mandell GL, Bennett JE, Dolin R, editors. Principles and practice of infectious diseases. 5th edition. Philadelphia: Churchill Livingstone; 2000. p. 2685–95.

58. Chayakulkeeree M, Ghannoum MA, Perfect JR. Zygomycosis: the re-emerging fungal infection. Eur J Clin Microbiol Infect Dis 2006;25(4):215–29.

59. Gupta KL, Khullar DK, Behera D, et al. Pulmonary mucormycosis presenting as fatal massive haemoptysis in a renal transplant recipient. Nephrol Dial Transplant 1998;13(12):3258–60.

60. Rubin SA, Chaljub G, Winer-Muram HT, et al. Pulmonary zygomycosis: a radiographic and clinical spectrum. J Thorac Imaging 1992;7(4):85–90.

61. Chamilos G, Marom EM, Lewis RE, et al. Predictors of pulmonary zygomycosis versus invasive pulmonary aspergillosis in patients with cancer. Clin Infect Dis 2005;41(1):60–6.

62. Hachem RY, Kontoyiannis DP, Chemaly RF, et al. Utility of galactomannan enzyme immunoassay and (1,3) beta-D-glucan in diagnosis of invasive fungal infections: low sensitivity for *Aspergillus fumigatus* infection in hematologic malignancy patients. J Clin Microbiol 2009;47(1):129–33.

63. Perfect JR. Use of newer antifungal therapies in clinical practice: what do the data tell us? Oncology (Williston Park) 2004;18(13 Suppl 7):15–23.

64. Van Burik JH, Hare RS, Solomon HF, et al. Posaconazole is effective as salvage therapy in zygomycosis: a retrospective summary of 91 cases. Clin Infect Dis 2006;42:e61–5.

65. Spellberg B, Andes D, Perez M, et al. Safety and outcomes of open-label deferasirox iron chelation therapy for mucormycosis. Antimicrob Agents Chemother 2009;53(7):3122–5.

66. Gil-Lamaignere C, Simitsopoulou M, Roilides E, et al. Interferon-gamma and granulocyte macrophage colony-stimulating factor augment the activity of

polymorphonuclear leukocytes against medically important zygomycetes. J Infect Dis 2005;191(7):1180–7.

67. Lekakis LJ, Lawson A, Prante J, et al. Fatal rhizopus pneumonia in allogeneic stem cell transplant patients despite posaconazole prophylaxis: two cases and review of the literature. Biol Blood Marrow Transplant 2009;15(8):991–5.

68. Naggie S, Perfect JR. Molds: hyalohyphomycosis, phaeohyphomycosis and zygomycosis. Clin Chest Med 2009;30(2):337–53, vii–viii.

69. Saw SM, Ooi PL, Tan DT, et al. Risk factors for contact lens-related fusarium keratitis: a case-control study in Singapore. Arch Ophthalmol 2007;125(5):611–7.

70. Nucci M, Marr KA, Queiroz-Telles F, et al. *Fusarium* infection in hematopoietic stem cell transplant recipients. Clin Infect Dis 2004;38(9):1237–42.

71. Boutati EI, Anaissie EJ. *Fusarium*, a significant emerging pathogen in patients with hematologic malignancy: ten years' experience at a cancer center and implications for management. Blood 1997;90(3):999–1008.

72. Nucci M, Anaissie E. Fusarium infections in immunocompromised patients. Clin Microbiol Rev 2007;20(4):697–704.

73. Cimon B, Carrère J, Vinatier JF, et al. Clinical significance of *Scedosporium apiospermum* in patients with cystic fibrosis. Eur J Clin Microbiol Infect Dis 2000; 19(1):53–6.

74. Katragkou A, Dotis J, Kotsiou M, et al. *Scedosporium apiospermum* infection after near-drowning. Mycoses 2007;50(5):412–21.

75. Jacobson ES. Pathogenic roles for fungal melanins. Clin Microbiol Rev 2000; 13(4):708–17.

76. Lake FR, Froudist JH, McAleer R, et al. Allergic bronchopulmonary fungal disease caused by *Bipolaris* and *Curvularia*. Aust N Z J Med 1991;21(6):871–4.

77. Malde B, Greenberger PA. Allergic bronchopulmonary aspergillosis. Allergy Asthma Proc 2004;25(4 Suppl 1):S38–9.

78. Revankar SG. Phaeohyphomycosis. Infect Dis Clin North Am 2006;20(3):609–20.

79. Gugnani HC, Mitchell TG, Litvintseva AP, et al. Isolation of *Cryptococcus gattii* and *Cryptococcus neoformans* var *grubii* from the flowers and bark of Eucalyptus trees in India. Med Mycol 2005;43(6):565–9.

80. Hoang LM, Maguire JA, Doyle P, et al. *Cryptococcus neoformans* infections at Vancouver Hospital and Health Sciences Centre (1997–2002): epidemiology, microbiology and histopathology. J Med Microbiol 2004;53(Pt 9):935–40.

81. Pappas PG, Perfect JR, Cloud GA, et al. Cryptococcosis in human immunodeficiency virus-negative patients in the era of effective azole therapy. Clin Infect Dis 2001;33(5):690–9.

82. Zinck SE, Leung AN, Frost M, et al. Pulmonary cryptococcosis: CT and pathologic findings. J Comput Assist Tomogr 2002;26(3):330–4.

83. Vilchez RA, Linden P, Lacomis J, et al. Acute respiratory failure associated with pulmonary cryptococcosis in non-AIDS patients. Chest 2001;119(6):1865–9.

84. Saag MS, Graybill RJ, Larsen RA, et al. Practice guidelines for the management of cryptococcal disease. Clin Infect Dis 2000;30(4):710–8.

85. Nadrous HF, Antonios VS, Terrell CL, et al. Pulmonary cryptococcosis in nonimmunocompromised patients. Chest 2003;124(6):2143–7.

86. Lee JH, Slifman NR, Gershon SK, et al. Life-threatening histoplasmosis complicating immunotherapy with tumor necrosis factor alpha antagonists infliximab and ethanercept. Arthritis Rheum 2002;46(10):2565–70.

87. Serrano JA, Novoa-Montero D. Review on human mycoses in South America. Rev Soc Ven Microbiol 2001;21(2):41–68. Available at: http://www.scielo.org.ve/

scielo.php?script=sci_arttext&pid=S1315-25562001000200015&lng=pt&nrm=iso&tlng=en. Accessed January 6, 2010.

88. Gugnani HC, Muotoe Okafor F. African histoplasmosis: a review. Rev Iberoam Micol 1997;14(4):155–9.
89. Randhawa HS. Occurrence of histoplasmosis in Asia. Mycopathologia 1970; 41(1):75–89.
90. Nissapatorn V, Lee CK, Rohela M, et al. Spectrum of opportunistic infections among HIV-infected patients in Malaysia. Southeast Asian J Trop Med Public Health 2004;35(Suppl 2):26–32.
91. Poonwan N, Imai T, Mekha N, et al. Genetic analysis of *Histoplasma capsulatum* strains isolated from clinical specimens in Thailand by a PCR-based random amplified polymorphic DNA method. J Clin Microbiol 1998;36(10):3073–6.
92. Harahap M, Nasution MA. Dermatomycoses in Indonesia. Int J Dermatol 1984; 23(4):273–4.
93. Hector R, Laniado-Laborin R. Coccidioidomycosis—a fungal disease of the Americas. PLoS Med 2005;2(1):e2.
94. Gatti F, De Broe M, Ajello L. Blastomycosis dermatitidis infection of the Congo. Report of a second autochthonous case. Am J Trop Med Hyg 1968;17:96–101.
95. Jerray M, Hayouni A, Benzarti M, et al. Blastomycosis in Africa: a new case from Tunisia. Eur Respir J 1992;5:365–7.

Emerging and Established Parasitic Lung Infestations

Vannan Kandi Vijayan, MD, PhD, DSc[a],*, Tarek Kilani, MD[b,c]

KEYWORDS

- Parasitic lung infections • Pulmonary amebiasis
- Pulmonary malaria • Tropical eosinophilia
- Pulmonary hydatidosis • Pulmonary paragonimiasis

Protozoal and helminthic parasitic diseases, although prevalent worldwide, are common in tropical regions of the world. A decline in parasitic infestations was observed in the last century, especially in developed countries, as a result of improved socioeconomic conditions with associated good hygiene practices. The increasing occurrence of immunosuppression in individuals due to human immunodeficiency virus (HIV) infection/acquired immunodeficiency syndrome (AIDS), organ transplantations, or the use of immunosuppressive drugs in the latter part of the last century and the beginning of this century have made these individuals prone to the development of parasitic infestations de novo from the environment, or recrudescence from dormant infestations.[1–3] In addition, increase in global travel and changes in climate have aggravated the situation.[2] Many protozoal and helminthic parasites cause clinically significant lung diseases.[4,5] The important parasitic lung infestations are listed in **Table 1**.[5] Although parasitic diseases are seen worldwide, the major geographic distribution of these diseases are given in **Table 2**.

PROTOZOAL PARASITES

Entamoeba histolytica, *Leishmania* spp (*Leishmania donovani*, *Leishmania tropica*, *Leishmania major* and *Leishmania infantum*), malarial parasites (*Plasmodium vivax*, *Plasmodium falciparum*, *Plasmodium malaria*, *Plasmodium ovale* and *Plasmodium knowlesi*), *Babesia* spp (*Babesia microti*, *Babesia divergens*) and *Toxoplasma gondii* are the important protozoal parasites that cause pulmonary diseases.

[a] Department of Respiratory Medicine, Vallabhbhai Patel Chest Institute, University of Delhi, Delhi 110007, India
[b] Department of Thoracic and Cardiovascular Surgery, Medical School, Tunis, Tunisia
[c] Department of Thoracic and Cardiovascular Surgery, Abderrahmane Mami Teaching Hospital, Ariana 2080, Tunisia
* Corresponding author.
E-mail address: vijayanvk@hotmail.com

Infect Dis Clin N Am 24 (2010) 579–602
doi:10.1016/j.idc.2010.04.002
0891-5520/10/$ – see front matter © 2010 Elsevier Inc. All rights reserved.

Table 1	
Established pulmonary diseases caused by parasitic infections	
Diseases	Parasites
Protozoa	
Pulmonary amebiasis	*Entamoeba histolytica*
Pulmonary leishmaniasis	*Leishmania donovani*
Pulmonary malaria	*Plasmodium vivax, Plasmodium falciparum Plasmodium ovale*
Pulmonary babesiosis	*Babesia microti, Babesia divergens*
Pulmonary toxoplasmosis	*Toxoplasma gondii*
Helminths	
(a) Cestodes	
Pulmonary hydatid disease	*Echinococcus granulosus Echinococcus multilocularis*
(b) Trematodes	
Pulmonary schistosomiasis	*Schistosoma haematobium Schistosoma mansoni Schistosoma japonicum*
Pulmonary paragonimiasis	*Paragonimus westermani*
(c) Nematodes	
Pulmonary ascariasis	*Ascaris lumbricoides*
Pulmonary ancylostomiasis	*Ancylostoma duodenale Necator americanus*
Pulmonary strongyloidiasis	*Strongyloides stercoralis*
Tropical pulmonary eosinophilia (pulmonary filariasis)	*Wuchereria bancrofti Brugia malayi*
Pulmonary dirofilariasis	*Dirofilaria immitis Dirofilaria repens*
Visceral larva migrans	*Toxocara canis Toxocara cati*
Pulmonary trichinellosis	*Trichinella spiralis*

Data from Vijayan VK. Parasitic lung infections. Curr Opin Pulm Med 2009;15(3):275.

Pulmonary Amebiasis

Pulmonary amebiasis is one of the most common parasitic infestations worldwide. Amebiasis has been reported mainly from the developing countries of Asia, Africa, and Central and South America, especially in malnourished, elderly, immunosuppressed, and alcoholic individuals and pregnant women. It has been estimated that approximately 50 million people worldwide suffer from invasive amebic infestation each year, with a mortality of up to 100,000 annually.[6,7] Ingestion of mature *E histolytica* cysts in fecally contaminated food, water, or from the hands causes infestation.[8] Evidence shows that invasive amebiasis is an emerging parasitic disorder in patients with HIV infection[9] and in men who have sex with men.[10] Pleuropulmonary amebiasis occurs mainly by cephalad extension from the amebic liver abscess.[11,12] The main symptoms are fever, cough, hemoptysis, right upper quadrant abdominal pain, and chest pain. Some patients may present with respiratory distress and shock. Lung abscess, hepatobronchial fistula, and bronchopleural fistula with pyopneumothorax have also been reported. Expectoration of anchovy sauce–like pus indicates amebiasis.[12]

Table 2
Major geographic distributions of parasitic diseases

	Disease	Geographic Distribution
1	Amebiasis	Asian subcontinent, Africa, Asian Pacific region, South and Central America
2	Visceral leishmaniasis	India, South America, central Asia, the Middle East, Africa
3	Malaria	Africa, South and Central America, central Asia, southwest Asia, southeast Europe, Indian subcontinent, Pacific islands
4	Babesiosis	United States, Europe
5	Toxoplasmosis	France, Central America
6	Ascariasis	Tropical and subtropical regions, southeast United States
7	Hookworm disease	
	Ancylostoma duodenale	Europe, North Africa, the Middle East, South America
	Necator americanus	Southern United States, central Asia, the Caribbean, northern South America, sub-Saharan Africa, southern Asia, the Far East
	Ancylostoma ceylanicum	India, Taiwan, Philippines, Papua New Guinea
8	Strongyloidiasis	Indo-China, Central America, southern United States, Africa, tropical Australia, Pacific Islands, Papua New Guinea, rural Italy
9	Tropical pulmonary eosinophilia	India, Sri Lanka, Malaysia, southeast Asia, the Caribbean, South America, Africa, Polynesia
10	Dirofilariasis	Tropical and subtropical areas, southern Europe, United States, Mediterranean, Australia, Puerto Rico
11	Visceral larva migrans	Worldwide
12	Trichinellosis	Worldwide, most common in parts of Europe and United States
13	Hydatid disease	
	Cystic hydatid disease	Mediterranean countries, Middle East, Balkans, South America, Australia, New Zealand, central Europe
	Alveolar echinococcosis	The Northern Hemisphere
14	Schistosomiasis	
	S haematobium	Africa, Arabia, the Middle East, Iran
	S mansonii	Africa, South America, the Caribbean, the Middle East
	S japonicum	The Far East (China, Philippines, Japan)
15	Paragonimiasis	South America, Africa, southeast Asia

Diagnosis of pleuropulmonary amebiasis is suggested by the findings of increased hemidiaphragm, tender hepatomegaly, pleural effusion, and basal pulmonary involvement. Active trophozoites of *E histolytica* can be found in sputum or pleural pus. Microscopic examination of stool samples may reveal cysts or trophozoites of amebae. The presence of amebae in the stool does not indicate that the disease is due to pathogenic *E histolytica* because 2 other nonpathogenic species found in humans (*Entamoeba dispar* and *Entamoeba moshkovskii*) are indistinguishable morphologically.[13] A nonpathogenic *Entamoeba gingivalis*, which is present in the oral cavity, has to be differentiated from *E histolytica* in sputum samples. The diagnostic tests for amebiasis include culture of *E histolytica* and serologic tests. A combination of serologic tests with detection of the parasite by antigen detection by polymerase chain reaction (PCR) is the best approach to diagnosis.[14] Invasive amebiasis is treated with nitroimidazoles (metronidazole or tinidazole).[3,8] Metronidazole is given in a dosage of 750 mg orally 3 times a day for 7 to 10 days, and tinidazole in a dosage of 800 mg orally 3 times a day for 5 days.[8] Treatment with nitroimidazole should be followed by a luminal amebicidal drug (paromomycin or diloxanide furoate) to cure intestinal luminal infection. Paromomycin is given as 25 to 35 mg/kg per day in 3 divided doses for 7 days, or diloxanide furoate in a dosage of 500 mg orally 3 times a day for 10 days.[8] It has been shown in an in vitro study that ivermectin has activity against trophozoites of E histolytica.[15]

Pulmonary Leishmaniasis

Although there are 20 species belonging to the genus Leishmania that are pathogenic to humans, the important protozoan parasites that cause leishmaniasis are L donovani, L tropica, L major, and L infantum.[3] Various species of female Phlebotomus (sand fly) transmit infection to humans.[16] Leishmaniasis is endemic in Asia, Africa, Central and South America, and the Mediterranean area. It has been estimated that nearly 12 million people are presently infected worldwide and 2 million new cases occur annually.[17] Leishmaniasis and HIV infections coexist in a deadly synergy, and leishmaniasis accelerates the onset of AIDS in persons infected with HIV.[18] Visceral leishmaniasis is characterized by irregular fever, weight loss, enlargement of liver and spleen, and anemia. Pneumonitis, septal fibrosis, pleural effusion, and mediastinal adenopathy are reported in patients coinfected with HIV.[19,20] Leishmaniasis has also been reported in lung transplant patients.[21] Leishmania amastigotes can be found in the alveoli, pulmonary septa, and bronchoalveolar lavage (BAL) fluid.[22] Diagnosis of leishmaniasis is by the presence of the parasites in bone marrow aspirates and by the identification of specific DNA sequences in tissues by molecular biology techniques.[23] Treatment of leishmaniasis includes amphotericin B (especially the liposome formulations) and pentavalent antimonials.[24] Liposomal amphotericin B is prescribed in a dosage of 3 mg/kg/d intravenously on days 1 to 5, 15, and 21. Sodium stibogluconate is given in a dosage of 20 mg/kg daily intravenously or intramuscularly for 28 days.[3] Miltefosine, the first oral drug for the treatment of visceral leishmaniasis, is prescribed in a dosage of 2.5 mg/kg daily orally for 28 days, and the maximum daily dose is 150 mg.[3,25]

Pulmonary Malaria

Malaria is caused by obligate intraerythrocytic protozoa of the genus Plasmodium and is primarily transmitted by the bite of an infected female Anopheles mosquito.[26] Five species of malarial parasites (P vivax, P falciparum, P malaria, P ovale, and P knowlesi) infect humans.[27] It has been estimated that 3.3 billion people are at risk of malarial infection, and there are around 250 million cases annually, leading to approximately 1 million deaths in 2006.[26] The main symptoms of malaria include fever, headache, and vomiting, usually manifesting 10 to 15 days after the mosquito bite. Falciparum malaria is the most deadly type (Fig. 1). The pulmonary manifestations in falciparum malaria range from cough to severe and rapidly fatal noncardiogenic pulmonary edema and acute respiratory distress syndrome (ARDS).[28] Acute lung injury and ARDS have also been reported to occur in infestations with P vivax and P ovale.[29–31]

The diagnosis of malaria is based on the examination by light microscopy of stained thick and thin blood smears. Radiological findings in severe falciparum malaria include

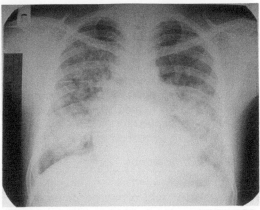

Fig. 1. Chest skiagram showing bilateral fluffy shadows in a patient presenting with acute respiratory distress syndrome due to severe falciparum malaria.

lobar consolidation, diffuse interstitial edema, pulmonary edema, and pleural effusion. A PCR detection of *P falciparum* in human urine and saliva samples has been described.[32] The drugs used for treatment of severe malaria are quinine dihydrochloride, quinidine gluconate, and injectable artemisinin derivatives. Artemisinin-based combination therapies (artemether + lumefantrine, artesunate + amodioquine, artesunate + mefloquine, or artesunate + sulfadoxine-pyrimethamine) are the best antimalarial drugs.[33] Patients presenting with ARDS require invasive mechanical ventilation with intensive care management.[34]

Pulmonary Babesiosis

Babesiosis is caused by intraerythrocytic protozoal parasites, *B microti* and *B divergens*.[35] Cattle and wild rodents are the principal reservoirs of babesiosis. Humans acquire the infection by the bite of an infected tick, *Ixodes scapularis* and can also be infected from a contaminated blood transfusion.[36] The parasites attack the red blood cells and can be misdiagnosed as *Plasmodium*. The risk factors for systemic infection are immunosuppression, advanced age, and splenectomy. The symptoms are fever, drenching sweats, cough, tiredness, loss of appetite, myalgia, and headache. ARDS occurring a few days after initiation of medical therapy is the important pulmonary manifestation.[37] Chest radiological features include bilateral infiltrates with an alveolar pattern and thickening of the septa. Specific diagnosis is made by examination of a Giemsa-stained thin blood smear, DNA amplification using PCR, or detection of specific antibody.[35] The peripheral blood smears may show, in addition to ring forms, tetrads inside the red blood cells. These tetrads, known as Maltese cross formations, are pathognomonic of babesiosis because they are not seen in malaria.[38] Treatment is with a combination of clindamycin (600 mg every 6 hours) and quinine (650 mg every 8 hours) for 7 to 10 days or atovaquone (750 mg every 12 hours) and azithromycin (500–600 mg on the first day and 250–600 mg on subsequent days) for 7 to 10 days.[39,40]

Pulmonary Toxoplasmosis

Toxoplasmosis is caused by a single-celled protozoan parasite, *T gondii*. Cats are the primary carriers of the organism.[41] Humans acquire the infection by eating raw or undercooked meat, vegetables, or milk products contaminated with the parasitic cysts. The symptoms of toxoplasmosis are flu-like syndrome, enlarged lymph nodes, or myalgia. Pulmonary toxoplasmosis has been reported with increasing frequency in patients with HIV infection. Toxoplasma pneumonia can manifest as interstitial pneumonia/diffuse alveolar damage or necrotizing pneumonia.[42] Diagnosis of toxoplasmosis is based on the detection of the protozoa in body tissues. A real-time PCR-based assay in BAL fluid has been reported in immunocompromised HIV-positive patients.[42,43] Toxoplasmosis can be treated with a combination of pyrimethamine (25–100 mg per day orally) and sulfadiazine (1–1.5 g 4 times a day orally) for 3 to 4 weeks.[3]

Emerging Pulmonary Protozoal Infestations

Many protozoal parasites that are known to be nonpathogenic to humans are reported to cause pulmonary diseases, especially in immunocompromised individuals.[3] *Acanthamoeba* species can cause systemic disease with pulmonary manifestations of nodular infiltrates, pneumonitis, and respiratory failure in immunocompromised patients.[44] *Cryptosporidium parvum* infection produces interstitial pulmonary infiltrates and focal areas of consolidation in AIDS patients.[45] Pneumonitis, lung abscess, and bronchiectasis due to recurrent aspiration from secondary megaesophagus have been reported in *Trypanosoma cruzi* infection (Chagas disease).[46] Cardiogenic pulmonary edema and pulmonary hypertension secondary to cardiac failure and dilated cardiomyopathy have also been reported in Chagas disease.[47] *Trypanosoma brucei rhodesiense* can cause noncardiogenic pulmonary edema and ARDS in the acute stage. Rare pulmonary protozoal infections that have been reported in immunocompromised individuals are listed in **Table 3**.[5]

HELMINTHIC PARASITES

Helminthic parasites that cause human diseases belong to the genera *Nematodes*, *Cestodes*, and *Trematodes*.

Nematodes

Pulmonary diseases caused by nematode parasites are pulmonary ascariasis, pulmonary ancylostomiasis, pulmonary strongyloidiasis, tropical pulmonary eosinophilia (TPE), pulmonary dirofilariasis, visceral larva migrans (VLM), and pulmonary trichinellosis. These diseases usually induce blood and tissue eosinophilia.

Pulmonary ascariasis

Ascariasis caused by *Ascaris lumbricoides* is the most common intestinal helminthic infection and approximately 1.5 billion individuals worldwide are infected.[48] The infection occurs through soil contamination of hands or food with eggs that are then swallowed.[48] The eggs hatch into larvae in the small intestine. The larvae penetrate the wall of the intestine and travel via capillaries and lymphatics to the hepatic circulation and to the right side of the heart and then the lungs. Pulmonary migration of larvae is usually asymptomatic. *Ascaris suum* has also been reported to cause pulmonary eosinophilia.[49] Patients may present with general symptoms of malaise, loss of appetite, fever lasting 2 to 3 days, headache, and myalgia. The respiratory symptoms include chest pain, cough with mucoid sputum, hemoptysis, shortness of breath, and wheezing. Acute severe eosinophilic pneumonia requiring ventilation has also been reported in ascariasis.[50,51] Leucocytosis, particularly eosinophilia, is an important laboratory finding. Chest radiographs show unilateral or bilateral, transient, migratory, nonsegmental opacities of various sizes.[52] A diagnosis of pulmonary disease due

Table 3	
Emerging pulmonary protozoal infections	
Diseases	**Parasites**
Pulmonary acanthamebiasis	*Acanthamoeba castellanii*
	Acanthamoeba polyphaga
Pulmonary balamuthiasis	*Balamuthia mandrillaris*
Pulmonary naegleriasis	*Naegleria fowleri*
Pulmonary trichomoniasis	*Trichomonas vaginalis*
	Trichomonas tenax
	Trichomonas hominis
Pulmonary lophomoniasis	*Lophomonas blattarum*
Pulmonary trypanosomiasis	*Trypanosoma cruzi*
	Trypanosoma brucei gambiense
	Trypanososma brucei rhodesiense
Pulmonary cryptosporidiosis	*Cryptosporidium parvum*
	Cryptosporidium hominis
	Cryptosporidium meleagridis
Pulmonary cyclosporidiasis	*Cyclospora cayetanensis*
Pulmonary encephalitozoonosis	*Encephalitozoon cuniculi*
	Encephalitozoon hellem
	Encephalitozoon intestinalis
Pulmonary entercytozoonosis	*Enterocytozoon bieneusi*
Pulmonary balantidiasis	*Balantidium coli*

Data from Vijayan VK. Parasitic lung infections. Curr Opin Pulm Med 2009;15(3):280.

to ascariasis can be made in an endemic region in a patient who presents with dyspnea, dry cough, fever, and eosinophilia. Stool examination usually does not show *Ascaris* eggs and stool samples may be negative until 2 to 3 months after respiratory symptoms occur, unless the patient was previously infected. Larvae can sometimes be found in respiratory or gastric secretions.[53]

Pulmonary disease due to ascariasis is a self-limiting disease. However, the persistence of gastrointestinal ascariasis may result in repeated episodes of respiratory symptoms due to larval migration. To eradicate *A lumbricoides* from the intestine, mebendazole is given in a dose of 100 mg twice a day for 3 days or as a single dose of 500 mg.[54] Albendazole can also be given as a single dose of 400 mg. The safety of mebendazole and albendazole during pregnancy has not been established. Other drugs are pyrantel pamoate (11 mg/kg, maximum dose 1 g) as a single dose and piperazine citrate (50–75 mg/kg/d for 2 days). Pediatric dose is the same as the adult dose. Ivermectin has also been found to be useful.[55]

Pulmonary ancylostomiasis

Ancylostomiasis, or hookworm disease, is caused by 3 parasite species, *Ancylostoma duodenale*, *Necator americanus*, and *Ancylostoma ceylanicum*. Humans are the only definitive host. Eggs containing segmented ova with 4 blastomers are passed in the feces. The filariform larva formed in the soil penetrates the intact skin. These larvae reach the pulmonary circulation through the lymphatics and venules. During pulmonary larval migration, patients may present with fever, cough, wheezing, and transient pulmonary infiltrates in chest radiographs.[1,4] Bronchitis and bronchopneumonia can occur when the larvae break through the pulmonary capillaries to enter the alveolar spaces. This stage is associated with blood and pulmonary eosinophilia. A direct microscopic examination of stools shows the presence of characteristic hookworm eggs. Mebendazole is given as 100 mg twice daily for 3 days, and albendazole as a single dose of 400 mg. Pyrantel pamoate at a dose of 11 mg/kg orally (maximum 1 g) as a single dose has also been found to be useful.

Pulmonary strongyloidiasis

Strongyloides stercoralis is seen worldwide, but is common in South America, southeast Asia, sub-Saharan Africa, and the Appalachian region of the United States.[56] It infects 30 million people in 70 countries.[57] The unique feature of *S stercoralis* is that it can complete its life cycle in the human host or in the soil. The filariform larvae produced in the intestine can penetrate the intestinal epithelium or the perianal skin without leaving the host. This ability is responsible for autoinfection and for persistence of infection for 20 to 30 years in persons who have left the endemic areas.[58] The filariform larvae that are produced in the soil can penetrate directly through the skin, invade the tissues, penetrate into the venous or lymphatic channels, and be carried by the blood stream to the heart and then to the lungs.[59] When there is immunosuppression, autoinfection is enhanced and leads to hyperinfection. In this situation, the number of migrating larvae increases greatly and they disseminate into many organs including lungs, meninges, brain, lymph nodes, and kidneys.[60] Patients infected with HIV are at a higher risk of dissemination.[60] *Strongyloides* hyperinfection syndrome has been reported in lung transplant individuals.[61] During migration of filariform larvae through the lungs, bronchopneumonia and hemorrhages in the alveoli can occur. The inflammation following such invasion of larvae leads to disseminated strongyloidiasis that is usually fatal. As the larvae penetrate the intestinal mucosa, gram-negative bacteria from the gut are carried by the larvae on their cuticles. As a result of invasion of bacteria along with the larvae, diffuse and patchy bronchopneumonia and pulmonary abscess can occur.

The lung signs and symptoms include cough, shortness of breath, wheezing, and hemoptysis.[62] In patients at high risk for strongyloidiasis, adult respiratory distress syndrome and septicemia can occur.[59,60] The diagnosis of strongyloidiasis by examination of a single stool specimen using conventional techniques usually fails to detect larvae in up to 70% of cases.[57] The diagnostic yield can be increased by examination of several stool specimens on consecutive days. In disseminated disease, larvae and adult parasites can be seen in sputum, urine, BAL fluid, and other body fluids.[63,64] Treatment is with ivermectin at a dosage of 200 μg/kg orally for 1 or 2 days, or thiabendazole at 25 mg/kg twice a day for 2 days. Albendazole 400 mg twice a day for 5 days has also been found to be useful in the treatment of strongyloidiasis.[65] In immunocompromised individuals with disseminated strongyloidiasis, the dose of thiabendazole has to be doubled and the duration of treatment may be several weeks. In addition, appropriate treatment of bacterial infection has to be instituted. Corticosteroids should not be prescribed to such patients and, if they have already been prescribed, they must be tapered off and discontinued.

TPE (pulmonary filariasis)

TPE is caused by immunologic hyperresponsiveness to the human filarial parasites *Wuchereria bancrofti* and *Brugia malayi*.[66–69] A pseudo-tuberculosis condition associated with eosinophilia was described in 1940 in a group of patients with bilateral miliary mottling and massive blood eosinophilia not responding to antituberculosis treatment,[70] and the name tropical eosinophilia for this entity was coined by Weingarten.[71] It is prevalent in filarial endemic regions of the world, especially the

Indian subcontinent, south east Asia, and the South Pacific islands.[67-69] As a result of the global increase in travel by individuals from filarial endemic regions to nonendemic regions, TPE is being increasingly reported from countries to which filarial infection is not endemic.[72] Conversely, individuals from nonendemic areas visiting filarial endemic regions are more prone to develop TPE because they do not have natural immunity against filarial infection to the same degree as endemic normal subjects.[73,74] BAL studies have shown an intense eosinophilic inflammatory process in the lower respiratory tract.[75,76] Electron microscopic examination of lung eosinophils have shown eosinophils in an activated state.[75] Patients with TPE show marked increases of filaria-specific immunoglobulin G (IgG), immunoglobulin M (IgM), and immunoglobulin E (IgE) antibodies in peripheral blood and lung epithelial lining fluid.[77] If untreated, partially treated, or treated late, TPE may lead to the development of interstitial lung disease.[67,74]

The lung is the main organ involved in TPE, but other organs, such as liver, spleen, lymph nodes, brain, and gastrointestinal tract, may also be involved.[67,78] The male/female ratio is 4:1 and it is mainly seen in older children and young adults between the ages of 15 and 40 years.[67] The systemic symptoms include fever, weight loss, and fatigue. The respiratory symptoms are paroxysmal cough, breathlessness, and nocturnal wheezing and chest pain. Leucocytosis with an absolute increase in eosinophils in the peripheral blood is the hallmark of TPE. Absolute eosinophil counts are usually more than 3000 cells/μm and may range from 5000 to 80,000.[79] The chest radiological features of TPE include reticulonodular shadows predominantly seen in mid and lower zones (**Fig. 2**). In patients with a long-standing history, a few patients have honeycomb lungs.[67] Lung function tests reveal mainly a restrictive ventilation defect with superimposed airways obstruction.[80,81] Single-breath carbon monoxide transfer factor is reduced in 88% of untreated patients with TPE.[82]

The treatment recommended for treatment of TPE is oral diethylcarbamazine citrate (DEC) 6 mg/kg per day for 3 weeks.[83] However, there is an incomplete reversal of clinical, hematologic, radiological, and physiologic changes in TPE 1 month after a 3-week course of DEC.[84] A chronic mild interstitial lung disease has been found to persist in TPE despite treatment.[85]

Pulmonary dirofilariasis

Pulmonary dirofilariasis is a zoonotic infection caused by the filarial nematodes *Dirofilaria immitis* and *Dirofilaria repens*. Humans are accidental hosts of this parasite, which

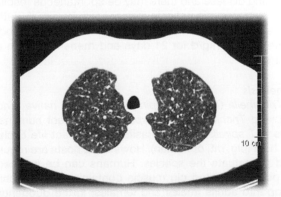

Fig. 2. HRCT scan of a patient with TPE showing bilateral nodular shadows.

is transmitted to humans by the mosquito. The parasite is a vascular parasite[86] and is usually seen in the pulmonary artery where they produce a pulmonary nodule or coin lesion.[87] Nearly 50% of subjects infected with dirofilariasis are asymptomatic. Clinical symptoms are chest pain, cough, fever, hemoptysis, and dyspnea. Computerized tomography (CT) may show a well-defined nodule with smooth margin connected to an arterial branch.[88] Rarely, cavity formation in the lung has also been reported.[89] A PCR-based diagnosis of *D repens* in human pulmonary dirofilariasis is available.[90] A definitive histopathologic diagnosis of pulmonary dirofilariasis can be made in tissue specimens obtained by wedge biopsy, video-assisted thoracoscopy, or, rarely, by fine needle biopsy. There is no specific treatment of human dirofilariasis.

Pulmonary VLM

Certain nematode parasites entering an unnatural host (eg, humans) may not be able to complete their life cycle and their progress is arrested. VLM occurs when the parasite enters the body via the oral route.[91] The common parasites that cause VLM in humans are a dog ascarid (*Toxocara canis*) and, less commonly, a cat ascarid (*Toxocara cati*). The animals acquire the infection by ingestion of eggs of the parasites from contaminated soil. The life cycle is then completed in the definitive hosts (dogs and cats). Eggs are passed by the animals in feces and embryonate in the soil. When ingested by an intermediate host (eg, humans), these embryonated *Toxocara* eggs hatch into infective larvae in the intestine. The infective larvae penetrate the intestinal wall and are carried by the circulation to many organs including liver, lungs, muscles, central nervous system, and eye. The progress of the larvae is arrested in these sites of the intermediate host by the formation of a granulomatous lesion. In humans, the larvae never develop into adult worms. Therefore, infected humans never excrete toxocara eggs in the feces. VLM is characterized by leucocytosis and eosinophilia. Most children infected with *Toxocara* spp are asymptomatic. The main symptoms in patients with VLM are fever, cough, wheezing, seizures, anemia, and fatigue. Pulmonary manifestations are reported in 80% of cases, and patients may present with severe asthma. Chest skiagram may reveal focal, patchy infiltrates. In some cases, severe eosinophilic pneumonia may lead to respiratory distress.[92,93] Other clinical features include generalized lymph node enlargement, hepatomegaly, and splenomegaly. Serologic tests by enzyme-linked immunosorbent assay (ELISA) using excretory-secretary proteins obtained from cultured *T canis* may be useful in the diagnosis.[94] Because humans are not the definitive host of *Toxocara* spp, eggs or larvae cannot be found in the feces.

VLM is a self-limiting disease and there may be spontaneous resolution. Therefore, mild to moderately symptomatic patients may not require any drug therapy. Patients with severe VLM can be treated with DEC, thiabendazole, or mebendazole. DEC can be given in a dose of 6 mg/kg/d for 21 days and mebendazole in a dose of 20 to 25 mg/kg/d for 21 days.[95]

Pulmonary trichinellosis

Five species of *Trichinella* (*Trichinella spiralis*, *Trichinella nativa*, *Trichinella nelsoni*, *Trichinella britovi*, and *Trichinella pseudospiralis*) can infect humans, and the most important species is *T spiralis*.[96] The parasite has a direct life cycle with complete development in 1 host (pig, rat, or human). However, 2 hosts are required to complete the life cycle and perpetuate the species. Humans can be infected from raw and partially cooked pork, if infected pig muscle containing larval trichinellae is eaten. The larvae develop into adults (males and females) in the duodenum and jejunum. The newborn larvae produced by female parasites pass through the lymphatics or blood vessels to reach the striated muscles.[97] The larvae undergo encystment in the muscle and a host capsule develops around the larvae. Later, it may become calcified. The life cycle is completed when infected muscle is ingested by a suitable host.

The common symptoms of trichinellosis are muscle pain, periorbital edema, fever, and diarrhea.[98] Pulmonary symptoms include dyspnea, cough, and pulmonary infiltrates. Dyspnea may be due to the involvement of the diaphragm. Leucocytosis, eosinophilia, and increased levels of serum muscle enzymes are important laboratory findings. A definitive diagnosis can be made by muscle biopsy (usually deltoid muscle) that may show larvae of *T spiralis*.[99] Symptomatic treatment of trichinellosis includes analgesics and corticosteroids. Specific treatment is with mebendazole at a daily dose of 5 mg/kg in 2 doses, or with albendazole at 800 mg/d (15 mg/kg/d) in 2 doses.[100] Mebendazole is prescribed in higher doses (up to 20–25 mg/kg/d in 3 doses) in some countries.[100] Both drugs are prescribed for 10 to 15 days. The treatment cycle may be repeated after 5 days.[100] Trichinellosis can be prevented by only consuming properly cooked pork.

Cestodes

Hydatidosis is caused by the larval stage of taeniid tapeworms of the *Echinococcus* genus: *Echinococcus granulosus* and *Echinococcus multilocularis*. The adult worm lives in the intestine of canids, which are the definitive hosts. The canids are infected by eating contaminated organs of the intermediate hosts, herbivores. Humans are accidental hosts, and are infected from food, drinks, or hands contaminated by embryonated eggs that have been excreted in the feces of canids. The larvae reach the blood and lymphatic circulation of intestines and are transported to the liver, which is the main target. The lungs and other organs may also be affected.

Pulmonary cystic hydatidosis

Cystic hydatidosis or hydatid cyst caused by *E granulosus* is a serious health problem in most parts of the world, particularly in sheep-raising areas of the Mediterranean countries, the Middle East, the Balkans, South America, Australia, and New Zealand, where it is endemic in rural areas. There are about 65 million infected people in approximately 100 countries. The incidence of hydatidosis varies from less than 1/100,000 to more than 15/100,000, with a tendency to increase in some regions (Balkans, Kazakhstan, China) suggesting that it is a re-emerging disease.[101] Dogs are the definitive hosts and sheep the main intermediate host. The liver is the primary location in 55% to 70% of cases, followed by the lung in 18% to 35%.[102] Typically, larvae that pass through or bypass the liver filter are trapped in pulmonary arterial capillaries. The entrapped larvae develop into hydatid cysts that grow gradually and often create complications by rupturing in the airway or, less commonly, in the pleural space.

Secondary pulmonary hydatidosis is exceptional. Secondary metastatic pulmonary hydatidosis may occur by the rupture of a liver cyst in vena caval circulation or a heart cyst in the right ventricular cavity. Secondary bronchogenic pulmonary hydatidosis may occur by the rupture of a primary lung cyst in the bronchi and then seeding of the protoscolices along the bronchial tree.

In most cases (72%–82%), primary lung hydatidosis is single. Multiple hydatidosis (20%) may be unilateral or bilateral. Patients are asymptomatic in the initial stages of infection. Chest pain, hemoptysis, dyspnea, or allergic reaction may occur subsequently. Giant cysts in childhood may be manifested by developmental disturbances or dysmorphic deviation of the thorax. Bronchial rupture of the cyst is observed in 30% of cases and can result in vomiting of the contents of hydatid cysts, hemoptysis, and infection of the cysts. Intrapleural rupture may be the initial manifestation in 3.5% to

6% of cases. This rupture may be acute, leading to hydropneumothorax or empyema (**Fig. 3**), or insidious with delayed development of secondary pleural hydatidosis.[103,104] Secondary metastatic hydatidosis can rapidly be fatal or may lead to the development of secondary disseminated metastatic pulmonary hydatidosis, often associated with obstruction of pulmonary artery branches resulting in chronic hydatic cor pulmonale.[104–106]

Secondary bronchogenic hydatidosis leads to disseminated lesions as grapes of small multilocular hydatids. It may be seen after spontaneous rupture of a primary cyst or observed after surgical cyst removal and perioperative inoculation (**Fig. 4**). Vomiting of small entire hydatids is a specific sign called hydatidoptysis.[104–108]

Diagnosis of pulmonary hydatid cyst is still based on radiography, and a noncomplicated cyst presents as a well-defined homogenous hydrous round (cannonball) opacity that may be lobulated by contiguous bronchovascular axes (**Fig. 5**). Fissured or ruptured cyst in the bronchi may have the characteristic findings of air crescent, pneumocyst, floating membrane, ring within a ring, or completely empty cavity images. The dry membrane retention image may have a polymorphous aspect and may mimic a tumor. Complicated cases may have atypical presentation with heterogeneous images or associated atelectasis.[109–111] Thoracic ultrasonography may be useful if the cyst is accessible to ultrasound examination. It may confirm the cystic

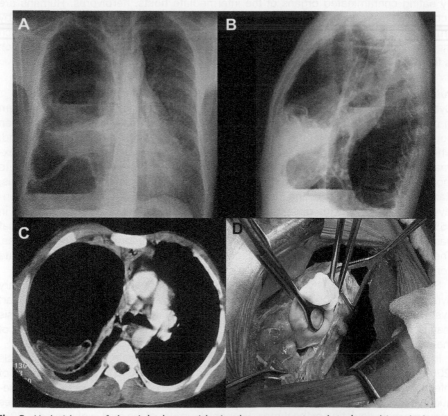

Fig. 3. Hydatid cyst of the right lung with simultaneous rupture into bronchi and pleura: chest radiographs (*A*, *B*) showing hydropneumothorax, CT (*C*) with the retracted membrane in the cystic cavity, and operative view (*D*).

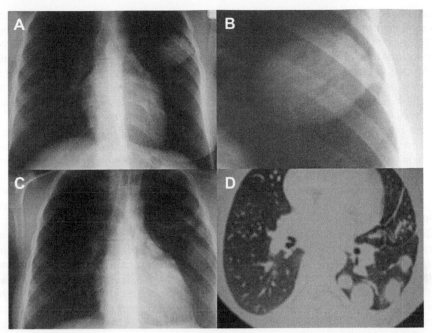

Fig. 4. Postoperative secondary bronchogenic hydatidosis: (*A, B*) preoperative chest radiographs showing complicated hydatid cyst of the left upper lobe with retracted membrane. (*C, D*) Chest radiographs and CT 14 months after surgery showing disseminated secondary bronchogenic hydatidosis in the left lower lobe.

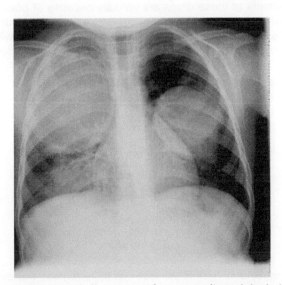

Fig. 5. Bilateral typical cannonball images of noncomplicated hydatid cysts on chest radiographs.

structure, showing the characteristic double-contour aspect (the pericyst and the parasite membrane endocyst) in nonruptured cysts (**Fig. 6**). Detached or retracted membrane may be observed in ruptured cysts. Daughter cysts are rarely observed in lung hydatidosis. Liver and abdomen ultrasound study is generally systematically performed to search for associated abdominal hydatid cysts.[112,113] CT is helpful in doubtful cases, because the internal structure of the cyst can be analyzed and its density measured; the state of the neighboring parenchyma and the whole thorax and abdomen can be evaluated for associated cystic lesions or anomalies.[114,115] Laboratory tests are complementary to clinical and imaging investigations. Eosinophils can be slightly increased in complicated cysts. Serologic tests are less sensitive in patients with lung hydatidosis (65%) than in those localized in liver (80%–94%).[116,117] False-positive tests may be observed in patients suffering from other helminthic infestations. Immunologic tests may be helpful to confirm the hydatic origin of a cystic lesion and permit the serologic monitoring of medically or surgically treated patients.

Surgery is the main treatment of pulmonary hydatidosis and aims to remove the parasite and treat associated parenchymal, bronchial, or pleural disease. During surgery, spillage of hydatid fluid must be avoided to prevent secondary hydatidosis. Relapse rates up to 11.3% have been reported. Parasite extraction may be achieved by the removal of intact hydatid (**Fig. 7**) or by hydatid fluid aspiration with or without the use of scolicidal agents. Surgery must be as conservative as possible and resection is necessary in case of severe and irremediable lung damage. Lung resection rates vary from 7% to 16%. Bilateral lung hydatidosis, present in 4% to 26% of operated cases, may be treated in 1-stage or 2-stage surgery by bilateral thoracotomy or sternotomy. Video-assisted thoracoscopic surgery (VATS) can be safely used in selected cases with the same surgical rules as in open surgery.[102,118–121] If there are associated cysts, especially in the liver, these may be treated in the same operation or separately. Long-term treatment with benzoimidazole carbamates (albendazole or mebendazole) has not been found to be effective in lung hydatidosis. Treatment with benzoimidazole has been suggested to prevent recurrences, although there is no evidence of its efficacy.[121,122] The effects of these drugs are variable because of poor absorption and low drug availability in blood and in the cyst despite 6 to 12 months of treatment. Treatment with these drugs has also been found to be associated with alopecia and

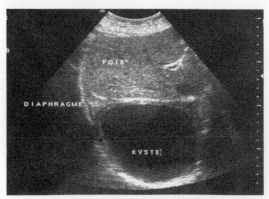

Fig. 6. Ultrasound study of a right lower lobe cyst by retrograde transhepatic and transdiaphragmatic approach with typical double contour aspect of the cyst (*black arrow*) (FOIE, liver, KYSTE, cyst).

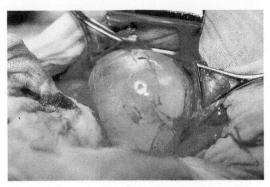

Fig. 7. Operative view of entire hydatid delivery after pericyst incision.

hepatic and hematologic toxicity. Therefore medical therapy must be reserved for inoperable or complex cases.[123–125] Surgery is the main treatment in most cases, with a low mortality (0%–5%) and morbidity (0%–13%).[102,118–122] Percutaneous treatment by puncture-aspiration-injection-reaspiration (PAIR) or percutaneous thermal ablation is used in hepatic hydatidosis. PAIR has rarely been used for lung hydatidosis because of the risk of anaphylactic shock, pneumothorax with pleural spillage, and bronchopleural fistulae.[116,122,126] Hydatidosis remains endemic in many parts of the world and preventive programs to break the parasite cycle remain hard to realize in sheep-raising countries. Immunologic and parasite antigen detection studies are in progress to produce an efficient vaccine for dogs and sheep.[116,122]

Pulmonary alveolar echinococcosis
Alveolar echinococcosis is a rare but severe, highly pathogenic, and potentially fatal form of echinococcosis. Wild canines, especially foxes, are the definitive hosts, and other hosts are dogs, cats, and wolves. Small animals (mainly rodents) are the intermediate hosts. Alveolar echinococcosis is restricted to the Northern Hemisphere (Europe, North America, some regions of China, and Japan) with a tendency to extend to endemic zones because of the increase in fox populations, especially in cities, leading to an urban cycle of the parasite.[101,116,127] The liver is the first target of the parasite, with a silent and long incubation period (5–15 years). Exogenous proliferation causes infiltration of adjacent tissues and pressure necrosis. It can metastasize to distant organs; mainly lungs, brain, and bones. Lung involvement results from metastatic dissemination or direct extension through the diaphragm of hepatic echinococcosis with intrathoracic rupture into the bronchial tree, pleural cavity, or mediastinum. Direct extension to the right atrium through the inferior vena cava with recurrent episodes of pulmonary embolism has also been reported. Imaging studies with radiography, ultrasonography, CT, and magnetic resonance imaging (MRI), may help in the diagnosis of metastatic lung disease. Biopsy may be needed to confirm the diagnosis.[128,129] Serologic tests (ELISA, indirect hemagglutination assay [IHA]), are available and are of great value for early detection in endemic areas to confirm diagnosis and to plan early surgery.[116,130] Radical resection of localized lesions is the only curative technique for alveolar echinococcosis but it is rarely possible in invasive and disseminated disease. Medical treatment is with mebendazole 40 to 50 mg/kg/d in 3 divided doses, or with albendazole 10 to 15 mg/kg/d orally in 2 divided doses for a long period (minimum of 2 years) after radical surgery, or life-time treatment of nonresectable or incompletely resected lesions.[116,123]

Trematodes

Pulmonary schistosomiasis and pulmonary paragonimiasis are the important diseases caused by trematodes.

Pulmonary schistosomiasis

Schistosomiasis (bilharziasis) affects more than 200 million people around the world in more than 70 countries. It is the third most common endemic parasitic disease after malaria and amebiasis.[131] Three important species of schistosoma that may cause pulmonary disease are Schistosoma haematobium (Africa, Arabia), Schistosoma mansonii (Africa, Arabia, Antilles, and South America), and Schistosoma japonicum (Japan, China). Infected humans excrete schistosoma eggs in urine or feces. The intermediate host, snails, ingest the eggs, which go through several multiplication cycles to produce the infective form, cercaria. Cercaria are found in water and are able to penetrate human skin or intestinal mucosa after ingestion. Swimming in contaminated water is the common mode of transmission. After penetration of the skin, the young form of the parasite, called schistosomula, migrate to the lung and later to the liver. Adult forms migrate in groups to mesenteric or pelvic veins.

Acute pulmonary manifestations are observed 3 to 8 weeks after skin penetration and present as an acute febrile illness with wheezing, dry cough, and shortness of breath due to an immunologic reaction in which eosinophils are sequestrated in the lungs (Katayama syndrome). Urticaria, headache, hepatosplenomegaly, and marked eosinophilia are generally observed in the acute form.[132-134] Chest radiography and CT show small, ill-defined nodular lesions, reticulonodular lesions, or diffuse ground-glass opacity. Chronic pulmonary schistosomiasis results from a granulomatous reaction to eggs or worms embolized from pelvic veins in small pulmonary vessels through the inferior vena cava for S haematobium, or from mesenteric veins through portacaval anastomosis in patients with portal hypertension (S Mansonii and S japonicum). At this stage, pulmonary schistosomiasis is frequently asymptomatic with different radiographic findings: nodules, miliary forms, pseudo-tumoral forms, or cavitary lesions. Pulmonary arterial hypertension (PAH) may develop after many years and may lead to chronic cor pulmonale in 2% to 6% of cases. Recent studies have shown an incidence of PAH of 6.3% to 13.5% in patients with schistosomiasis, and it is the most prevalent cause of PAH in endemic zones such as Brazil.[135,136] PAH associated with schistosomiasis was believed to be related to mechanical vascular obstruction by the parasites and was classified in group 4 of the Venice Clinical Classification of Pulmonary Hypertension in 2003. Recent studies have found that mechanical obstruction is not the main factor and have suggested that inflammation and vasospastic factors play a significant role; this has been confirmed by necropsy studies of lung specimens with vascular lesions indistinguishable from those of idiopathic PAH. Therefore, pulmonary hypertension associated with schistosomiasis is now classified in group 1 of the Updated Clinical Classification of PAH.[136,137]

Diagnosis of schistosomiasis may be made by stool and urine examination for parasite eggs, or by rectal biopsy. The sensitivity of these tests is low for early infection. In chronic schistosomiasis without portacaval hypertension, rectal biopsy has 80% positivity and parasitologic examination about 50%. Serologic tests (ELISA to be confirmed by enzyme-linked immunoelectro transfer blot) are positive 2 weeks after infestation, and may aid in the diagnosis if associated with eosinophilia in the acute phase. They remain positive for years, and are not helpful for determining the prognosis, and cannot differentiate a current disease from former infection. Lung biopsy may show the bilharzial granuloma surrounding the parasite egg.[133-138]

Treatment is with praziquantel 40 mg/kg daily. Treatment may cause a reactive pneumonitis to dying eggs or worms. Acute pneumonia can be observed 2 weeks after treatment, which is believed to be related to lung embolization by detached adult worms in pelvic veins.[139] Patients with PAH are treated with specific PAH treatment along with antiparasitic medication. It is not found to have a significant hemodynamic effect on PAH.[136] Studies are in progress to develop a vaccine against schistosomiasis.[140]

Pulmonary paragonimiasis (lung flukes)

Paragonimiasis is a food-borne zoonosis caused by *Paragonimus westermani* or other species of *Paragonimus*. It is endemic in east and southeast Asia, Africa, and South America. The parasite is transmitted via snails to freshwater crabs or crayfish, and then to humans or other mammals (cats, dogs, tigers). Human infection occurs by ingestion of raw or incompletely cooked freshwater crabs or crayfish infected with the metacercaria. The ingested metacercaria excyst in the duodenum and then migrate through the intestinal wall into the abdominal cavity in 3 to 6 hours and, after several days, they penetrate the diaphragm into the pleural cavity and lungs, reaching the bronchioles where they develop into adult worms. The eggs produced by the adult worms are expectorated in sputum or passed out in feces if bronchial secretions are swallowed. The lung is the main target organ and ectopic locations may be the central nervous system or skin.[141–143]

Pulmonary manifestations include fever, chest pain, chronic cough with blood-tinged sputum, or hemoptysis that may mimic tuberculosis. Pleural effusion or pneumothorax may be the first manifestation during intrapleural migration of the juvenile worms.[141,142] Chest radiography or CT may show patchy airspace consolidation due to exudative or hemorrhagic pneumonia that may cavitate. Worm cysts may be seen as solitary or multiple nodules or gas-filled cysts with ring shadows and crescent shaped areas within the cyst that represent worms attached to the wall of the cavity.[144,145] Diagnosis is confirmed by the detection of eggs in the sputum or BAL 2 to 3 months after infection. Eggs or worms may be detected in a subcutaneous lump or in pleural effusion. Intradermal and serologic tests are also available (ELISA, dot immunogold filtration assay [DIGFA], indirect hemagglutination, indirect fluorescent antibody tests, and immunoblot). Differentiation of paragonimiasis from tuberculosis may be difficult.[141,142]

Praziquantel and triclabendazole are the drugs recommended to treat paragonimiasis. Praziquantel is administered at a total dose of 150 mg/kg, 3 doses per day for 2 days with a cure rate of 80% to 90%. Triclabendazole is administered at a dose of 20 mg/kg/d in 2 divided doses with a cure rate of up to 98.5%. Other drugs, such as mebendazole and bithionol, have been tried with cure rates of 70% and 50% to 60% respectively. Surgical removal of parasites and infected tissues may be indicated in selected cases, especially cerebral and spinal paragonimiasis.[140,141] The most efficient way to prevent and control the disease is to avoid consumption of undercooked crabs, shrimps, and crayfish.

SUMMARY

Many lung infestations from established and newly emerging parasites have been reported as a result of the emergence of HIV/AIDS, the increasing use of immunosuppressive drugs, increasing organ transplantations, the increase in global travel, and climate change. A renewed interest in parasitic lung infections has been observed recently because many protozoal and helminthic parasites cause clinically significant lung diseases. The diseases caused by these parasites may mimic common and complicated lung diseases ranging from asymptomatic disease to ARDS requiring critical care management. The availability of new molecular diagnostic methods and antiparasitic drugs enables early diagnosis and prompt treatment to avoid the morbidity and mortality associated with these infestations. Good hygiene practices, improvement in socioeconomic conditions, vector control measures, and consumption of hygienically prepared and properly cooked food are essential to reduce the occurrence of parasitic infestations.

REFERENCES

1. Vijayan VK. Tropical parasitic lung diseases. Indian J Chest Dis Allied Sci 2008; 50(1):49–66.
2. Vijayan VK. Is the incidence of parasitic lung diseases increasing, and how may this affect modern respiratory medicine? Expert Rev Respir Med 2009;3(4): 339–44.
3. Martinez-Giron R, Estiban JG, Ribas A, et al. Protozoa in respiratory pathology: a review. Eur Respir J 2008;32(5):1354–70.
4. Vijayan VK. How to diagnose and manage common parasitic pneumonias? Curr Opin Pulm Med 2007;13(3):218–24.
5. Vijayan VK. Parasitic lung infections. Curr Opin Pulm Med 2009;15(3):274–82.
6. Petri WA Jr, Singh U. Enteric amoebiasis. In: Guerrant RL, Walker DH, Weller PF, editors. Tropical infectious diseases: principles, pathogenesis and practice. 2nd edition. Philadelphia: Elsevier Churchill Livingstone; 2006. p. 967–83.
7. Ravdin JI, Stauffer WN. *Entamoeba histolytica* (amoebiasis). In: Mandell GL, Bennett JE, Dolin R, editors. Mandell, Douglas and Bennette's principles and practice of infectious diseases. 6th edition. Philadelphia: Churchill Livingstone; 2005. p. 3097–111.
8. Haque R, Huston CD, Hughes M, et al. Amoebiasis. N Engl J Med 2003;348(16): 1565–73.
9. Hsu M-S, Hsieh S-M, Chen M-Y, et al. Association between amoebic liver abscess and human immunodeficiency virus infection in Taiwanese subjects. BMC Infect Dis 2008;8:48.
10. Stark D, van Hal SJ, Matthews G, et al. Invasive amoebiasis in men who have sex with men, Australia. Emerg Infect Dis 2008;14(7):1141–3.
11. Ackers JP, Mirelman D. Progress in research on *Entamoeba histolytica* pathogenesis. Curr Opin Microbiol 2006;9(4):367–73.
12. Shamsuzzaman SM, Hashiguchi Y. Thoracic amoebiasis. Clin Chest Med 2002; 23(2):479–92.
13. Hamzah Z, Petmitr S, Mungthin M, et al. Differential detection of *Entamoeba histolytica*, *Entamoeba dispar* and *Entamoeba moshkovskii* by a single-round PCR assay. J Clin Microbiol 2006;44(9):3196–200.
14. Tanyuksel M, Petri WA Jr. Laboratory diagnosis of amoebiasis. Clin Microbiol Rev 2003;16(4):713–29.
15. Gonzalez-Salazar F, Mata-Cardenas BD, Vargas-Villareal J. Sensibility of *Entamoeba histolytica* trophozoites to Ivermectin. Medicina (B Aires) 2009; 69(3):318–20.
16. Piscopo TV, Mallia AC. Leishmaniasis. Postgrad Med J 2006;82(972):649–57.
17. Leishmaniasis: background information. World Health Organization website. Available at: http://www.who.int/leishmaniasis/en/. Accessed August 12, 2009.
18. Desjeux P, Alvar J. Leishmania/HIV co-infection: epidemiology in Europe. Ann Trop Med Parasitol 2003;97(Suppl 1):3–15.

19. Marshall BG, Kropf P, Murray K, et al. Bronchopulmonary and mediastinal leishmaniasis: an unusual clinical presentation of *Leishmania donovani* infection. Clin Infect Dis 2000;30(5):764–9.
20. Chenoweth CE, Singal S, Pearson RD, et al. Acquired immunodefiency syndrome-related visceral leishmaniasis presenting in a pleural effusion. Chest 1993;103(2):648–9.
21. Antinori S, Cascio A, Parravicini C, et al. Leishmaniasis among organ transplant recipients. Lancet Infect Dis 2008;8(3):191–9.
22. Jopikii L, Salmela K, Saha H, et al. Leishmaniasis diagnosed from bronchoalveolar lavage. Scand J Infect Dis 1992;24(5):677–81.
23. Guddo F, Gallo E, Cillari E, et al. Detection of *Leishmania infantum* kinetoplast DNA in laryngeal tissue from an immunocompetent patient. Hum Pathol 2005; 36(10):1140–2.
24. Sunder S, Rai M. Treatment of visceral leishmaniasis. Expert Opin Pharmacother 2005;6(16):2821–9.
25. Jha TK, Sunder S, Thakur CP, et al. Miltefosine, an oral agent, for the treatment of Indian visceral leishmaniasis. N Engl J Med 1999;341(24):1795–800.
26. World Health Organization. Estimated burden of malaria in 2006. In: World Malaria report 2008. Geneva (Switzerland): WHO; 2008. p. 9–15.
27. Freedman DO. Malaria prevention in short-term travelers. N Engl J Med 2008; 359(6):603–12.
28. Rosenthal PJ. Artesunate for the treatment of severe falciparum malaria. N Engl J Med 2008;358(17):1829–36.
29. Tan LK, Yacoub S, Scott S, et al. Acute lung injury and other serious complications of *Plasmodium vivax* malaria. Lancet Infect Dis 2008;8(7): 449–54.
30. Rojo-Marcos G, Cuadros-Gonzalez J, Mesa-Latorre JM. Acute respiratory distress syndrome in a case of *Plasmodium ovale*. Am J Trop Med Hyg 2008; 79(3):391–3.
31. Anstey NM, Russell B, Yeo TW, et al. The pathophysiology of vivax malaria. Trends Parasitol 2009;25(5):220–7.
32. Mharakurwa S, Simoloka C, Thuma PE, et al. PCR detection of *Plasmodium falciparum* in human urine and saliva samples. Malar J 2006;5:103.
33. World Health Organization. Guidelines for the treatment of malaria. Geneva (Switzerland): World Health Organization; 2006. p. 1–266.
34. Talwar A, Fein AM, Ahluwalia G. Pulmonary and critical care aspects of severe malaria. In: Sharma OP, editor. Lung biology in health and disease: tropical lung diseases. 2nd edition. New York: Taylor & Francis; 2006. p. 255–77.
35. Krause PJ. Babesiosis. Med Clin North Am 2002;86(2):361–73.
36. Swanson SJ, Neitzel D, Reed KD, et al. Co-infections acquired from *Ixodes* ticks. Clin Microbiol Rev 2006;19(4):708–27.
37. Boustani MR, Lepore TJ, Gelfand JA, et al. Acute respiratory failure in patients treated for babesiosis. Am J Respir Crit Care Med 1994;149(6):1689–91.
38. Noskoviak K, Broome E. Babesiosis. N Engl J Med 2008;358(17):e19.
39. Krause PJ. Babesiosis diagnosis and treatment. Vector Borne Zoonotic Dis 2003;3(1):45–51.
40. Raju M, Salazar JC, Leopold H, et al. Atovaquone and azithromycin treatment for babesiosis in an infant. Pediatr Infect Dis J 2007;26(2):181–3.
41. Dodds EM. Toxoplasmosis. Curr Opin Ophthalmol 2006;17(6):557–61.

42. Petersen E, Edvinsson B, Lundgren B, et al. Diagnosis of pulmonary infection with *Toxoplasma gondii* in immunocompromised HIV-positive patients by real-time PCR. Eur J Clin Microbiol Infect Dis 2006;25(6):401–4.
43. Contini C. Clinical and diagnostic management of toxoplasmosis in the immuno-compromised patient. Parassitologia 2008;50(1–2):45–50.
44. Duarte AG, Sattar F, Granwehr B, et al. Disseminated acanthamebiasis after lung transplantation. J Heart Lung Transplant 2006;25(2):237–40.
45. Corti M, Villafane MF, Muzzio E, et al. Pulmonary cryptosporidiosis in AIDS patients. Rev Argent Microbiol 2008;40(2):106–8.
46. Bethlem NM, Lemle A, Saad EA. Pulmonary manifestations in Chagas' disease. In: Sharma OP, editor. Lung disease in the tropics. New York: Marcel Dekker; 1991. p. 251–77.
47. Lemle A. Chagas' disease. Chest 1999;115(3):906.
48. Crompton DWT. How much human helminthiasis is there in the world? J Parasitol 1999;85(3):397–403.
49. Hirakawa E, Suetsugu T, Tanoue A, et al. Pulmonary eosinophilia caused by visceral larva due to *Ascaris suum*. Nippon Naika Gakkai Zasshi 2009;98(1): 144–6.
50. Lau SK, Woo PC, Wong SS, et al. Ascaris-induced eosinophilic pneumonia in an HIV-infected patient. J Clin Pathol 2007;60(2):202–3.
51. Aggarwal B, Sharma M, Singh T. Acute eosinophilic pneumonia due to round worm infestation. Indian J Pediatr 2008;75(3):296–7.
52. Sarinas PS, Chitkara RK. Ascariasis and hookworm. Semin Respir Infect 1997; 12(2):130–7.
53. St Georgiev V. Pharmacotherapy of ascariasis. Expert Opin Pharmacother 2001; 2(2):223–39.
54. Belizaro VY, Amarillo ME, de Leon WU, et al. A comparison of the efficacy of single dose of albendazole, ivermectin and diethylcarbamazine alone or in combination against *Ascaris* and *Trichuris* spp. Bull World Health Organ 2003; 81(1):35–42.
55. Scowden EB, Schaffner W, Stone WJ. Overwhelming strongyloidiasis: an unappreciated opportunistic infection. Medicine (Baltimore) 1978;57(6): 527–44.
56. Genta RM. Global prevalence of strongyloidiasis: critical review with epidemio-logic insights into the prevention of disseminated disease. Rev Infect Dis 1989; 11(5):755–67.
57. Neva FA. Biology and immunology of human strongyloidiasis. J Infect Dis 1986; 153(3):397–406.
58. Siddiqui AA, Berk SL. Diagnosis of *Strongyloides stercoralis* infection. Clin Infect Dis 2001;33(7):1040–7.
59. Casati A, Cornero G, Muttini S, et al. Hyperacute pneumonitis in a patient with overwhelming *Strongyloides stercoralis* infection. Eur J Anaesthesiol 1996; 13(5):498–501.
60. Lessman KD, Can S, Talavera W. Disseminated *Strongyloides stercoralis* in human immunodeficiency virus-infected patients: treatment failure and review of literature. Chest 1993;104(1):119–22.
61. Balagopal A, Mills L, Shah A, et al. Detection and treatment of *Strongyloides* hyper infection syndrome following lung transplantation. Transpl Infect Dis 2009;11(2):149–54.
62. Nwokolo C, Imohiosen E. Strongyloidiasis of respiratory tract presenting as "asthma". Br Med J 1973;2(5859):153–4.

63. Williams J, Ninley D, Dralle W, et al. Diagnosis of pulmonary strongyloidiasis by bronchoalveolar lavage. Chest 1988;94(3):643–4.
64. Graspa D, Petrakakou E, Botsoli-Stergiou E, et al. *Strongyloides stercoralis* in bronchial washing specimens processed as conventional and Thin-Prep smears; report of a case and a review of the literature. Diagn Cytopathol 2009;37(12):903–5.
65. Datry A, Hilmarsdottir I, Mayorga-Sagastume R, et al. Treatment of *Strongyloides stercoralis* infection with ivermectin compared with albendazole: results of an open study of 60 cases. Trans R Soc Trop Med Hyg 1994;88(3):344–5.
66. Ottesen EA, Nutman TB. Tropical pulmonary eosinophilia. Annu Rev Med 1992; 43:417–24.
67. Udwadia FE. Tropical eosinophilia. In: Herzog H, editor. Pulmonary eosinophilia: progress in respiration research. Basel (Switzerland): S. Karger; 1975. p. 35–155.
68. Vijayan VK. Immunopathogenesis and treatment of eosinophilic lung diseases in the tropics. In: Sharma OP, editor. 2nd edition, Tropical lung disease (Lung biology in health and disease), vol. 211. New York: Marcel Dekker Inc; 2006. p. 195–239.
69. Johnson S, Wilkinson R, Davidson RN. Tropical respiratory medicine. IV: acute tropical infection and the lung. Thorax 1994;49(7):714–8.
70. Frimodt-Moller C, Barton RM. A pseudo-tuberculosis condition associated with eosinophilia. Ind Med Gaz 1940;75(12):607–13.
71. Weingarten RJ. Tropical eosinophilia. Lancet 1943;241(6230):103–5.
72. Hayashi K, Horiba M, Shindou J, et al. Tropical eosinophilia in a man from Sri Lanka. Nihon Kyobu Shikkan Gakkai Zasshi 1996;34(12):1411–5.
73. Jiva TM, Israel RH, Poe RH. Tropical pulmonary eosinophilia masquerading as acute bronchial asthma. Respiration 1996;63(1):55–8.
74. Vijayan VK. Tropical pulmonary eosinophilia. Curr Opin Pulm Med 2007;13(5): 428–33.
75. Pinkston P, Vijayan VK, Nutman TB, et al. Acute tropical pulmonary eosinophilia: characterization of the lower respiratory tract inflammation and its response to therapy. J Clin Invest 1987;80(1):216–25.
76. O'Bryan L, Pinkston P, Kumaraswami V, et al. Localized eosinophil degranulation mediates disease in tropical pulmonary eosinophilia. Infect Immun 2003;71(3): 1337–42.
77. Nutman TB, Vijayan VK, Pinkston P, et al. Tropical pulmonary eosinophilia: analysis of antifilarial antibody localized to the lung. J Infect Dis 1989;160(6): 1042–50.
78. Webb JK, Job CK, Gault EW. Tropical eosinophilia. Demonstration of microfilariae in lung, liver and lymph nodes. Lancet 1960;1(7129):835–42.
79. Cooray JH, Ismail MM. Re-examination of the diagnostic criteria of tropical pulmonary eosinophilia. Respir Med 1999;93(9):655–9.
80. Vijayan VK, Kuppurao KV, Sankaran K, et al. Tropical eosinophilia: clinical and physiological response to diethylcarbamazine. Respir Med 1991;85(1):17–20.
81. Poh SC. The course of lung function in treated tropical pulmonary eosinophilia. Thorax 1974;29(6):710–2.
82. Vijayan VK, Kuppurao KV, Sankaran K, et al. Pulmonary membrane diffusing capacity and capillary blood volume in tropical eosinophilia. Chest 1990; 97(6):1386–9.
83. Final Report. Joint WPRO/SEARO working group on Brugian filariasis. Manila (Philippines): WHO; 1979. p. 1–47.

84. Vijayan VK, Sankaran K, Venkatesan P, et al. Effect of diethylcarbamazine on the alveolitis of tropical eosinophilia. Respiration 1991;58(5–6):255–9.

85. Rom WN, Vijayan VK, Cornelius MJ, et al. Persistent lower respiratory tract inflammation associated with interstitial lung disease in patients with tropical pulmonary eosinophilia following treatment with diethylcarbamazine. Am Rev Respir Dis 1990;142(5):1088–92.

86. Theis JH. Public health aspects of dirofilariasis in the United States. Vet Parasitol 2005;133(2–3):157–80.

87. Miyoshi T, Tsubouchi H, Iwasaki A, et al. Human pulmonary dirofilariasis: a case report and review of the recent Japanese literature. Respirology 2006;11(3): 343–7.

88. Oshiro Y, Murayama S, Sunagawa U, et al. Pulmonary dirofilariasis: computed tomographic findings and correlation with pathologic features. J Comput Assist Tomogr 2004;28(6):796–800.

89. Takayama Y, Nakamur Y, Hamai K, et al. Case of pulmonary dirofilariasis with cavity formation in a young woman. Nihon Kokyuki Gakkai Zasshi 2009;47(5): 372–5.

90. Rivasi F, Boldorini R, Criante P, et al. Detection of *Dirofilaria (Nochtiella) repens* DNA by polymerase chain reaction in embedded paraffin tissues from two human pulmonary locations. APMIS 2006;114(7–8):567–74.

91. Magnaval JF, Glickman LT, Dorchies P, et al. Highlights of human toxocariasis. Korean J Parasitol 2001;39(1):1–11.

92. Feldman GJ, Parker HW. Visceral larva migrans associated with the hypereosinophilic syndrome and the onset of severe asthma. Ann Intern Med 1992; 116(10):838–40.

93. Bartelink AK, Kortbeek LM, Huidekoper HJ, et al. Acute respiratory failure due to toxocara infections. Lancet 1993;342(8881):1234.

94. Spieser F, Gottstein B. A collaborative study on larval excretory/secretary antigens of *Toxocara canis* for immunodiagnosis of human toxocariasis with ELISA. Acta Trop 1984;41(4):361–72.

95. Magnaval JF. Comparative efficacy of diethylcarbamazine and mebendazole for the treatment of human toxocariasis. Parasitology 1995;110(Pt 5): 529–33.

96. Pozio E, La Rosa G, Murrell KD, et al. Taxonomic revision of the genus *Trichinella*. J Parasitol 1992;78(4):654–9.

97. Despommier DD. How does *Trichinella spiralis* make itself at home? Parasitol Today 1998;14(8):318–23.

98. Capo V, Despommier DD. Clinical aspects of infections with *Trichinella* spp. Clin Microbiol Rev 1996;9(1):47–54.

99. Bruschi F, Murrell K. Trichinellosis. In: Guerrant RL, Walker DH, Weller PF, editors. Tropical infectious diseases: principles, pathogens and practice, vol. 2. Philadelphia: Churchill Livingstone; 1999. p. 917–25.

100. Dupouy-Camet J, Bruschi F. Management and diagnosis of human trichinellosis. In: Dupouy-Camet J, Murell KD, editors. Food and Agriculture Organization (FAO)/World Health Organization/World Organisation for Animal Health (OIE) Guidelines for the surveillance, management, prevention and control of trichinellosis. Paris: FAO/WHO/OIE; 2007. p. 52–4.

101. Eckert J, Conraths FJ, Tackman K. Echinococcosis: an emerging or re-emerging zoonosis? Int J Parasitol 2000;30(12):1283–94.

102. Kilani T, El Hammami S. Pulmonary hydatid and other lung parasitic infections. Curr Opin Pulm Med 2002;8(3):218–23.

103. Kilani T, Ben Safta Z, Jamoussi M, et al. Les complications pleurales du kyste hydatique du poumon: à propos de 16 cas. Ann Chir 1988;42(12):145–8.
104. Deve F. L'échinococcose secondaire. Paris: Masson; 1946. p. 70–7, 96–122, 137–51.
105. Talmoudi T, Jouven JC, Malmejac C, et al. L'embolie pulmonaire hydatique. Etude de 2 observations personnelles et revue de la littérature. Ann Chir Thorac Cardiovasc 1980;34(3):245–50.
106. Kilani T, Mechmeche R, Daoues A, et al. Endocavitary rupture of heart hydatid cyst - 5 cases. Tunis Med 1991;69(3):139–42.
107. Kilani T, Horchani H, Daoues A. Secondary bronchogenic pulmonary hydatido-sis. Ann Chir 1992;42(2):160–4.
108. Chafik A, El Maslout A, Khallafi S, et al. Bronchogenic dissemination of pulmo-nary hydatid cyst. Rev Mal Respir 2001;18(3):333–4.
109. Pedrosa I, Saiz A, Arrazola J, et al. Hydatid disease: radiologic and pathologic features and complications. Radiographics 2000;20(3):795–817.
110. Zidi A, Ben Miled-M'rad K, Hantous-Zannad S, et al. Kyste hydatique du pou-mon ouvert dans les bronches: apport de la tomodensitométrie. J Radiol 2007;88(1 Pt 1):59–64.
111. Bouhaouala MH, Hendaoui L, Charfi MR, et al. Hydatidose thoracique. Paris: EMC (Elsevier Masson SAS); 2007. Radiodiagnostic- Cœur-poumon; 32-470-A-20.
112. Meyer P, Blezat C, Bretagnolle M, et al. Aspects echographiques des kystes hydatiques du poumon chez l'enfant. Ann Radiol 1982;25(4):249–53.
113. Ben Miled-M'rad K, Bouricha A, Hantous S, et al. Ultrasonographic, CT and MRI findings of chest wall hydatidosis. J Radiol 2003;84(2 Pt 1):143–6.
114. Khannous M, Ferretti G, Ranchoup Y, et al. Hydatidose intrathoracique apport de la TDM. J Radiol 1993;74(11):541–8.
115. Koul PA, Koul AN, Wahid A, et al. CT in pulmonary hydatid disease: unusual appearances. Chest 2000;118(6):1645–7.
116. Eckert J, Deplazes P. Biological, epidemiological, and clinical aspects of echi-nococcosis, a zoonosis of increasing concern. Clin Microbiol Rev 2004;17(1): 107–35.
117. Biava MF, Dao A, Fortier B. Laboratory diagnosis of cystic hydatid disease. World J Surg 2001;25(1):10–4.
118. Safioleas M, Misiakos EP, Dosios T, et al. Surgical treatment for lung hydatid disease. World J Surg 1999;23(11):1181–5.
119. Shehatha J, Alizzi A, Alward M, et al. Thoracic hydatid disease: a review of 763 cases. Heart Lung Circ 2008;17(6):502–4.
120. Kuzucu A, Soysal O, Ozgel M, et al. Complicated hydatid cysts of the lung: clin-ical and therapeutic issues. Ann Thorac Surg 2004;77(4):1200–4.
121. Ramos G, Orduna A, Garcia-Yuste M. Hydatid cyst of the lung: diagnosis and treatment. World J Surg 2001;25(1):46–57.
122. Junghanns T, Menezes Da Silva A, Horton J, et al. Clinical management of cystic echinococcosis: state of the art, problems and perspectives. Am J Trop Med Hyg 2008;79(3):301–11.
123. World Health Organization Informal Working Group on Echinococcosis. Guide-lines for treatment of cystic and alveolar echinococcosis in humans. Bull World Health Organ 1996;74(3):231–42.
124. Davis A, Dixon H, Pawlowski ZS. Multicenter clinical trials of benzimidazole-carbamates in human cystic echinococcosis (phase 2). Bull World Health Organ 1989;67(5):503–8.

125. Horton RJ. Chemotherapy of *Echinococcus* infection in man with albendazole. Trans R Soc Trop Med Hyg 1989;83(1):97–102.
126. Mawhorter S, Temeck B, Chang R, et al. Nonsurgical therapy for pulmonary hydatid cyst disease. Chest 1997;112(5):1432–6.
127. Craig P. *Echinococcus multilocularis*. Curr Opin Infect Dis 2003;16(5):437–44.
128. Kayacan SM, Vatansever S, Temiz S, et al. Alveolar echinococcosis localized in the liver, lung and brain. Chin Med J 2008;121(1):90–2.
129. Ozkok A, Gul E, Okumus G, et al. Disseminated alveolar echinococcosis mimicking a metastatic malignancy. Intern Med 2008;47(16):1495–7.
130. Carmena D, Benito A, Eraso E. The immunodiagnosis of *Echinococcus multilocularis* infection. Clin Microbiol Infect 2007;13(5):460–75.
131. Engels D, Chitsulo L, Montresor A, et al. The global epidemiological situation of schistosomiasis and new approaches to control and research. Acta Trop 2002; 82(2):139–46.
132. Schwartz E. Pulmonary schistosomiasis. Clin Chest Med 2002;23(2):433–43.
133. Schwartz E, Rozenman J, Perelman M. Pulmonary manifestations of early schistosome infection among non immune travelers. Am J Med 2000;109(9):718–22.
134. Bethlem EP, Schettino GP, Carvalho CR. Pulmonary schistosomiasis. Curr Opin Pulm Med 1997;3(5):361–5.
135. Pereira GA Jr, Bestetti RB, Leite MP, et al. Porto pulmonary hypertension syndrome in *Schistosomiasis mansonii*. Trans R Soc Trop Med Hyg 2002; 96(4):427–8.
136. Lapa M, Dias B, Jardim C, et al. Cardiopulmonary manifestations of hepatosplenic schistosomiasis. Circulation 2009;119(11):1518–23.
137. Simonneau G, Robbins IM, Beghetti M, et al. Updated clinical classification of pulmonary hypertension. J Am Coll Cardiol 2009;54(Suppl 1):S43–54.
138. Bierman WF, Wetsteyn JC, Van Gool T. Presentation and diagnosis of imported schistosomiasis: relevance of eosinophilia, microscopy for ova and serology. J Travel Med 2005;12(1):9–13.
139. Sersar SI, Elnahas HA, Saleh AB, et al. Pulmonary parasitosis: applied clinical and therapeutic issues. Heart Lung Circ 2006;15(1):24–9.
140. El Ridi R, Tallima H. *Schistosoma mansonii* ex vivo lung-stage larvae excretory-secretory antigens as vaccine candidates against schistosomiasis. Vaccine 2009;27(5):666–73.
141. Liu Q, Wei F, Liu W, et al. Paragonimiasis: an important food-borne zoonosis in China. Trends Parasitol 2008;24(7):318–23.
142. Strobel M, Veasna D, Saykham M, et al. Pleuro-pulmonary paragonimiasis. Med Mal Infect 2005;35(10):476–81.
143. Im JG, Kong Y, Shin YM, et al. Pulmonary paragonimiasis: clinical and experimental studies. Radiographics 1993;13(3):575–86.
144. Im JG, Whang HY, Kim WS, et al. Pleuropulmonary paragonimiasis: radiologic findings in 71 patients. AJR Am J Roentgenol 1992;159(1):39–43.
145. Kim TS, Han J, Shim SS, et al. Pleuropulmonary paragonimiasis: CT findings in 31 patients. AJR Am J Roentgenol 2005;185(3):616–21.

Emerging, Novel, and Known Influenza Virus Infections in Humans

Julian W. Tang, PhD, MRCP, FRCPath[a,b,*],
Nandini Shetty, MSc, MD, FRCPath[c], Tommy T.Y. Lam, PhD[d],
K.L. Ellis Hon, MD, FCCM[e]

KEYWORDS

- Influenza - Pandemic - H1N1 - Transmission
- Treatment - Epidemiology

INFLUENZA VIRUSES

Influenza viruses belong to the family of Orthomyxoviridae, which are lipid-enveloped, single-stranded, negative-sense, 8-segmented RNA viruses (**Fig. 1**). Of the 3 known serotypes of influenza (A, B, and C), only types A and B cause frequent and occasionally severe diseases in humans. There is only 1 type of influenza B, whereas influenza A has multiple subtypes, characterized by a combination of the 16 known hemagglutinin (HA) and 9 neuraminidase (NA) genes that code for these viral envelope or surface proteins. These proteins play a role in viral entry and egress from human respiratory epithelial cells within which the virus replicates. Of these 16 HA subtypes, 6 have been found in human infections (H1, H2, H3, H5, H7, and H9). It is generally accepted that the human immune response is mainly targeted at the HA protein epitope of the

Funding: no specific funding was involved in the writing of this article.
[a] Division of Microbiology, Department of Laboratory Medicine, National University Hospital, 5 Lower Kent Ridge Road, Singapore 119074, Singapore
[b] Molecular Diagnosis Centre, Department of Laboratory Medicine, National University Hospital, 5 Lower Kent Ridge Road, Singapore 119074, Singapore
[c] Department of Clinical Microbiology, University College London Hospitals, 1st floor, Windeyer Institute of Medical Sciences, 46 Cleveland Street, London W1T 4JF, UK
[d] School of Biological Sciences, Kadoorie Biological Sciences Building, The University of Hong Kong, Pokfulam Road, Hong Kong Special Administrative Region, China
[e] Department of Paediatrics, The Chinese University of Hong Kong, Shatin, Hong Kong Special Administrative Region, China
* Corresponding author. Division of Microbiology, Department of Laboratory Medicine, National University Hospital, 5 Lower Kent Ridge Road, Singapore 119074, Singapore.
E-mail address: julian_wt_tang@nuhs.edu.sg

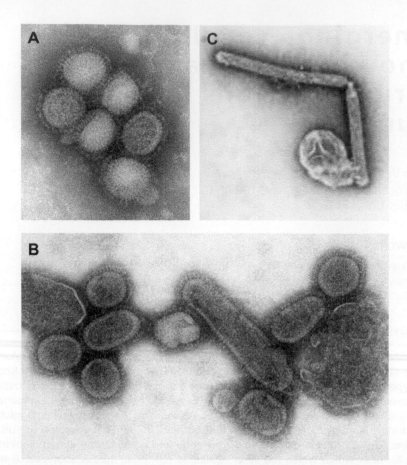

Fig. 1. Negatively stained transmission electron micrographs showing some of the ultrastructural morphology of (*A*) the recently emerged pandemic influenza A (H1N1) 2009 virus of swine origin (strain: A/CA/4/09), (*B*) the recreated 1918 pandemic influenza A (H1N1) virus grown in Madin-Darby canine kidney cell culture, and (*C*) 2 avian influenza A (H5N1) viruses (magnification ×108,000) showing the stippled appearance of the roughened surface of the proteinaceous coat encasing each virion. It should be noted that although these images show different views of these influenza viruses, electron microscopy generally cannot distinguish among the different influenza virus types, subtypes, or strains. (*Data from* The Centers for Disease Control Public Health Images Library. Available at http://phil.cdc.gov/phil/home.asp. Accessed April 17, 2010; #11,212 [*A*], #8243 [*B*], and #8038 [*C*].)

virus, which is why the seasonal influenza vaccine is mainly characterized by its HA (rather than its NA) composition for influenza A.

So far, only 3 subtypes of HA (H1, H2, H3) and 2 subtypes of NA (N1, N2) have caused pandemics in humans. Traditional pandemic surveillance has focused on monitoring the antigenic shift, that is, the reassortment of HA and/or NA genes between human and zoonotic influenza A viruses during rare events of dual infections in a human or an intermediate host. For the surveillance of currently circulating seasonal influenza viruses, most recently the A (H3N2) and A (H1N1) viruses, viral isolates are collected throughout the year to determine the most appropriate seasonal influenza vaccine composition for the coming influenza seasons in the northern and southern hemispheres.

Avian Influenza A (H5N1)

A zoonotic virus (ie, originating from animals and spreading to humans), avian influenza A (H5N1) emerged for the first time in Hong Kong in 1997 from chickens to infect humans, infecting 18 people and killing 6 of them—a high mortality rate of more than 30%.[1]

Originally discovered to be circulating on geese farms in 1996 in Guangdong, China, this highly pathogenic avian influenza A (H5N1) virus soon spread to Hong Kong, causing outbreaks among poultry in 1997. It was eventually eradicated from Hong Kong after a mass cull of all poultry, but it apparently continued to circulate asymptomatically amongst birds in southern China,[2] from where it eventually reemerged in the human population in 2002 to 2003 and has been causing ongoing sporadic human infection and disease, with a high mortality (close to 60%) till present. As of August 31, 2009, the World Health Organization has reported 440 cases of sporadic H5N1 human infection, of which 262 were lethal (a 60% case-fatality rate).[3]

In addition, sporadic, generally mild (although there has been at least 1 recorded death because of H7N7) human infections resulting from occasional bird-to-human transmissions, with low pathogenic avian influenza strains (eg, subtypes H9N2, H7N7, H7N2, and H7N3) have been ongoing since 1997, when heightened surveillance for avian influenza viruses began (**Fig. 2**).[4] So far, all these low pathogenic avian influenza viruses isolated from these sporadic human infections have been genetically similar to the corresponding avian influenza viruses circulating in birds. Thus, so far and within the limits of current surveillance, there seems to have been no further reassortment of these viruses with either human or swine influenza viruses. Until recently, avian influenza A (H5N1) was considered the prime virus subtype candidate for causing the next influenza pandemic.

However, the recent unexpected emergence of the pandemic Influenza A (H1N1) 2009 virus (also referred to as H1N1v) of swine origin from Mexico has demonstrated that even influenza subtypes that have been encountered in previous Influenza pandemics may constitute new pandemic threats.[5]

INFLUENZA PANDEMICS

Before the emergence of the recent pandemic influenza A (H1N1) 2009 virus, there were 3 pandemics during the twentieth century: in 1918 (the Spanish flu), 1957 (the Asian flu), and 1968 (the Hong Kong flu). These incidents have been widely studied with the help of available (and sometimes extensive) epidemiologic records and any preserved, archived viral isolates or infected tissue specimens.

The first of these pandemics in 1918 coincided with World War I and infected an estimated one-third of the world's population (approximately 500 million people), with approximately 50 million deaths. In contrast, the subsequent 1957 and 1968 pandemics (now shown to have originated in Asia) resulted in a lower morbidity and mortality but still had a significant global effect. Perhaps most importantly, the occurrence of these subsequent pandemics gave rise to the concept that such pandemics could and would recur.

Pandemic influenza viruses are thought to arise when there is frequent human contact with certain animal species that can be infected with their own specific influenza viruses and when these viruses develop the ability to jump the species barrier to infect humans. This crossing is made possible in the presence of certain gene mutations permitting the binding of such animal influenza viruses to surface proteins on human respiratory epithelial cell receptors.[6]

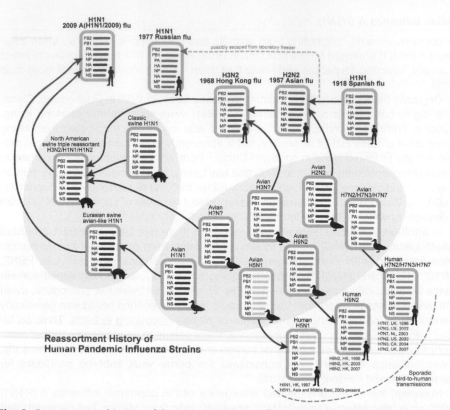

Fig. 2. Reassortment history of human pandemic influenza strains. Each influenza gene segment is represented by a colored horizontal bar. The 1918 Spanish flu influenza and classic swine influenza probably originated from an avian influenza virus population at some point in the past, but arrows indicating their origins have been omitted here because the exact species-crossing events cannot be defined for certain and remain controversial. The reassortment events generating the H3N2 Hong Kong flu pandemic strain have been simplified here because of space constraints. Sporadic bird-to-human transmission events are also shown in the bottom right corner.

Birds are the natural reservoir for influenza A viruses, although other animals such as pigs and horses have also acquired and maintained their own separate genetic lineages of influenza.[7] The origin of the 1918 A (H1N1) pandemic influenza virus has become more controversial recently, and there is a debate over whether it was derived from a human influenza strain existing before 1918,[8] or directly from a purely avian influenza strain from around 1918,[9] or whether it was generated by the reassortment or recombination between human and avian influenza viruses cocirculating around that time. The reason for this controversy is that there are very few viral isolates available for analysis from around this time (before 1918); therefore, the complete diversity of avian influenza viruses circulating then cannot be known.

In contrast, the origins of the 1957 and 1968 influenza pandemics have been more clearly defined (see **Fig. 2**). The 1957 pandemic was caused by an A (H2N2) reassortant strain admixing HA, NA, and polymerase basic protein 1 (PB1) gene segments from avian influenza strains, with the remaining gene segments from the A (H1N1) human pandemic influenza virus subtype that had been circulating since its emergence in 1918.[10] The strain A (H2N2) eventually replaced A (H1N1); then A (H2N2) was itself replaced by the 1968 A (H3N2) pandemic subtype. The 1968 A (H3N2) virus was also a reassortant strain in which the HA and PB1 gene segments from an avian influenza strain reassorted with the then currently circulating A (H2N2) virus.[10] Since 1977, this A (H3N2) virus has been cocirculating with an A (H1N1) strain similar to the 1918 A (H1N1) pandemic virus, which was accidentally released from a laboratory.[11] Thus, these 2 viruses have now become familiar to us as the seasonal influenza A subtypes for more than 30 years. Analyses of the viruses that caused the 1957 and 1968 influenza pandemics therefore proved that zoonotic transmissions of influenza viruses (ie, from animals to man) with gene reassortment were capable of generating antigenically new influenza strains, novel to human immunity, with significant effects on the public health.

Pandemic Influenza A (H1N1) 2009

The emergence of the first influenza pandemic virus in April 2009 in more than 40 years caught the world by surprise. It was a surprise not just because of the zoonotic origin of the virus (ie, swine rather than avian) but also because of the geographic origins (ie, the Americas rather than Southeast Asia).[12] However, the pandemic preparedness that was already in place to combat the more expected avian influenza pandemic has been used to good effect. The stockpiling of antivirals and a lot of basic and applied research into developing vaccines against novel influenza viruses had already commenced.

Apart from the clinical preparedness, a lot of groundwork has also already been done on the development and application of mathematical models for describing and predicting how the pandemic will evolve,[13,14] as well as identifying and prioritizing public health interventions.[15] This approach has been stimulated greatly by the severe acute respiratory syndrome outbreaks of 2003, and it was easy to apply these techniques to influenza. These mathematical models included not just the traditional epidemiologic models but also the newer approach of phylogenetic analysis applied to partial or whole viral genomes. In some recent analyses of the novel pandemic influenza A (H1N1) virus, this latter approach has been used to give unique insights into the evolution of this new virus.[16]

CLINICAL FEATURES, DIAGNOSIS, AND MANAGEMENT OF INFLUENZA

Case definitions form the cornerstone of the investigation and management of individual patients and outbreaks, although the different influenza subtypes may present in slightly different ways. However, these differences, although statistically noticeable in comparative case series, may not be necessarily useful when faced with individual patients. Ultimately, laboratory diagnosis will always be required to distinguish among the different infecting subtypes.

Clinical Presentation

Seasonal influenza viruses
Clinically, influenza is usually a self-limiting disease. After an average incubation period of around 1 to 2 days, onset of illness is characterized by an abrupt onset of fever and chills accompanied by headache, generalized myalgia, rhinorrhea, sore throat, and cough. Gastrointestinal symptoms such as vomiting, abdominal pain, and diarrhea are often reported. The most common cause of hospitalization is lower respiratory tract infection, including croup, bronchitis, bronchiolitis, and pneumonia. Manifestations involving the central nervous system may be observed, including encephalopathy, postinfluenza encephalitis, transverse myelitis, Guillain-Barré

syndrome, and acute necrotizing encephalitis. Myositis often occurs 3 days (range, 0–18 days) after onset of illness. In young infants, influenza can mimic generalized sepsis. Myocarditis is a rare complication. Epidemiologically, most deaths occur in infants and the elderly (>65 years old) during the annual influenza epidemics as a result of decreased immunity against influenza virus infection. The mortality curve typically presents with a U shape when age-specific excess mortality caused by pneumonia and seasonal influenza is plotted.[17]

Avian influenza A (H5N1) virus

The incubation period for this virus has been estimated to be up to 7 days, but it is more commonly 2 to 5 days after the last known exposure to sick or dead poultry. In cases where limited human-to-human transmission likely occurred, the incubation period was estimated to be between 2 and 10 days.[18]

Analyses of the human A (H5N1) infections in Hong Kong, Vietnam, Thailand, and Cambodia revealed that fever and cough were the most common initial symptoms. Gastrointestinal symptoms including vomiting, diarrhea, and abdominal pain were reported early in the course of illness in some cases.[19] Others reported pleuritic pain and bleeding from the nose and gums. Generally, patients with H5N1 virus infection were hospitalized 4 to 6 days after onset of illness.[18]

Common laboratory findings in patients with A (H5N1) infection at the time of hospital admission include leukopenia, lymphopenia, and mild-to-moderate thrombocytopenia.[19] However, for patients with a clinically mild illness, there was no decrease in the white cell count. Chest radiographic findings included patchy, interstitial, lobar, and/or diffuse infiltrates; consolidation; pleural effusion; and pneumothorax. In fatal A (H5N1) cases, the median time from onset to death was 9 days.[18]

The fatality rate among hospitalized patients has been high and varies considerably between countries (33%–100%), although the true rate maybe much lower because of an unknown number of milder nonfatal infections in the community.[20] Acute respiratory distress syndrome complicated 76.5% (13 in 17) of cases in Thailand and 44.4% (8 in 18) of cases in Hong Kong. Multiple organ failure, with signs of renal dysfunction and sometimes cardiac compromise, was often noted. In the severe human A (H5N1) infections in Hong Kong, reactive hemophagocytic syndrome was a unique pathologic feature in 3 fatal cases, as were increased blood levels of interferon-α, tumor necrosis factor α, and other cytokines, providing evidence that cytokine responses contributed to the pathogenesis of human H5N1 infections.[21]

Exactly how the severity of illness varies by clade or subclade of H5N1 virus infection, by age, or by immunologic, genetic, or other factors is unknown.[18] Most patients who died did not have a preexisting disease, in contrast to situations where other subtypes of human influenza virus infections caused epidemics during interpandemic periods. However, patients with underlying cardiovascular, pulmonary, or renal diseases were, as expected, still more susceptible to severe influenza infection.[20]

Pandemic influenza A (H1N1) 2009 virus

An analysis of 18 cases of pneumonia with confirmed A (H1N1) 2009 infection among 98 patients hospitalized for acute respiratory illness in Mexico City, Mexico, showed that more than 50% of them were between ages 13 and 47 years and only 8 had preexisting medical conditions. All patients had fever, cough, dyspnea or respiratory distress, increased serum lactate dehydrogenase levels, and bilateral patchy pneumonia (**Fig. 3**). Other common findings were an increased creatine kinase level (in 62% of the patients) and lymphopenia (in 61%). Twelve patients required mechanical ventilation, and 7 died. Within 7 days after contact with the initial case patients, a mild or moderate influenzalike illness developed in 22 health care workers, none of whom required hospitalization.[22]

In a study of 642 confirmed cases of human A (H1N1) 2009 infection identified from the rapidly evolving US outbreak in April 2009, the age of patients ranged from 3 months to 81 years; 60% of patients were 18 years old or younger. Of patients with available data, 18% had recently traveled to Mexico and 16% were identified from

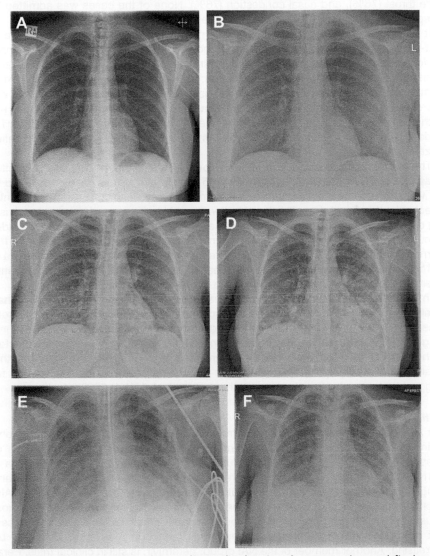

Fig. 3. A series of consecutive chest radiographs showing the progression and final resolution of an adult woman aged 22 years infected with pandemic influenza A (H1N1) 2009. The initial appearance is suggestive of a developing viral pneumonitis, which then seems to resolve (*A–C*), but then the patient probably developed a secondary bacterial infection (although not proven conclusively) (*D*) that necessitated a transfer to the intensive care unit (*E*) before finally resolving (*F*). The patient was finally discharged feeling well, with no long-term sequelae. (*Courtesy of* University College London Hospitals NHS Trust, London, UK.)

school outbreaks of A (H1N1) 2009 infection. The most common presenting symptoms were fever (94%), cough (92%), and sore throat (66%); 25% of patients had diarrhea, and 25% had vomiting. Of the 399 patients for whom hospitalization status was known, 36 (9%) required hospitalization and 2 died.[12]

A Canadian study also reported cough in 90% of patients but fever in only 59% of confirmed and probable cases. Other common symptoms included headache (83%), sore throat (76%), and nasal congestion (76%). None of the cases was admitted to hospital. No deaths were associated with the cluster.[23]

It is now becoming clear that most cases of A (H1N1) 2009 infection are mild and self-limiting and present in a manner that is indistinguishable from seasonal influenza. As for seasonal influenza, those with preexisting medical conditions such as the traditional chronic diseases (eg, diabetes, asthma, renal or cardiac failure, and any form of immunosuppression) seem to be at greater risk of severe disease and death (and are therefore routinely targeted for the annual seasonal influenza immunization). Even so, with this virus, it has been suggested that obesity may be an additional risk factor for serious disease,[24] as is pregnancy,[25] which is also a recognized risk in seasonal influenza infection.

The age distribution of infection with this novel virus also differs from seasonal influenza. For example, the older age groups (>65 years) have always been considered to be vulnerable to seasonal influenza infection, but they seem to be less frequently infected by this novel virus. This trend is now thought to be caused by some preexisting cross-reacting immunity to this virus as a result of their past exposure to the older circulating seasonal influenza A (H1N1) strains that have been more similar to the current pandemic A (H1N1) 2009 virus. The current circulating seasonal influenza A (H1N1) virus and its corresponding seasonal influenza vaccine antigen components seem to not provide any cross-immunity to the pandemic strain.[26]

In the more frequently targeted younger adult age groups, an unusual feature has been observed; more patients in this group progress to more serious respiratory disease, whereas there is also a significant gastrointestinal component (nausea, vomiting, and diarrhea in 10%–50% of cases) involved.[12] In addition, in children infected with A (H1N1) 2009, the incidence of seizures seems to be prominent. Although this is also seen with seasonal influenza,[27] the few recent case reports available so far suggest that outcomes are better with the pandemic A (H1N1) 2009 infection.[28]

Antivirals
For all these influenza subtypes, apart from the usual respiratory support and monitoring, there are only a few specific antiviral drugs for treatment. In the cases of seasonal influenza A (H3N2), avian influenza A (H5N1), and pandemic influenza A (H1N1) 2009, virtually all these viruses are resistant to treatment with the adamantane drugs (amantadine and rimantadine) but still susceptible to the NA inhibitors (NAIs) such as oseltamivir and zanamivir. In the case of seasonal influenza A (H1N1), most viruses are resistant to oseltamivir (although zanamivir is still effective in most cases) but still susceptible to the adamantane drugs, although resistance seems to be increasing. Another member of the NAI group, peramivir, is still in clinical trials. Peramivir has an advantage over oseltamivir (taken orally) and zanamivir (taken by inhalation) in that it can be given intravenously. Combination therapy with oseltamivir and rimantadine can be given empirically if the influenza subtype is unknown, and some patients infected with A (H1N1) 2009 have been given this combination as initial empiric therapy.[28]

According to the manufacturer's information, oseltamivir is generally well tolerated and its adverse effects are mild and mainly gastrointestinal (ie, nausea, vomiting, diarrhea). However, reports from the use of oseltamivir as postexposure prophylaxis (75 mg once daily for 10 days) in primary and secondary school children (age, 4–12 years) have described additional symptoms such as feeling sick, headaches, stomach aches, difficulty sleeping, nightmares, and poor concentration.[29,30]

Table 1 shows the currently recommended NAI doses for treatment and postexposure prophylaxis for patients of different ages. Treatment is recommended for 5 days, whereas prophylaxis is recommended for at least 2 weeks or a minimum of 7 days (eg, at least 10 days as per CDC recommendations in **Table 1**) after contact with the last infected individual and onset of illness. Pediatric dosing is based on weight for those weighing less than 40 kg and older than 1 year. For children younger than 1 year, oseltamivir is not licensed to be administered; however, it can be used on an "emergency authorization use" basis, for which the recommended dosing regimen is also shown in **Table 1**. There should be careful monitoring for adverse effects when the drug is used in this younger age group outside its licensure.

The treatment of pregnant women infected with A (H1N1) 2009 is considered a priority, because there seems to be an increased risk (although this is relative) of complications in this population.[25] A recent study suggests that, so far, treatment with oseltamivir appears to be safe in pregnancy[31] and that, on this basis, it should be commenced as soon as possible after the onset of symptoms,[32] as well as being offered for postexposure prophylaxis.[33] However, as always, the actual application of these recommendations is left to the individual decision and risk assessment of the patient and the doctor.

Table 1
Recommended antiviral dosing regimens (for oseltamivir and zanamivir) for the treatment and prophylaxis of influenza A (H1N1) 2009 virus

	Recommended Dose for Treatment	Recommended Dose for Prophylaxis
Oseltamivir (treatment, 5 d; prophylaxis, at least 10 d[a])		
Adults	75 mg twice daily	75 mg once daily
Children aged <12 mo		
<3 mo	12 mg twice daily	Not recommended unless critically ill because of limited data in this age group.
3–5 mo	20 mg twice daily	20 mg once daily
6–11 mo	25 mg twice daily	25 mg once daily
Children aged ≥ 12 mo and based on weight		
15 kg or less	60 mg/d, divided into 2 doses	30 mg once daily
16–23 kg	90 mg/d, divided into 2 doses	45 mg once daily
24–40 kg	120 mg/d, divided into 2 doses	60 mg once daily
>40 kg	150 mg/d, divided into 2 doses	75 mg once daily
Zanamivir		
Adults	Two 5-mg inhalations (10 mg total) twice per day	Two 5-mg inhalations (10 mg total) once per day
Children	Two 5-mg inhalations (10 mg total) twice per day (7 y or older)	Two 5-mg inhalations (10 mg total) once per day (5 y or older)

[a] As recommended in the manufacturer's fact sheet on oseltamivir for health care providers at http://www.cdc.gov/h1n1flu/EUA/pdf/tamiflu-hcp.pdf.

Adapted from the Centers for Disease Control and Prevention Web site. Available at: http://www.cdc.gov/h1n1flu/recommendations.htm. Accessed August 28, 2009.

Resistance to oseltamivir arising in patients treated with it has been reported in a few cases so far. The most commonly reported resistance mutation, H275Y, occurs in the NA gene.[34,35] The incidence and prevalence of oseltamivir-resistant A (H1N1) 2009 viruses is likely to increase, given the continued widespread use of the drug for treatment. However, oseltamivir should be used for treating only severely ill cases of A (H1N1) 2009 infection (as per seasonal influenza use recommendations) and not for postexposure prophylaxis unless vulnerable groups have been exposed.[32] There has been one case of oseltamivir resistance reported in an individual with no history of oseltamivir use.[36] The issue of worry then is whether such resistant viruses will eventually become fit enough to transmit efficiently in the population (perhaps displacing the wild-type susceptible virus), making the worldwide stockpiles of oseltamivir effectively useless.

Treatment

Antibiotics

There is increasing evidence and conviction that a significant proportion (20%–30%) of deaths caused by past influenza pandemics may have been a result of secondary bacterial infections. Recent analyses of the 1918 pandemic mortality figures suggest that a significant number of deaths were caused by secondary infections with *Haemophilus influenzae*, *Streptococcus pneumoniae*, *Streptococcus pyogenes*, and/or *Staphylococcus aureus*.[37] These findings suggest that antibiotics and antibacterial vaccines may be important in the management of influenza infections.[38]

PUBLIC HEALTH ISSUES: PREVENTION AND CONTROL

There are several approaches to prevent infection by the pandemic influenza A (H1N1) 2009 virus, although not all of them are currently available and the evidence supporting the use of some approaches is limited or controversial.

At the individual and population level (ie, in terms of increasing overall herd immunity), immunization with a specific A (H1N1) 2009 vaccine is one of the most effective ways to prevent infection. There are multiple ongoing vaccine trials,[39,40] and recently, a specific live attenuated vaccine (indicated for children and adults, aged 2 to 49 years) has been approved by the US Food and Drug Administration, as of September 15, 2009. Other countries are in the process of approving the vaccine, and it is likely that vaccines against the pandemic influenza virus will be widely available in most countries by the time this article is published. The rapid licensing of this new vaccine has only been made possible by the urgency of the pandemic situation and the application of existing seasonal influenza vaccine manufacturing regulations that do not require annual changes in influenza antigen composition of the seasonal influenza vaccine to undergo relicensing each year. To make the limited supply of these vaccines go further, lower antigenic doses and different adjuvants are being tested to immunize as much of the population as required.[41]

In addition, individual vaccination benefits the population as a whole by reducing the number of susceptible individuals who can be infected by the virus. Given the currently accepted relatively low value for the reproductive number (R_o) of 1 to 2,[13,14] less than 60% (where required vaccine coverage, V_c, is estimated by the formula $V_c = 1 - 1/R_o$) of the population requires vaccination to curtail the onward transmission of influenza. However, there are significant technical (ie, how to make and deliver such a huge amount of vaccine in a short time), moral, and economic (ie, who gets vaccinated first and for what price) challenges that will be faced by the planned global immunization program against the pandemic A (H1N1) 2009 influenza virus.[42,43] With such large populations being vaccinated, there needs to be careful monitoring for common and rarer (eg, Guillan-Barré syndrome) adverse effects.[44]

Postexposure prophylaxis with oseltamivir for those in close contact with confirmed cases has already been discussed. The disadvantage of mass prophylaxis has been seen in school children when the incidence of adverse effects may be greater than the incidence of secondary infections.[29,30] This situation becomes more relevant with lower estimates of influenza transmissibility (ie, the lower the value of R_o), although this may be higher in certain situations, such as the dense crowding seen in schools and other public entertainment venues.

Simple surgical and N95 masks are probably effective to a certain extent either in preventing the noninfected wearer (eg, health care workers) from inhaling influenza-containing droplets (from either a close or more distant source) or in containing the infectious exhaled air from an infected wearer (eg, patients). The problem with wearing masks for either purpose tends to mainly be that of

---

Box 1
Nonpharmaceutical public health interventions

Human surveillance

- Case reporting
- Early rapid viral diagnosis
- Disinfection
- Hand hygiene
- Respiratory etiquettes
- Surgical and N95 masks
- Other personal protective equipment[a]

Community restrictions

- School closures
- Workplace closures
- Cancellation of group events
- International and domestic travel restrictions[b]

Patient management

- Isolation of sick individuals
- Provision of social support services to the isolated

Contact management

- Quarantine[c]
- Voluntary sheltering[d]
- Contact tracing

[a] Gowns, gloves, and protective eye covers.
[b] Exit and entry screening, travel advisories.
[c] Separating exposed individuals from others.
[d] Voluntary sequestration of healthy persons to avoid exposure.
Data from Aledort JE, Lurie N, Wasserman J, et al. Non-pharmaceutical public health interventions for pandemic influenza: an evaluation of the evidence base. BMC Public Health 2007;7:208.

maintaining an effective mask position on the face for long periods of time.[45] Sweating and contact irritation can combine to cause mask displacement or removal (noncompliance). It may be particularly difficult when patients suffering from coughing or sneezing are made to wear masks to contain their infection as a form of infection control.

Social distancing has received much attention because of its potential to mitigate and perhaps even curtail the widespread transmission of pandemic influenza. One well-investigated example of this has been the effects of school closure on the subsequent progression of an influenza pandemic. Various mathematical modeling studies have suggested that, although there may be some delay in the spread of the pandemic from closing schools, this measure will only be effective if the subsequent behavior of children outside the school does not result in a similar number of contacts and that such relative isolation is prolonged during the pandemic period. However, the social and economic disruption for the working parents with such a strategy may be difficult to overcome because at least one parent will have to take time off work to look after young children at home. In particular, school closure has to be part of an overall mitigation strategy, including the treatment and home isolation of infected individuals to reduce further contacts.[15]

Air travel can rapidly transport infections between different destinations around the world and also act as a source for generating new infections within the crowded confines of modern passenger planes. Various mathematical modeling tools have been used to assess the effect of restricting air travel on the spread of pandemic influenza. However, the benefits may be fairly minor and may not be worth the inevitable and serious social and economic disruption this will cause.[46]

The possible nonpharmaceutical public health interventions are summarized in **Box 1.**[47]

SUMMARY

The understanding of how novel influenza viruses arise (usually from animal reservoirs) has increased at an incredible rate assisted by the rapid advances in sequencing technologies and phylogenetic methods. Such understanding allows more effective public health surveillance of seasonal human influenza viruses, as well as candidate pandemic viruses that may cross the species barrier from animals to humans. Development in antiviral drugs for influenza is still slow (compared with rapid advances and the variety in the case of anti–human immunodeficiency virus drugs), but this is counterbalanced by the effective and highly organized and regulated vaccine-manufacturing base that is already in existence for the seasonal influenza vaccines. Unlike infectious agents that infect humans only (such as smallpox and measles), influenza viruses, being zoonotic (with animal and human reservoirs), will continue to pose a persistent and variable threat to human health for the foreseeable future. It is therefore important that systems are in place, in health care institutions and in the general community, to react and adapt quickly to limit human morbidity and mortality caused by this ever-changing pathogen.

REFERENCES

1. Subbarao K, Klimov A, Katz J, et al. Characterization of an avian influenza A (H5N1) virus isolated from a child with a fatal respiratory illness. Science 1998; 279(5349):393–6.
2. Webster RG, Guan Y, Peiris M, et al. Characterization of H5N1 influenza viruses that continue to circulate in geese in southeastern China. J Virol 2002;76(1):118–26.

3. World Health Organization. Confirmed human cases of avian influenza A(H5N1). Available at: http://www.who.int/csr/disease/avian_influenza/country/en/. Accessed August 31, 2009.

4. Wong SS, Yuen KY. Avian influenza virus infections in humans. Chest 2006; 129(1):156–68.

5. Gatherer D. The 2009 H1N1 influenza outbreak in its historical context. J Clin Virol 2009;45(3):174–8.

6. Yamada S, Suzuki Y, Suzuki T, et al. Haemagglutinin mutations responsible for the binding of H5N1 influenza A viruses to human-type receptors. Nature 2006; 444(7117):378–82.

7. Webster RG, Bean WJ, Gorman OT, et al. Evolution and ecology of influenza A viruses. Microbiol Rev 1992;56(1):152–79.

8. Taubenberger JK, Morens DM. 1918 influenza: the mother of all pandemics. Emerg Infect Dis 2006;12(1):15–22.

9. Fanning TG, Slemons RD, Reid AH, et al. 1917 avian influenza virus sequences suggest that the 1918 pandemic virus did not acquire its hemagglutinin directly from birds. J Virol 2002;76(15):7860–2.

10. Kawaoka Y, Krauss S, Webster RG. Avian-to-human transmission of the PB1 gene of influenza A viruses in the 1957 and 1968 pandemics. J Virol 1989;63(11):4603–8.

11. Kendal AP, Noble GR, Skehel JJ, et al. Antigenic similarity of influenza A (H1N1) viruses from epidemics in 1977–1978 to "Scandinavian" strains isolated in epidemics of 1950–1951. Virology 1978;89(2):632–6.

12. Dawood FS, Jain S, Finelli L, et al. Emergence of a novel swine-origin influenza A (H1N1) virus in humans. N Engl J Med 2009;360(25):2605–15.

13. Pourbohloul B, Ahued A, Davoudi B, et al. Initial human transmission dynamics of the pandemic (H1N1) 2009 virus in North America. Influenza Other Respi Viruses 2009;3(5):215–22.

14. Fraser C, Donnelly CA, Cauchemez S, et al. Pandemic potential of a strain of influenza A (H1N1): early findings. Science 2009;324(5934):1557–61.

15. Cauchemez S, Ferguson NM, Wachtel C, et al. Closure of schools during an influenza pandemic. Lancet Infect Dis 2009;9(8):473–81.

16. Smith GJ, Vijaykrishna D, Bahl J, et al. Origins and evolutionary genomics of the 2009 swine-origin H1N1 influenza A epidemic. Nature 2009;459(7250):1122–5.

17. Hsieh YC, Wu TZ, Liu DP, et al. Influenza pandemics: past, present and future. J Formos Med Assoc 2006;105(1):1–6.

18. Uyeki TM. Human infection with highly pathogenic avian influenza A (H5N1) virus: review of clinical issues. Clin Infect Dis 2009;49(2):279–90.

19. Tran TH, Nguyen TL, Nguyen TD, et al. Avian influenza A (H5N1) in 10 patients in Vietnam. N Engl J Med 2004;350(12):1179–88.

20. Beigel JH, Farrar J, Han AM, et al. Avian influenza A (H5N1) infection in humans. N Engl J Med 2005;353(13):1374–85.

21. Peiris JS, Yu WC, Leung CW, et al. Re-emergence of fatal human influenza A subtype H5N1 disease. Lancet 2004;363(9409):617–9.

22. Perez-Padilla R, de la Rosa-Zamboni D, Ponce de Leon S, et al. Pneumonia and respiratory failure from swine-origin influenza A (H1N1) in Mexico. N Engl J Med 2009;361(7):680–9.

23. Cutler J, Schleihauf E, Hatchette TF, et al. Investigation of the first cases of human-to-human infection with the new swine-origin influenza A (H1N1) virus in Canada. CMAJ 2009;181(3–4):159–63.

24. Vaillant L, La Ruche G, Tarantola A, et al. Epidemiology of fatal cases associated with pandemic H1N1 influenza 2009. Euro Surveill 2009;14(33):1–6.

25. Jamieson DJ, Honein MA, Rasmussen SA, et al. H1N1 2009 influenza virus infection during pregnancy in the USA. Lancet 2009;374(9688):451–8.

26. Hancock K, Veguilla V, Lu X, et al. Cross-reactive antibody responses to the 2009 pandemic H1N1 influenza virus. N Engl J Med 2009;361(20):1945–52.

27. Weitkamp JH, Spring MD, Brogan T, et al. Influenza A virus-associated acute necrotizing encephalopathy in the United States. Pediatr Infect Dis J 2004; 23(3):259–63.

28. Neurologic complications associated with novel influenza A (H1N1) virus infection in children-Dallas, Texas, 2009. MMWR Morb Mortal Wkly Rep 2009;58(28):773–8.

29. Kitching A, Roche A, Balasegaram S, et al. Oseltamivir adherence and side effects among children in three London schools affected by influenza A(H1N1)v, May 2009-an internet-based cross-sectional survey. Euro Surveill 2009;14(30):19287.

30. Wallensten A, Oliver I, Lewis D, et al. Compliance and side effects of prophylactic oseltamivir treatment in a school in South West England. Euro Surveill 2009; 14(30):19285.

31. Tanaka T, Nakajima K, Murashima A, et al. Safety of neuraminidase inhibitors against novel influenza A (H1N1) in pregnant and breastfeeding women. CMAJ 2009;181(1–2):55–8.

32. World Health Organization. WHO 2009 treatment guide. Available at: http://www.who.int/csr/resources/publications/swineflu/h1n1_guidelines_pharmaceutical_mngt.pdf. Accessed August 28, 2009.

33. Novel influenza A (H1N1) virus infections in three pregnant women-United States, April-May 2009. MMWR Morb Mortal Wkly Rep 2009;58(18):497–500.

34. Oseltamivir-resistant 2009 pandemic influenza A (H1N1) virus infection in two summer campers receiving prophylaxis-North Carolina, 2009. MMWR Morb Mortal Wkly Rep 2009;58(35):969–72.

35. Oseltamivir-resistant novel influenza A (H1N1) virus infection in two immunosuppressed patients-Seattle, Washington, 2009. MMWR Morb Mortal Wkly Rep 2009; 58(32):893–6.

36. Center of Disease Control and Prevention. Hong Kong oseltamivir resistance. Available at: http://www.cdc.gov/h1n1flu/HAN/070909.htm. Accessed August 28, 2009.

37. Brundage JF, Shanks GD. Deaths from bacterial pneumonia during 1918–19 influenza pandemic. Emerg Infect Dis 2008;14(8):1193–9.

38. Gupta RK, George R, Nguyen-Van-Tam JS. Bacterial pneumonia and pandemic influenza planning. Emerg Infect Dis 2008;14(8):1187–92.

39. Clark TW, Pareek M, Hoschler K, et al. Trial of influenza A (H1N1) 2009 monovalent MF59-adjuvanted vaccine – preliminary report. N Engl J Med 2009;361(25):2424–35.

40. Greenberg ME, Lai MH, Hartel GF, et al. Response after one dose of a monovalent influenza A (H1N1) 2009 vaccine—preliminary report. N Engl J Med 2009; 361(25):2405–13.

41. Neuzil KM. Pandemic influenza vaccine policy—considering the early evidence. N Engl J Med 2009;361(25):e59.

42. Neuzil KM, Bright RA. Influenza vaccine manufacture: keeping up with change. J Infect Dis 2009;200(6):835–7.

43. Yamada T. Poverty, wealth, and access to pandemic influenza vaccines. N Engl J Med 2009;361(12):1129–31.

44. Evans D, Cauchemez S, Hayden FG. "Prepandemic" immunization for novel influenza viruses, "swine flu" vaccine, Guillain-Barre syndrome, and the detection of rare severe adverse events. J Infect Dis 2009;200(3):321–8.

45. MacIntyre CR, Cauchemez S, Dwyer DE, et al. Face mask use and control of respiratory virus transmission in households. Emerg Infect Dis 2009;15(2): 233–41.
46. Hollingsworth TD, Ferguson NM, Anderson RM. Frequent travelers and rate of spread of epidemics. Emerg Infect Dis 2007;13(9):1288–94.
47. Aledort JE, Lurie N, Wasserman J, et al. Non-pharmaceutical public health interventions for pandemic influenza: an evaluation of the evidence base. BMC Public Health 2007;7:208.

Severe Acute Respiratory Syndrome and Coronavirus

David S.C. Hui, MD(UNSW), FRACP, FRCP[a],*, Paul K.S. Chan, MD, FRCPath[b]

KEYWORDS

- SARS • Clinical features • Pathogenesis
- Treatment • Outcome

Severe acute respiratory syndrome (SARS) emerged unexpectedly in 2003 and posed an enormous threat to international health and economy.[1–4] By the end of the epidemic in July 2003, 8098 probable cases were reported in 29 countries and regions with a mortality of 774 (9.6%).[5] SARS re-emerged at small scales in late 2003 and early 2004 in South China after resumption of wild animal trading activities in markets.[6,7]

THE VIRUS AND ITS ORIGIN

Members of the Coronaviridae family are classified into 3 groups based on serologic and, more recently, genetic similarity. Coronaviruses (CoVs) are found in a wide range of animal species including cat, dog, pig, rabbit, cattle, mouse, rat, chicken, pheasant, turkey, whale, as well as humans. Before the SARS epidemic, the only recognized coronaviruses causing respiratory tract infection in humans were HCoV-OC43 and HCoV-229E. In 2003, a previously unrecognized CoV was detected from SARS patients,[8–15] and was confirmed to be the causative agent for SARS; it became known as SARS-CoV. Retrospective serologic surveys suggested that cross-species transmission of SARS-CoV or its variants from various animal species to humans might have occurred frequently in the wet market, as a high seroprevalence was detected among animal handlers who had no notable SARS-like illnesses.[16]

The role of masked palm civets in transmitting SARS-CoV to humans was first suspected in 2003 when a closely related variant of SARS-CoV was detected from palm

[a] Division of Respiratory Medicine, Stanley Ho Center for Emerging Infectious Diseases, Prince of Wales Hospital, The Chinese University of Hong Kong, Prince of Wales Hospital, 30-32 Ngan Shing Street, Shatin, New Territories, Hong Kong, China
[b] Department of Microbiology, The Chinese University of Hong Kong, Prince of Wales Hospital, 32 Ngan Shing Street, Shatin, New Territories, Hong Kong, China
* Corresponding author.
E-mail address: dschui@cuhk.edu.hk

Infect Dis Clin N Am 24 (2010) 619–638
doi:10.1016/j.idc.2010.04.009
0891-5520/10/$ – see front matter © 2010 Elsevier Inc. All rights reserved.

civets in Dongmen market, Shenzhen.[17] Further epidemiologic evidence was obtained during a small-scale outbreak in late 2003 and early 2004, in which 3 of the 4 patients had direct or indirect contact with palm civets.[6,18] Subsequent sequence analysis suggested that the SARS-CoV–like virus has not been circulating among market masked civets for a long period, and therefore the true natural reservoir for SARS-CoV was sought. In 2005, CoVs that are similar to SARS-CoV were found in horseshoe bats by 2 independent research teams.[19,20] These bat SARS-like CoVs share 88% to 92% sequence homology with human or civet isolates, but with key differences found in the region encoding spike (S) protein that is critical in determining host range and tissue tropism.[21] The data suggest that bats could be a natural reservoir of a close ancestor of SARS-CoV, and that the CoVs seem to have used an entirely new receptor when they crossed species from bats to palm civets and humans.

In addition to masked palm civets and bats, other animal species might have been involved in the evolution and emergence of SARS-CoV. At least 7 animal species can harbor SARS-CoV in certain circumstances, including raccoon dog, red fox, Chinese ferret, mink, pig, wild boar, and rice field rat.[21]

EPIDEMIOLOGY

In November 2002, there was an unusual epidemic of severe pneumonia of unknown origin in Foshan, Guangdong Province in southern China, with a high rate of transmission to health care workers (HCWs).[22,23] A retrospective analysis of 55 patients admitted to a chest hospital with atypical pneumonia in Guangzhou between January 24 and February 18 2003 showed positive SARS-CoV in the nasopharyngeal aspirates (NPA), whereas 48 (87%) patients had positive antibodies to SARS-CoV in their convalescent sera. Genetic analysis showed that the SARS-CoV isolates from Guangzhou had the same origin as those in other countries, with a phylogenetic pathway that matched the spread of SARS to other parts of the world.[24]

A 64-year-old physician from southern China, who had visited Hong Kong (HK) on 21 February 2003 and died 10 days later of severe pneumonia, was the source of infection causing subsequent outbreaks of SARS in HK and several other countries.[1–3,25] At least 16 hotel guests or visitors were infected by the Guangdong physician while they were visiting friends or staying on the same floor of Hotel M, where the physician had stayed briefly. Through international air travel, these visitors spread the infection globally within a short period.

SARS seems to spread by close person-to-person contact via droplet transmission or fomite.[26] The high infectivity of this viral illness is shown by the 138 patients (many of whom were HCWs) who were hospitalized with SARS within 2 weeks as a result of exposure to a single patient (a visitor to Hotel M), who was admitted with community-acquired pneumonia (CAP) to a general medical ward at the Prince of Wales Hospital (PWH) in HK.[1,27] This super-spreading event was believed to be related to the use of a jet nebulizer, driven by air at 6 L/min, for the administration of aerosolized salbutamol to an index patient, together with overcrowding and poor ventilation in the hospital ward.[1,28] SARS-CoV was also detected in respiratory secretions, feces, urine, and tears of infected individuals.[28] In addition, there was evidence to suggest that SARS might have spread by airborne transmission in a major community outbreak at the Amoy Garden, a private residential complex in HK.[29] Higher nasopharyngeal viral load was found in patients living in adjacent units of the same block inhabited by the index patient at the Amoy Garden, whereas a lower, but detectable, nasopharyngeal viral load was found in patients living further away from the index patient.[30] Air samples obtained from a room occupied by a SARS patient and swab samples taken from frequently touched surfaces in rooms and in a nurses' station were positive by polymerase chain reaction (PCR) testing.[31] The temporal-spatial spread of SARS among inpatients in the index medical ward of the PWH in HK was also consistent with airborne transmission.[32] These data support SARS having the potential to be converted from droplet to airborne droplet transmission,[27–32] and they emphasize the need for adequate respiratory protection in addition to strict contact and droplet precautions when managing SARS patients.

CLINICAL FEATURES

The estimated mean incubation period was 4.6 days (95% confidence interval [CI] 3.8–5.8 days), whereas the mean time from symptom onset to hospitalization varied between 2 and 8 days, decreasing in the course of the epidemic. The mean time from onset to death was 23.7 days (CI 22.0–25.3 days), whereas the mean time from onset to discharge was 26.5 days (CI 25.8–27.2 days).[33] The major clinical features on presentation include persistent fever, chills/rigor, myalgia, dry cough, headache, malaise, and dyspnea. Sputum production, sore throat, coryza, nausea and vomiting, dizziness, and diarrhea are less common features (**Table 1**).[1–4,34]

Watery diarrhea was a prominent extrapulmonary symptom in 40% to 70% of patients with SARS 1 week into the clinical course of the illness.[35,36] Intestinal biopsy specimens taken by colonoscopy or autopsy revealed evidence of secretory diarrhea with minimal architectural disruption, but there was evidence of active viral replication within the small and large intestines.[36] Reactive hepatitis was a common complication of SARS-CoV infection, with 24% and 69% of patients respectively having increased alanine aminotransferase (ALT) levels on admission and during the subsequent course of the illness. Those with severe hepatitis had worse clinical outcomes, but chronic hepatitis B itself was not associated with disease severity.[37]

SARS-CoV was detected in the cerebrospinal fluid and serum samples of 2 cases with status epilepticus.[38,39] The data suggest that a severe acute neurologic syndrome might occasionally accompany SARS.

Table 1
Clinical features of SARS on presentation

Symptom	% of Patients with Symptom
Persistent fever >38°C	99–100
Nonproductive cough	57–75
Myalgia	45–61
Chills/rigor	15–73
Headache	20–56
Dyspnea	40–42
Malaise	31–45
Nausea and vomiting	20–35
Diarrhea	20–25
Sore throat	13–25
Dizziness	4.2–43
Sputum production	4.9–29
Rhinorrhea	2.1–23
Arthralgia	10.4

Data from Refs. [1–4,25]

Older subjects might have atypical presentation such as decrease in general well-being, poor feeding, fall/fracture,[40] and, in some cases, delirium, without the typical febrile response (temperature >38°C).[40–42] In contrast, young children (<12 years of age) often ran a more benign clinical course mimicking other viral upper respiratory tract infections, whereas teenagers tended to have a clinical course similar to that of adults.[1,43] There was no reported fatality in young children and teenage patients,[43–46] but SARS in pregnancy carried a significant risk of mortality.[47] Orchitis was reported as a complication in male patients.[48] A meta-analysis showed overall seroprevalence rates of 0.1% for the general population and 0.23% for HCWs, although the true incidence of asymptomatic infection remains unknown.[49]

A case-control study involving 124 medical wards in 26 hospitals in Guangzhou and HK has identified 6 independent risk factors of super-spreading nosocomial outbreaks of SARS (Box 1): minimum distance between beds less than 1 m, performance of resuscitation, staff working while experiencing symptoms, SARS patients requiring oxygen therapy or noninvasive positive pressure ventilation (NPPV), whereas availability of washing or changing facilities for staff was a protective factor.[50] Experimental studies have shown that the exhaled air particle dispersion distances from patients receiving oxygen via a simple oxygen mask and a jet nebulizer were 0.4 m and at least 0.8 m, respectively.[51,52] Exhaled air distances from NPPV via the different face masks could range from 0.4 m to 1 m, with more diffuse room contamination for face masks that require connection to the whisper swivel exhalation device.[53,54] These data have important clinical implications in preventing any future nosocomial outbreaks of SARS and other respiratory infections. HCWs should take adequate respiratory precautions when managing patients with CAP of unknown cause that is complicated by respiratory failure within these distances.

The clinical course of SARS generally followed a typical pattern[35]: phase I (viral replication) was associated with increasing viral load and was clinically characterized by fever, myalgia, and other systemic symptoms that generally improved after a few days; phase II (immunopathologic injury) was characterized by recurrence of fever, hypoxemia, and radiological progression of pneumonia with reductions in viral load. The high morbidity of SARS was highlighted by the observation that, even when there was only 12% of total lung field involved by consolidation on chest radiographs, 50% of patients would require supplemental oxygen to maintain satisfactory oxygenation greater than 90%,[55] whereas about 20% of patients would progress into acute respiratory distress syndrome (ARDS) necessitating invasive ventilatory support.[34] Peiris and colleagues[35] showed a progressive decrease in rates of viral shedding from

---

Box 1
Independent risk factors of super-spreading nosocomial outbreaks of SARS

Minimum distance between beds <1 m (odds ratio [OR] 6.98, 95% CI 1.68–28.75, $P = .008$)

Washing or changing facilities for staff (OR 0.12, 95% CI 0.02–0.97, $P = .05$)

Performance of resuscitation (OR 3.81, 95% CI 1.04–13.87, $P = .04$)

Staff working while experiencing symptoms (OR 10.55, 95% CI 2.28–48.87, $P = .003$)

SARS patients requiring oxygen therapy (OR 4.30, 95% CI 1.00–18.43, $P = .05$)

SARS patients requiring NPPV (OR 11.82, 95% CI 1.97–70.80, $P = .007$)

Data from Yu IT, Xie ZH, Tsoi KK, et al. Why did outbreaks of severe acute respiratory syndrome occur in some hospital wards but not in others? Clin Infect Dis 2007;44:1017–25.

nasophargynx, stool, and urine from day 10 to day 21 after symptom onset in 20 patients who had serial measurements with reverse transcriptase (RT)-PCR. Thus, clinical worsening during phase II was most likely the result of immune-mediated lung injury as a result of an overexuberant host response and could not be explained by uncontrolled viral replication.[35]

LABORATORY FEATURES

Lymphopenia, low-grade disseminated intravascular coagulation (thrombocytopenia, prolonged activated partial thromboplastin time, increased D-dimer), increased lactate dehydrogenase (LDH), and creatinine phosphokinase (CPK) were common laboratory features of SARS.[1–3,56,57] Absolute lymphopenia occurred in 98% of cases of SARS during the clinical course of the disease. The CD4 and CD8 T lymphocyte counts declined early in the course of SARS, whereas low counts of CD4 and CD8 at presentation were associated with adverse clinical outcome.[58] The CD3 and CD4 T cell percentages were reported to be negatively correlated with the appearance of immunoglobulin G (IgG) antibody against SARS-CoV.[59]

A retrospective study in Toronto found that all laboratory variables except absolute neutrophil count (ANC) showed fair to poor discriminatory ability in distinguishing SARS from other causes of CAP, and that routine laboratory tests may not be reliable in the diagnosis of SARS.[60] Nevertheless, when evaluating patients with CAP and no immediate alternative diagnosis who are epidemiologically at high risk, a low ANC on presentation, along with poor clinical and laboratory responses after 72 hours of antibiotic treatment, may raise the index of suspicion for SARS and indicate a need to perform SARS-CoV testing.[61] Scoring systems may help identify patients who should receive more specific tests for influenza or SARS.[62]

RADIOLOGICAL FEATURES

Radiographic features of SARS generally resemble those found in other causes of CAP.[63] The more distinctive radiographic features of SARS include the predominant involvement of lung periphery and the lower zone in addition to the absence of cavitation, hilar lymphadenopathy, or pleural effusion.[1,63] Radiographic progression from unilateral focal air-space opacity to multifocal or bilateral involvement during the second phase of the disease, followed by radiographic improvement with treatment, is commonly observed.[1,63] In a case series, 12% of patients developed spontaneous pneumomediastinum, and 20% of patients developed evidence of ARDS in a period of 3 weeks.[35] The incidence of barotrauma (26%) in intensive care unit (ICU) admissions was high despite the application of low-volume and low-pressure mechanical ventilation.[64] High-resolution computed tomography (HRCT) of thorax was useful in detecting lung opacities in cases with a high index of clinical suspicion of SARS but unremarkable chest radiographs. Common HRCT features included ground-glass opacification, sometimes with consolidation, and interlobular septal and intralobular interstitial thickening, with predominantly a peripheral and lower lobe involvement (**Fig. 1**).[65]

PATHOGENESIS

The route of entry for SARS-CoV in humans is through the respiratory tract, mainly via droplet transmission. Although human intestinal cells have proven to be susceptible to SARS-CoV replication, the role of the intestinal tract as a portal of entry remains uncertain.[66] Similarly, although infectious viruses were found in stool samples, there was

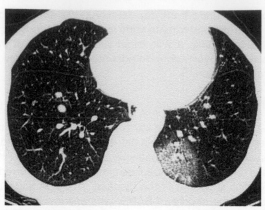

Fig. 1. Thoracic HRCT of a patient with SARS showing typical early changes with solitary ground-glass opacification at the left lower lobe.

insufficient evidence to support the fecal-oral route of transmission for SARS-CoV infection.

The surface envelop S protein of SARS-CoV seems to play a key role in establishing infection and determining the cell and tissue tropism. The SARS-CoV S protein has 3 domains: the N-terminal half (S1) contains a receptor-binding domain (RBD), and the C-terminal half (S2) contains a fusion peptide. Entry of the virus requires receptor binding, followed by conformational change of the S protein, and then cathepsin L–mediated proteolysis within the endosome.[67–69] The angiotensin-converting enzyme 2 (ACE2) is the receptor for SARS-CoV,[70] and is expressed on a wide variety of tissues including lungs, intestine, kidneys, and blood vessels. The presence of ACE2 seems not to be the sole determinant for tropism of SARS-CoV. For instance, SARS-CoV has been found in colonic enterocytes and hepatocytes that lack ACE2, whereas SARS-CoV has not been detected in endothelial cells of blood vessels and smooth muscle cells of intestine, despite their expression of ACE2.[36,71,72]

There are some data to suggest that, in addition to ACE2, 2 other surface molecules play a critical role in establishing SARS-CoV infection in human cells. DC-SIGN (CD209) dendritic cell–specific intercellular adhesion molecule–grabbing nonintegrin, is a type 2 transmembrane adhesion molecule that recognizes a variety of microorganisms. DC-SIGN is expressed in macrophages and dendritic cells including those found in skin, lungs, intestine, rectum, cervix, placenta, and lymph node. However, the binding of SARS-CoV to DC-SIGN does not lead to entry of viruses into dendritic cells; instead it facilities the transfer of viruses to other susceptible cells. In this way, the dendritic cells play an important role in virus dissemination within the infected host.[73–75] L-SIGN (CD209L or DC-SIGNR) is a homolog of DC-SIGN, which is expressed in liver, lymph node, and placenta. L-SIGN acts in conjunction with the liver and lymph node sinusoidal endothelial cell C-type lectin (LSECtin) to enhance SARS-CoV infection. There is evidence to show that L-SIGN serves as an alternative receptor to mediate the entry of SARS-CoV.[73,76,77]

Once infection can be established, the mechanisms by which SARS-CoV causes disease can be separated into (1) direct lytic effects on host cells and (2) indirect consequences resulting from the host immune response. Clinically, SARS is characterized by a pronounced systemic illness, but the pathology of SARS, as revealed from fatal cases, was mainly confined to the lungs, where diffuse alveolar damage was the most prominent feature. Multinucleated syncytial giant cells, although characteristic, were rarely seen. In cases without secondary infection, a lack of immune response was observed at this late terminal stage. Apart from those related to end-stage multiorgan failure, the pathologies of gastrointestinal tract, urinary system, liver, and other organ systems were unremarkable.[78–82] Lungs and intestinal tract are the only 2 organ systems that support high levels of SARS-CoV replication.[72,83]

At least 2 mechanisms of direct injury in infected lungs have been revealed. First, in addition to being the host receptor mediating the entry of SARS-CoV, the ACE2 probably contributes to the diffuse alveolar damage. ACE2 is a negative regulator of the local renin-angiotensin system, where its imbalance leads to the development of diffuse alveolar damage. Data from animal studies suggest that the diffuse alveolar damage seen in SARS is mediated by the S protein-ACE2-renin-angiotensin pathway.[84,85] The second direct injury mechanism is by the induction of apoptosis. The SARS-CoV–encoded 3a and 7a proteins have been shown to be a strong inducer of apoptosis in cell lines derived from different organs including lungs, kidneys, and liver.[86–88]

IMMUNOBIOLOGY

Clinically, SARS is characterized by a phase of cytokine storm. The intense immune response to infection, as reflected by the increase in chemokines and cytokines, results in the pathology seen in cases that run a severe course of illness. In postmortem lung tissues, chemokine C-X-C motif ligand (CXCL)-10 (or interferon [IFN]-inducible protein [IP] 10) and interleukin (IL)-18 were found to be increased.[78] During the first 2 weeks, a variety of cytokines/chemokines were found to be increased in the peripheral circulation, including CXCL-9 (chemokine C-X-C motif ligand 2 or monokine induced by γ-IFN), CXCL-10 (or IP-10), and C-C motif ligand (CCL)-2 or monocyte chemoattractant protein-1 [MCP-1]), IL-1β, IL-6, IL-8 (CXCL-8), IL-12, IFN-γ, transforming growth factor (TGF)-β, monokine induced by IFN-γ (MIG, CXCL-9).[89–93] Among these increased cytokines/chemokines, increased levels of IP-10, MIG, and IL-8 during the first week after the onset of fever and increase of MIG during the second week were associated with poor outcome.[92]

Several host genetic markers have been reported to have an association with the outcome of SARS.[94] An association of HLA-B*4601 with SARS infection was revealed from a cohort of patients from Taiwan, but the finding was not reproduced in HK patients.[95,96] In the latter HK study, HLA-B*0703 was found to be associated with an increased susceptibility, whereas HLA-DRB1*0301 was protective against SARS-CoV infection.[96] In another study based on patients from HK, it was shown that the human Fc γ-receptor genotype, FcγRIIA-R/R131 and CD14-159CC were associated with more severe outcome of SARS.[97,98] RANTES-28 CG and GG genotypes were found to be associated with an increased susceptibility to SARS.[99] In a cohort study of SARS patients in HK, an association between CLEC4M homozygosity and protection against SARS was found.[100] However, the observation could not be reproduced in 2 other studies in HK and Beijing, respectively.[101,102]

TREATMENT
Ribavirin

Ribavirin, a nucleoside analogue that has activity against several viruses in vitro, was widely used for treating SARS patients after recognizing the lack of clinical response to broad-spectrum antibiotics and oseltamivir.[1–3,25,35] Nevertheless, it is now known that ribavirin has no significant in vitro activity against SARS-CoV.[103–105] Hemoglobin levels in about 60% of patients dropped by 2 g/dL after 2 weeks of oral ribavirin therapy, at a dose of 1.2 g 3 times a day.[106] The use of ribavirin for SARS in Toronto was based on the higher dosage used for treating hemorrhagic fever, which led to more toxicity, including increased liver transaminases and bradycardia.[3] Furthermore, addition of ribavirin did not have any useful effect on the serum SARS-CoV viral load of pediatric SARS patients.[107] Therefore, it is unlikely that ribavirin alone has any significant clinical benefits in the treatment of SARS.

Protease Inhibitors

Genomic analysis of the SARS-CoV has revealed several enzymatic targets including protease.[13,14,108] Lopinavir and ritonavir in combination is a boosted protease inhibitor regimen widely used in the treatment of human immunodeficiency virus (HIV) infection. In vitro activity against SARS-CoV was shown for lopinavir and ribavirin at 4 μg/mL and 50 μg/mL, respectively. Inhibition of in vitro cytopathic effects was achieved down to a concentration of 1 μg/mL of lopinavir combined with 6.25 μg/mL of ribavirin. Therefore, the data suggest that this combination might be synergistic against SARS-CoV in vivo.[109] The addition of lopinavir 400 mg/ritonavir 100 mg (LPV/r) as initial therapy was associated with significant reduction in overall death rate (2.3% vs 15.6%) and intubation rate (0% vs 11%) compared with a matched historical cohort that received ribavirin alone as the initial antiviral therapy.[110] Other reported beneficial effects include a reduction in corticosteroid use, fewer nosocomial infections, a decreasing viral load, and rising peripheral lymphocyte count.[110]

In contrast, the outcome of the subgroup who had received LPV/r as rescue therapy after receiving pulsed methylprednisolone (MP) treatment of worsening respiratory symptoms was not better than the matched cohort.[110] The improved clinical outcome in patients who received LPV/r as part of the initial therapy may be the result of peak (9.6 μg/mL) and trough (5.5 μg/mL) serum concentrations of lopinavir inhibiting the virus.[111] Nelfinavir, another protease inhibitor commonly used for HIV infection, was shown to inhibit replication of SARS-CoV in Vero cell culture.[112]

IFNs

Type 1 IFNs, such as IFN-α, are produced early as part of the innate immune response to virus infections. Type 1 IFNs inhibit a wide range of RNA and DNA viruses including SARS-CoV in vitro.[104,105,113] Complete inhibition of cytopathic effects of SARS-CoV in culture was observed for IFN subtypes, β-1b, α-n1, α-n3, and human leukocyte IFN-α.[98] IFN-α showed an in vitro inhibitory effect on SARS-CoV starting at concentrations of 1000 IU/mL,[105] whereas recombinant human IFN-β 1a potently inhibited SARS-CoV in vitro.[114] IFN-β and IFN-γ can synergistically inhibit the replication of SARS-CoV in vitro.[115] In addition, a combination of ribavirin and IFN-β has been shown to have synergistic effects in inhibiting SARS-CoV in animal and human cell lines,[116] whereas combinations of ribavirin with IFN-β 1a or IFN-α also show synergistic effects in vitro.[117]

In experimentally infected cynomolgus macaques, prophylactic treatment with pegylated IFN-α significantly reduced viral replication and excretion, viral antigen expression by type 1 pneumocytes, and pulmonary damage, compared with untreated macaques, whereas postexposure treatment with pegylated IFN-α yielded intermediate results.[118] Use of IFN-α 1 plus corticosteroids was associated with improved oxygen saturation, more rapid resolution of radiographic lung opacities, and lower levels of CPK in SARS patients.[119] These findings support clinical testing of approved IFNs for the treatment of SARS.

Human Monoclonal Antibody

There is evidence that SARS-CoV infection is initiated through binding of the SARS-CoV S protein to ACE2.[70] A high-affinity human monoclonal antibody (huMab) termed

80R has been identified against the SARS-CoV S protein and has potent neutralizing activity in vitro and in vivo.[120] HuMab 80R efficiently neutralized SARS-CoV and inhibited syncytia formation between cells expressing the S protein and those expressing the SARS-CoV receptor ACE2. HuMab 80R may be a useful viral entry inhibitor for the emergency prophylaxis and treatment of SARS.[120] HuMab was shown to prophylactically reduce replication of SARS-CoV in the lungs of infected ferrets and abolish shedding of viruses in pharyngeal secretions, in addition to completely preventing SARS-CoV–induced macroscopic lung pathology.[121]

Vaccines

An adenovirus-based vaccine was shown to induce strong SARS-CoV–specific immune responses in rhesus macaques, and holds promise for the development of a protective vaccine against SARS-CoV.[122] A DNA vaccine based on the S gene could induce the production of specific IgG antibody against SARS-CoV efficiently in mice, with a seroconversion rate of 75% after 3 doses of immunization.[123,124] Recombinant S proteins that exhibit antigenicity and receptor-binding ability are also good candidates for developing a SARS vaccine.[125] A recombinant attenuated vaccinia virus, Ankara, expressing the S protein of SARS-CoV can elicit protective immunity in mice.[126] Another recombinant attenuated parainfluenza virus expressing the S protein also produced immunity following intranasal inoculation to mice.[127] Synthetic peptide derived from the S protein is another target for vaccine development. Promising results have been obtained in vitro[128] and in vivo from rabbit and monkey models.[129]

Systemic Corticosteroids

During phase II of the clinical course, when patients progress to develop pneumonia and hypoxemia, intravenous administration of rescue pulsed MP has been shown to suppress cytokine induced lung injury.[1,35,106,109,130] The rationale could be that the progression of the pulmonary disease is mediated by the host inflammatory response.[35] Corticosteroids significantly reduced IL-8, MCP-1, and IFN-γ IP-10 concentrations from 5 to 8 days after treatment in 20 adult SARS patients.[89] Induction of IP-10 is believed to be a critical event in the initiation of immune-mediated lung injury and lymphocyte apoptosis.[90]

The use of rescue pulsed MP during clinical progression was associated with favorable clinical improvement with resolution of fever and lung opacities within 2 weeks.[1,106,130] However, a retrospective analysis showed that the use of pulsed MP was associated with an increased risk of 30-day mortality (adjusted OR 26.0, 95% CI 4.4–154.8).[131] This retrospective study could not establish whether a causal relationship existed between the use of MP and an increased risk of death, as clinicians were more inclined to give pulsed MP therapy in deteriorating patients. Nevertheless, complications such as disseminated fungal disease[132] and avascular necrosis of bone have been reported following prolonged corticosteroid therapy.[133] With the rescue pulsed MP approach, avascular necrosis of bone was found in 12 (4.7%) patients after screening 254 using magnetic resonance imaging. The risk of avascular necrosis was 0.6% for patients receiving less than 3 g, and was 13% for those receiving more than 3 g prednisolone–equivalent dose.[134] A randomized placebo-controlled study conducted at PWH, HK showed that plasma SARS-CoV RNA concentrations in the second and third weeks of illness were higher in patients given initial hydrocortisone (n = 10) than in those given normal saline (n = 7) during phase I of the clinical course of illness.[135] Despite the small sample size, the data suggest that pulsed MP given in the earlier phase might prolong viremia and thus it should only be given during the later phase for rescue purposes. Carefully designed clinical trials with larger sample sizes are required to determine the optimal timing and dosage of systemic steroid in the treatment of possibly immune-mediated lung injury in SARS.

Convalescent Plasma

Convalescent plasma, donated by patients who have recovered from SARS, contains neutralizing antibody and may be clinically useful for treating other SARS patients.[136,137]

Traditional Chinese Medicine

Glycyrrhizin, an active component of liquorice roots, was shown to inhibit the replication of SARS-CoV in vitro.[103] A controlled study comparing integrative Chinese and Western medicine with Western medicine alone suggested that the combination treatment given in phase I of SARS was more effective in reducing the number of patients with abnormal oxygen saturations.[138] However, it was not clear which of the Chinese medicine components was responsible for the benefit, and the dosage of steroid given to the groups was not clear.

Intravenous Gammaglobulin and Pentaglobulin

Intravenous gammaglobulin (IVIg) has immunomodulatory properties and may down-regulate cytokine expression.[139] It was used extensively in Singapore during the SARS outbreak in 2003. However, it was noted that one-third of critically ill patients developed venous thromboembolism, including pulmonary embolism, despite prophylactic use of low-molecular-weight heparin.[140] There was evidence of pulmonary embolism in 4 out of 8 postmortem cases.[141] In addition, there were 5 cases of large artery ischemic stroke, of which 3 cases had been given IVIg.[142]

Pentaglobulin (IgM enriched Ig) was administered to 12 patients with SARS who continued to deteriorate despite pulsed steroid and ribavirin, and its use was associated with subsequent improvement in oxygenation and radiographic scores. It was difficult to judge its effects because the study was uncontrolled and pulsed steroid was used concurrently.[143] Pulmonary artery thrombosis was reported in a patient with SARS who had been treated with ribavirin, steroid, kaletra, IVIg, and pentaglobulin.[144] It is possible that IVIg- or pentaglobulin-induced increase in viscosity may be consequential in patients with hypercoagulable states such as SARS.[145]

Nitric Oxide

Inhaled nitric oxide (NO) was reported to have beneficial effects in SARS. In a controlled study comparing the use of NO (n = 6) and supportive treatment (n = 8) for severe respiratory failure, there was improvement in oxygenation after inhaled NO was administered, and this allowed ventilatory support to be discontinued. The beneficial effects persisted after termination of NO inhalation.[146] NO has been shown to inhibit the replication cycle of SARS-CoV in vitro.[147]

OUTCOMES
Short-term

Based on the data received by the World Health Organization, the case fatality rate for SARS was less than 1% for patients aged 24 years or younger, 6% for 25 to 44 years, 15% for 45 to 64 years, and more than 50% for patients aged 65 years or older.[148] Poor prognostic factors for more severe disease included advanced age,[1,35,149,150] chronic hepatitis B treated with lamivudine,[35] severe hepatitis,[37] high initial LDH,[150] high peak LDH,[1] high neutrophil count on presentation,[1,150] diabetes mellitus or other comorbid conditions,[3,151] low CD4 and CD8 lymphocyte counts at presentation,[58] and a high initial SARS-CoV viral load.[107,152]

Long-term

Significant impairment of the diffusing capacity of carbon monoxide in the lung (DLCO) occurred in 15.5% and 23.7% of SARS survivors at the PWH cohort at 6 and 12 months, respectively.[153,154] Although significant improvement in serial chest radiography was observed among the SARS survivors, 27.8% still had abnormal radiographic scores at 12 months.[154] Despite the presence of extensive parenchymal changes revealed by computer tomography during the early convalescent period, most SARS survivors had lung function test indices within normal limits. However, their exercise ability (6-minute walk distance) at 12 months after illness onset was lower than the general population.[154] The functional disability seems out of proportion to the degree of lung function impairment and might be caused by extrapulmonary factors such as muscle deconditioning and steroid myopathy.[153,154] Critical illness associated polyneuropathy/mypoathy was also observed in a few SARS survivors.[155] The reported incidence rates of avascular necrosis of bone among different cohorts in HK ranged from 4.7% to 15%,[156,157] whereas 1 study from Beijing reported a high incidence of 42%.[133]

Several other groups have shown that persistent lung function abnormalities occur in less than one-third of patients at 1 year and that there was significant impairment of health status among SARS survivors and their carers.[158–160] The physical impairment and the long period of isolation and extreme uncertainty during the SARS illness created enormous psychological stress[161] and mood disturbances.[162] In addition, steroid toxicity, personal vulnerability, and psychosocial stressors might have jointly contributed to the development of psychosis in some patients.[163]

VACCINE DEVELOPMENT

Various forms of SARS-CoV vaccine have been evaluated. Inactivated whole virus vaccines are immunogenic and protective in animal models. However, this approach requires the production of a large amount of infectious virus in a biosafety level 3 containment facility, which is not widely available among vaccine manufacturers. Because the S protein of SARS-CoV is responsible for receptor binding and membrane fusion, it is a priority target for the development of subunit vaccines. Full-length S protein delivered in the form of DNA vaccine, or expressed in attenuated vaccinia virus or recombinant baculovirus systems, have been to shown to induce T cell and neutralizing antibody responses, and have been found to be protective in challenge studies.[124,126,164,165] However, there are concerns about using full-length S protein as a vaccine, because harmful immune responses causing liver damage in vaccinated animals have been reported.[166] The possibility of enhanced disease, as observed in vaccinated cats on infection with feline infectious peritonitis virus, is also a concern.[167,168] Theoretically, antibodies present at low concentrations may form complexes with virions, and be taken up by macrophage via the Fc receptors expressed on its surface. This process enhances virus dissemination and may lead to adverse outcomes. Vaccines based on a partial S protein or other structural proteins of SARS-CoV have been explored. The greatest challenge to sustainable vaccine development is that SARS-CoV has disappeared from humans, and antigenic changes of the re-emergent strain, if it ever occurs, remain unknown.

SUMMARY

SARS is a highly infectious disease with a significant morbidity and mortality. Respiratory failure is the major complication, and 20% of patients may progress to ARDS. HCWs are particularly vulnerable to SARS as the viral loads of SARS-CoV in patients increase to peak levels during the second week after patients are hospitalized.[35,169] Because SARS has the potential to be converted from droplet to airborne transmission, HCWs should use adequate respiratory protection, in addition to strict contact and droplet precautions, when managing patients with SARS. Because there is currently no proven effective treatment of SARS, early recognition, isolation, and stringent infection control measures are the key to controlling this highly contagious disease. Isolation facilities, strict droplet and contact precautions (hand hygiene, gown, gloves, N95 masks, eye protection) for HCWs managing patients with SARS, avoidance of using jet nebulizers on general wards,[1,27,52] contact tracing, and quarantine isolation for close contacts are important measures in controlling the spread of the infection in hospitals and the community.

The presence of SARS-like CoVs in horseshoe bats implicates bats in previous and potentially future emergence of novel CoV infection in humans. Public health measures should be enforced to ban the trading of wild animals in wet markets in South China, where SARS-CoV infection started. When evaluating epidemiologically high-risk patients with community-acquired pneumonia and no immediate alternative diagnosis, a low ANC on presentation, along with poor responses after 72 hours of antibiotic treatment, may raise the index of suspicion for SARS. Further studies are needed to examine host genetic markers that may predict clinical outcome.

REFERENCES

1. Lee N, Hui DS, Wu A, et al. A major outbreak of severe acute respiratory syndrome in Hong Kong. N Engl J Med 2003;348:1986–94.
2. Hsu LY, Lee CC, Green JA, et al. Severe acute respiratory syndrome in Singapore: clinical features of index patient and initial contacts. Emerg Infect Dis 2003;9:713–7.
3. Booth CM, Matukas LM, Tomlinson GA, et al. Clinical features and short-term outcomes of 144 patients with SARS in the greater Toronto area. JAMA 2003; 289:2801–9.
4. Twu SJ, Chen TJ, Chen CJ, et al. Control measures for severe acute respiratory syndrome (SARS) in Taiwan. Emerg Infect Dis 2003;9:718–20.
5. WHO. Summary of probable SARS cases with onset of illness from 1 November to 31 July 2003. Available at: http://www.who.int/csr/sars/country/table2003_09_23/en. Accessed September 23, 2003.
6. Wang M, Yan M, Xu H, et al. SARS-CoV infection in a restaurant from palm civet. Emerg Infect Dis 2005;11:1860–5.
7. Che XY, Di B, Zhao GP, et al. A patient with asymptomatic severe acute respiratory syndrome (SARS) and antigenemia from the 2003–2004 community outbreak of SARS in Guangzhou, China. Clin Infect Dis 2006;43:e1–5.
8. Peiris JS, Lai ST, Poon LL, et al. Coronavirus as a possible cause of severe acute respiratory syndrome. Lancet 2003;361:1319–25.
9. Kuiken T, Fouchier RA, Schutten M, et al. Newly discovered coronavirus as the primary cause of severe acute respiratory syndrome. Lancet 2003;362:263–70.
10. Drosten C, Gunther S, Preiser W, et al. Identification of a novel Coronavirus in patients with severe acute respiratory syndrome. N Engl J Med 2003;348: 1967–76.

11. Ksiazek TG, Erdman D, Goldsmith CS, et al. A novel Coronavirus associated with severe acute respiratory syndrome. N Engl J Med 2003;348: 1953–66.

12. Fouchier RA, Kuiken T, Schutten M, et al. Aetiology: Koch's postulates fulfilled for SARS virus. Nature 2003;423:240.

13. Rota PA, Oberste MS, Monroe SS, et al. Characterization of a novel coronavirus associated with severe acute respiratory syndrome. Science 2003;300:1394–9.

14. Marra MA, Jones SJ, Astell CR, et al. The genome sequence of the SARS-associated coronavirus. Science 2003;300:1399–404.

15. Ruan YJ, Wei CL, Ee LA, et al. Comparative full-length genome sequence analysis of 14 SARS coronavirus isolates and common mutations associated with putative origins of infection. Lancet 2003;361:1779–85.

16. Du L, Qiu JC, Wang M, et al. Analysis on the characteristics of blood serum Ab-IgG detective result of severe acute respiratory syndrome patients in Guangzhou, China. Zhonghua Liu Xing Bing Xue Za Zhi 2004;25:925 8.

17. Guan Y, Zheng BJ, He YQ, et al. Isolation and characterization of viruses related to the SARS coronavirus from animals in Southern China. Science 2003;302: 276–8.

18. Song HD, Tu CC, Zhang, et al. Cross-host evolution of severe acute respiratory syndrome coronavirus in palm civet and human. Proc Natl Acad Sci U S A 2005; 102:2430–5.

19. Lau SK, Woo PC, Li KS, et al. Severe acute respiratory syndrome coronavirus-like virus in Chinese horseshoe bats. Proc Natl Acad Sci U S A 2005;102: 14040–5.

20. Li W, Shi Z, Yu M, et al. Bats are natural reservoirs of SARS-like coronaviruses. Science 2005;310:676–9.

21. Shi Z, Hu Z. A review of studies on animal reservoirs of the SARS coronavirus. Virus Res 2008;133:74–87.

22. Zhao Z, Zhang F, Xu M, et al. Description and clinical treatment of an early outbreak of severe acute respiratory syndrome (SARS) in Guangzhou, PR China. J Med Microbiol 2003;52:715–20.

23. Xu RH, He JF, Evans MR, et al. Epidemiologic clues to SARS origin in China. Emerg Infect Dis 2004;10:1030–7.

24. Zhong NS, Zheng BJ, Li YM, et al. Epidemiology and cause of severe acute respiratory syndrome in Guangdong, People's Republic of China, in 2003. Lancet 2003;362:1353–8.

25. Tsang KW, Ho PL, Ooi GC, et al. A cluster of cases of severe acute respiratory syndrome in Hong Kong. N Engl J Med 2003;348:1977–85.

26. Peiris JS, Yuen KY, Osterhaus AD, et al. The severe acute respiratory syndrome. N Engl J Med 2003;349:2431–41.

27. Wong RS, Hui DS. Index patient and SARS outbreak in Hong Kong. Emerg Infect Dis 2004;10:339–41.

28. Loon SC, Teoh SC, Oon LL, et al. The severe acute respiratory syndrome coronavirus in tears. Br J Ophthalmol 2004;88:861–3.

29. Yu IT, Li Y, Wong TW, et al. Evidence of airborne transmission of the severe acute respiratory syndrome virus. N Engl J Med 2004;350:1731–9.

30. Chu CM, Cheng VC, Hung IF, et al. Viral load distribution in SARS outbreak. Emerg Infect Dis 2005;11:1882–6.

31. Booth TF, Kournikakis B, Bastien N, et al. Detection of airborne severe acute respiratory syndrome (SARS) coronavirus and environmental contamination in SARS outbreak units. J Infect Dis 2005;191:1472–7.

32. Yu IT, Wong TW, Chiu YL, et al. Temporal-spatial analysis of severe acute respiratory syndrome among hospital inpatients. Clin Infect Dis 2005;40:1237–43.
33. Leung GM, Hedley AJ, Ho LM, et al. The epidemiology of severe acute respiratory syndrome in the 2003 Hong Kong epidemic: an analysis of all 1755 patients. Ann Intern Med 2004;141:662–73.
34. Hui DS, Wong PC, Wang C. Severe acute respiratory syndrome: clinical features and diagnosis. Respirology 2003;8:S20–4.
35. Peiris JS, Chu CM, Cheng VC, et al. Clinical progression and viral load in a community outbreak of coronavirus-associated SARS pneumonia: a prospective study. Lancet 2003;361:1767–72.
36. Leung WK, To KF, Chan PK, et al. Enteric involvement of severe acute respiratory syndrome-associated coronavirus infection. Gastroenterologist 2003;125: 1011–7.
37. Chan HL, Kwan AC, To KF, et al. Clinical significance of hepatic derangement in severe acute respiratory syndrome. World J Gastroenterol 2005;11:2148–53.
38. Hung EC, Chim SS, Chan PK, et al. Detection of SARS coronavirus RNA in the cerebrospinal fluid of a patient with severe acute respiratory syndrome. Clin Chem 2003;49:2108–9.
39. Lau KK, Yu WC, Chu CM, et al. Possible central nervous system infection by SARS coronavirus. Emerg Infect Dis 2004;10:342–4.
40. Wong KC, Leung KS, Hui M. Severe acute respiratory syndrome (SARS) in a geriatric patient with a hip fracture. A case report. J Bone Joint Surg Am 2003;85:1339–42.
41. Lee AK, Oh HM, Hui KP, et al. Atypical SARS in a geriatric patient. Emerg Infect Dis 2004;10:261–4.
42. Fisher DA, Lim TK, Lim YT, et al. Atypical presentations of SARS. Lancet 2003; 361:1740.
43. Hon KL, Leung CW, Cheng WT, et al. Clinical presentations and outcome of severe acute respiratory syndrome in children. Lancet 2003;561:1701–3.
44. Sit SC, Yau EKC, Lam YY, et al. A young infant with severe acute respiratory syndrome. Pediatrics 2003;112:e257–60.
45. Bitnun A, Allen U, Heurter H, et al. Children hospitalized with severe acute respiratory syndrome-related illness in Toronto. Pediatrics 2003;112:e261–8.
46. Chiu WK, Cheung PC, Ng KL, et al. Severe acute respiratory syndrome in children: experience in a regional hospital in Hong Kong. Pediatr Crit Care Med 2003;4:279–83.
47. Wong SF, Chow KM, Leung TN, et al. Pregnancy and perinatal outcomes of women with severe acute respiratory syndrome. Am J Obstet Gynecol 2004; 191:292–7.
48. Xu JL, Qi X, Chi J, et al. Orchitis: a complication of severe acute respiratory syndrome (SARS). Biol Reprod 2006;74:410–6.
49. Leung GM, Lim WW, Ho LM, et al. Seroprevalence of IgG antibodies to SARS-coronavirus in asymptomatic or subclinical population groups. Epidemiol Infect 2006;134:211–21.
50. Yu IT, Xie ZH, Tsoi KK, et al. Why did outbreaks of severe acute respiratory syndrome occur in some hospital wards but not in others? Clin Infect Dis 2007;44:1017–25.
51. Hui DS, Hall SD, Chan MT, et al. Exhaled air dispersion during oxygen delivery via a simple oxygen mask. Chest 2007;132:540–6.
52. Hui DS, Chow BK, Hall SD, et al. Exhaled air and aerosolized droplet dispersion during application of a jet nebulizer. Chest 2009;135:648–54.

53. Hui DS, Hall SD, Chan MT, et al. Non-invasive positive pressure ventilation: an experimental model to assess air and particle dispersion. Chest 2006;130: 730–40.
54. Hui DS, Chow BK, Hall SD, et al. Exhaled air dispersion distances during application of non-invasive ventilation via different Respironics face masks. Chest 2009;167:348–53.
55. Hui DS, Wong KT, Antonio GE, et al. Severe acute respiratory syndrome (SARS): correlation of clinical outcome and radiological features. Radiology 2004;233: 579–85.
56. Hui DS, Sung JJ. Severe acute respiratory syndrome. Chest 2003;124:12–5.
57. Wong GW, Hui DS. Severe acute respiratory syndrome: epidemiology, diagnosis and treatment. Thorax 2003;58:558–60.
58. Wong RS, Wu A, To KF, et al. Haematological manifestations in patients with severe acute respiratory syndrome: retrospective analysis. Br Med J 2003; 326:1358–62.
59. Chen X, Zhou B, Li M, et al. Serology of severe acute respiratory syndrome: implications for surveillance and outcome. J Infect Dis 2004;189:1158–63.
60. Muller MP, Tomlinson G, Marrie TJ, et al. Can routine laboratory tests discriminate between severe acute respiratory syndrome and other causes of community acquired pneumonia? Clin Infect Dis 2005;40:1079–86.
61. Lee N, Rainer TH, Ip M, et al. Role of laboratory variables in differentiating SARS-coronavirus from other causes of community-acquired pneumonia within the first 72 hrs of hospitalization. Eur J Clin Microbiol Infect Dis 2006;25:765–72.
62. Rainer TH, Lee N, Ip M, et al. Features discriminating SARS from other severe viral respiratory tract infections. Eur J Clin Microbiol Infect Dis 2007;26:121–9.
63. Wong KT, Antonio GE, Hui DS, et al. Severe acute respiratory syndrome: radiographic appearances and pattern of progression in 138 Patients. Radiology 2003;228:401–6.
64. Gomersall CD, Joynt GM, Lam P, et al. Short-term outcome of critically ill patients with severe acute respiratory syndrome. Intensive Care Med 2004;30: 381–7.
65. Wong KT, Antonio GE, Hui DS, et al. Thin section CT of severe acute respiratory syndrome: evaluation of 73 patients exposed to or with the disease. Radiology 2003;228:395–400.
66. Chan PK, To KF, Lo AW, et al. Persistent infection of SARS coronavirus in colonic cells in vitro. J Med Virol 2004;74:1–7.
67. Simmons G, Gosalia DN, Rennekamp AJ, et al. Inhibitors of cathepsin L prevent severe acute respiratory syndrome coronavirus entry. Proc Natl Acad Sci U S A 2005;102:11876–81.
68. Tripet B, Howard MW, Jobling M, et al. Structural characterization of the SARS-coronavirus spike S fusion protein core. J Biol Chem 2004;279:20836–49.
69. Hofmann H, Pöhlmann S. Cellular entry of the SARS coronavirus. Trends Microbiol 2004;12:466–72.
70. Li W, Moore MJ, Vasilieva N, et al. Angiotensin-converting enzyme 2 is a functional receptor for the SARS coronavirus. Nature 2003;426:450–4.
71. Hamming I, Timens W, Bulthuis ML, et al. Tissue distribution of ACE2 protein, the functional receptor for SARS coronavirus. A first step in understanding SARS pathogenesis. J Pathol 2004;203:631–7.
72. Tang JW, To KF, Lo AW, et al. Quantitative temporal-spatial distribution of severe acute respiratory syndrome-associated coronavirus (SARS-CoV) in post-mortem tissues. J Med Virol 2007;79:1245–53.

73. Yang ZY, Huang Y, Ganesh L, et al. pH-dependent entry of severe acute respiratory syndrome coronavirus is mediated by the spike glycoprotein and enhanced by dendritic cell transfer through DC-SIGN. J Virol 2004;78:5642–50.

74. Gramberg T, Hofmann H, Möller P, et al. LSECtin interacts with filovirus glycoproteins and the spike protein of SARS coronavirus. Virology 2005;340:224–36.

75. van Kooyk Y, Geijtenbeek TB. DC-SIGN: escape mechanism for pathogens. Nat Rev Immunol 2003;3:697–709.

76. Jeffers SA, Tusell SM, Gillim-Ross L, et al. CD209L (L-SIGN) is a receptor for severe acute respiratory syndrome coronavirus. Proc Natl Acad Sci U S A 2004;101:15748–53.

77. Marzi A, Gramberg T, Simmons G, et al. DC-SIGN and DC-SIGNR interact with the glycoprotein of Marburg virus and the S protein of severe acute respiratory syndrome coronavirus. J Virol 2004;78:12090–5.

78. Lo AW, Tang NL, To KF. How the SARS coronavirus causes disease: host or organism? J Pathol 2006;208:142–51.

79. Ng WF, To KF, Lam WW, et al. The comparative pathology of severe acute respiratory syndrome and avian influenza A subtype H5N1–a review. Hum Pathol 2006;37:381–90.

80. Gu J, Korteweg C. Pathology and pathogenesis of severe acute respiratory syndrome. Am J Pathol 2007;170:1136–47.

81. Cameron MJ, Bermejo-Martin JF, Danesh A, et al. Human immunopathogenesis of severe acute respiratory syndrome (SARS). Virus Res 2007;133:13–9.

82. Guo Y, Korteweg C, McNutt MA, et al. Pathogenetic mechanisms of severe acute respiratory syndrome. Virus Res 2007;133:4–12.

83. To KF, Tong JH, Chan PK, et al. Tissue and cellular tropisms of the coronavirus associated with severe acute respiratory syndrome-an in-situ hybridization study of fatal cases. J Pathol 2004;202:157–63.

84. Imai Y, Kuba K, Rao S, et al. Angiotensin-converting enzyme 2 protects from severe acute lung failure. Nature 2005;436:112–6.

85. Burrell LM, Johnston CI, Tikellis C, et al. ACE2, a new regulator of the renin-angiotensin system. Trends Endocrinol Metab 2004;15:166–9.

86. Wong SL, Chen Y, Chan CM, et al. In vivo functional characterization of the SARS-Coronavirus 3a protein in Drosophila. Biochem Biophys Res Commun 2005;337:720–9.

87. Law PT, Wong CH, Au TC, et al. The 3a protein of severe acute respiratory syndrome-associated coronavirus induces apoptosis in Vero E6 cells. J Gen Virol 2005;86:1921–30.

88. Tan YJ, Fielding BC, Goh PY, et al. Over expression of 7a, a protein specifically encoded by the severe acute respiratory syndrome coronavirus, induces apoptosis via a caspase-dependent pathway. J Virol 2004;78:14043–7.

89. Wong CK, Lam CW, Wu AK, et al. Plasma inflammatory cytokines and chemokines in severe acute respiratory syndrome. Clin Exp Immunol 2004;136:95–103.

90. Jiang Y, Xu J, Zhou C, et al. Characterization of cytokine/chemokine profiles of severe acute respiratory syndrome. Am J Respir Crit Care Med 2005;171:850–7.

91. Huang KJ, Su IJ, Theron M, et al. An interferon-gamma-related cytokine storm in SARS patients. J Med Virol 2005;75:185–94.

92. Tang NL, Chan PK, Wong CK, et al. Early enhanced expression of IP-10 (CXCL-10) and other chemokines predict adverse outcome in severe acute respiratory syndrome (SARS). Clin Chem 2005;51:2333–40.

93. Zhang Y, Li J, Zhan Y, et al. Analysis of serum cytokines in patients with severe acute respiratory syndrome. Infect Immun 2004;72:4410–5.

94. Lau YL, Peiris JS. Pathogenesis of severe acute respiratory syndrome. Curr Opin Immunol 2005;17:404–10.
95. Lin M, Tseng HK, Trejaut JA, et al. Association of HLA class I with severe acute respiratory syndrome coronavirus infection. BMC Med Genet 2003;4:9.
96. Ng MH, Lau KM, Li L, et al. Association of human-leukocyte-antigen class I (B∗0703) and class II (DRB1∗0301) genotypes with susceptibility and resistance to the development of severe acute respiratory syndrome. J Infect Dis 2004;190:515–8.
97. Yuan FF, Tanner J, Chan PK, et al. Influence of FcγRIIA and MBL polymorphisms on severe acute respiratory syndrome. Tissue Antigens 2005;66:291–6.
98. Yuan FF, Boehm I, Chan PK, et al. High prevalence of the CD14-159CC genotype in patients infected with severe acute respiratory syndrome-associated coronavirus. Clin Vaccine Immunol 2007;14:1644–5.
99. Ng MW, Zhou G, Chong WP, et al. The association of RANTES polymorphism with severe acute respiratory syndrome in Hong Kong and Beijing Chinese. BMC Infect Dis 2007;7:50.
100. Chan VS, Chan KY, Chen Y, et al. Homozygous L-SIGN (CLEC4M) plays a protective role in SARS coronavirus infection. Nat Genet 2006;38:38–46.
101. Tang NL, Chan PK, Hui DS, et al. Lack of support for an association between CLEC4M homozygosity and protection against SARS coronavirus infection. Nat Genet 2007;39:691–2.
102. Zhi L, Zhou G, Zhang H, et al. Lack of support for an association between CLEC4M homozygosity and protection against SARS coronavirus infection. Nat Genet 2007;39:692–4.
103. Cinatl J, Morgenstern B, Bauer G, et al. Glycyrrhizin, an active component of liquorice roots, and replication of SARS-associated coronavirus. Lancet 2003; 361:2045–6.
104. Tan EL, Ooi EE, Lin CY, et al. Inhibition of SARS coronavirus infection in vitro with clinically approved antiviral drugs. Emerg Infect Dis 2004;10:581–6.
105. Stroher U, DiCaro A, Li Y, et al. Severe acute respiratory syndrome-related coronavirus is inhibited by interferon-α. J Infect Dis 2004;189:1164–7.
106. Sung JJ, Wu A, Joynt GM, et al. Severe acute respiratory syndrome: report of treatment and outcome after a major outbreak. Thorax 2004;59:414–20.
107. Ng EK, Ng PC, Hon KL, et al. Serial analysis of the plasma concentration of SARS coronavirus RNA in pediatric patients with severe acute respiratory syndrome. Clin Chem 2003;49:2085–8.
108. Anand K, Ziebuhr J, Wadhwani P, et al. Coronavirus main proteinase (3Clpro) structure: basis for design of anti-SARS drugs. Science 2003;300:1763–7.
109. Chu CM, Cheng VC, Hung IF, et al. Role of lopinavir/ritonavir in the treatment of SARS: initial virological and clinical findings. Thorax 2004;59:252–6.
110. Chan KS, Lai ST, Chu CM, et al. Treatment of severe acute respiratory syndrome with lopinavir/ritonavir: a multicenter retrospective matched cohort study. Hong Kong Med J 2003;9:399–406.
111. Hurst M, Faulds D. Lopinavir. Drugs 2000;60:1371–81.
112. Yamamoto N, Yang R, Yoshinaka Y, et al. HIV protease inhibitor nelfinavir inhibits replication of SARS-associated coronavirus. Biochem Biophys Res Commun 2004;318:719–25.
113. Cinatl J, Morgenstern B, Bauer G, et al. Treatment of SARS with human interferons. Lancet 2003;362:293–4.
114. Hensley LE, Fritz LE, Jahrling PB, et al. Interferon-β 1a and SARS coronavirus replication. Emerg Infect Dis 2004;10:317–9.

115. Sainz B Jr, Mossel EC, Peters CJ, et al. Interferon-beta and interferon-gamma synergistically inhibit the replication of severe acute respiratory syndrome-associated coronavirus (SARS-CoV). Virology 2004;329:11–7.

116. Morgenstern B, Michaelis M, Baer PC, et al. Ribavirin and interferon-beta synergistically inhibit SARS-associated coronavirus replication in animal and human cell lines. Biochem Biophys Res Commun 2005;326:905–8.

117. Chen F, Chan KH, Jiang Y, et al. In vitro susceptibility of 10 clinical isolates of SARS coronavirus to selected antiviral compounds. J Clin Virol 2005;39:69–75.

118. Haagmans BL, Kuiken T, Martina BE, et al. Pegylated interferon-α protects type 1 pneumocytes against SARS coronavirus infection in macaques. Nat Med 2004;10:290–3.

119. Loutfy MR, Blatt LM, Siminovitch KA, et al. Interferon alfacon-1 plus corticosteroids in severe acute respiratory syndrome: a preliminary study. JAMA 2003;290:3222–8.

120. Sui J, Li W, Murakami A, et al. Potent neutralization of severe acute respiratory syndrome (SARS) coronavirus by a human mAb to S1 protein that blocks receptor association. Proc Natl Acad Sci U S A 2004;101:2536–41.

121. ter Meulen J, Bakker AB, van den Brink EN, et al. Human monoclonal antibody as prophylaxis for SARS coronavirus infection in ferrets. Lancet 2004;363:2139–41.

122. Gao W, Tamin A, Soloff A, et al. Effects of a SARS-associated coronavirus vaccine in monkeys. Lancet 2003;362:1895–6.

123. Zhao P, Ke JS, Qin ZL, et al. DNA vaccine of SARS-CoV S gene induces antibody response in mice. Acta Biochim Biophys Sin (Shanghai) 2004;36:37–41.

124. Yang ZY, Kong WP, Huang Y, et al. A DNA vaccine induces SARS coronavirus neutralization and protective immunity in mice. Nature 2004;428:561–4.

125. Ho TY, Wu SL, Cheng SE, et al. Antigenicity and receptor-binding ability of recombinant SARS coronavirus spike protein. Biochem Biophys Res Commun 2004;313:938–47.

126. Bisht H, Roberts A, Vogel L, et al. Severe acute respiratory syndrome coronavirus spike protein expressed by attenuated vaccinia virus protectively immunizes mice. Proc Natl Acad Sci U S A 2004;101:6641–6.

127. Bukreyev A, Lamirande EW, Buchholz UJ, et al. Mucosal immunisation of African green monkeys (Cercopithecus aethiops) with an attenuated parainfluenza virus expressing the SARS coronavirus spike protein for the prevention of SARS. Lancet 2004;363:2122–7.

128. Bosch BJ, Martina BE, van der Zee R, et al. Severe acute respiratory syndrome coronavirus (SARS-CoV) infection inhibition using spike protein heptad repeat-derived peptides. Proc Natl Acad Sci U S A 2004;101:8455–60.

129. Choy WY, Lin SG, Chan PK, et al. Synthetic peptide studies on the severe acute respiratory syndrome (SARS) coronavirus spike glycoprotein: perspective for SARS vaccine development. Clin Chem 2004;50:1036–42.

130. Ho JC, Ooi GC, Mok TY, et al. High dose pulse versus non-pulse corticosteroid regimens in severe acute respiratory syndrome. Am J Respir Crit Care Med 2003;168:1449–56.

131. Tsang OT, Chau TN, Choi KW, et al. Coronavirus-positive nasopharyngeal aspirate as predictor for severe acute respiratory syndrome mortality. Emerg Infect Dis 2003;9:1381–7.

132. Wang H, Ding Y, Li X, et al. Fatal aspergillosis in a patient with SARS who was treated with corticosteroids. N Engl J Med 2003;349:507–8.

133. Hong N, Du XK. Avascular necrosis of bone in severe acute respiratory syndrome. Clin Radiol 2004;59:602–8.
134. Griffith JF, Antonio GE, Kumta SM, et al. Osteonecrosis of hip and knee in patients with severe acute respiratory syndrome treated with steroids. Radiology 2005;235:168–75.
135. Lee N, Allen Chan KC, Hui DS, et al. Effects of early corticosteroid treatment on plasma SARS-associated Coronavirus RNA concentrations in adult patients. J Clin Virol 2004;31:304–9.
136. Cheng Y, Wong R, Soo YO, et al. Use of convalescent plasma therapy in SARS patients in Hong Kong. Eur J Clin Microbiol Infect Dis 2005;24:44–6.
137. Soo YO, Cheng Y, Wong R, et al. Retrospective comparison of convalescent plasma with continuing high-dose methylprednisolone treatment in SARS patients. Clin Microbiol Infect 2004;10:676–8.
138. Liu BY, Hu JQ, Xie YM, et al. Effects of integrative Chinese and Western medicine on arterial oxygen saturation in patients with severe acute respiratory syndrome. Chin J Integr Med 2004;10:117–22.
139. Ballow M. Mechanisms of action of intravenous immune serum globulin in autoimmune and inflammatory diseases. J Allergy Clin Immunol 1997;100:151–7.
140. Lew TW, Kwek TK, Tai D, et al. Acute respiratory distress syndrome in critically ill patients with severe acute respiratory syndrome. JAMA 2003;290:374–80.
141. Chong PY, Chui P, Ling AE, et al. Analysis of deaths during the severe acute respiratory syndrome (SARS) epidemic in Singapore: challenges in determining a SARS diagnosis. Arch Pathol Lab Med 2004;128:195–204.
142. Umapathi T, Kor AC, Venketasubramanian N, et al. Large artery ischaemic stroke in severe acute respiratory syndrome (SARS). J Neurol 2004;251:1227–31.
143. Ho JC, Wu AY, Lam B, et al. Pentaglobulin in steroid-resistant severe acute respiratory syndrome. Int J Tuberc Lung Dis 2004;8:1173–9.
144. Ng KH, Wu AK, Cheng VC, et al. Pulmonary artery thrombosis in a patient with severe acute respiratory syndrome. Postgrad Med J 2005;81:e3.
145. Dalakas MC, Clark WM. Strokes, thromboembolic events, and IVIg: rare incidents blemish an excellent safety record. Neurology 2003;60:1763–7.
146. Chen L, Liu P, Gao H, et al. Inhalation of nitric oxide in the treatment of severe acute respiratory syndrome: a rescue trial in Beijing. Clin Infect Dis 2004;39:1531–5.
147. Akerstrom S, Mousavi-Jazi M, Klingstrom J, et al. Nitric oxide inhibits the replication cycle of severe acute respiratory syndrome coronavirus. J Virol 2005;79:1966–9.
148. WHO. SARS case fatality ration, incubation period. Available at: http://www.who.int/csr/sars/archive/2003_05_07a/en/print.html. Accessed May 23, 2005.
149. Donnelly CA, Ghani AV, Leung GM, et al. Epidemiological determinants of spread of causal agent of severe acute respiratory syndrome in Hong Kong. Lancet 2003;361:1761–6.
150. Tsui PT, Kwok ML, Yuen H, et al. Severe acute respiratory syndrome: clinical outcome and prognostic correlates. Emerg Infect Dis 2003;9:1064–9.
151. Chan JW, Ng CK, Chan YH, et al. Short term outcome and risk factors for adverse clinical outcomes in adults with Severe acute respiratory syndrome (SARS). Thorax 2003;58:686–9.
152. Chu CM, Poon LL, Cheng VC, et al. Initial viral load and the outcomes of SARS. CMAJ 2004;171:1349–52.

153. Hui DS, Joynt GM, Wong KT, et al. Impact of severe acute respiratory syndrome (SARS) on pulmonary function, functional capacity and quality of life in a cohort of survivors. Thorax 2005;60:401–9.
154. Hui DS, Wong KT, Ko FW, et al. The one-year impact of severe acute respiratory syndrome (SARS) on pulmonary function, exercise capacity and quality of life in a cohort of survivors. Chest 2005;128:2247–61.
155. Tsai LK, Hsieh ST, Chao CC, et al. Neuromuscular disorders in severe acute respiratory syndrome. Arch Neurol 2004;61:1669–73.
156. Yu WC, Hui DS, Chan-Yeung M. Antiviral agents and corticosteroids in the treatment of SARS. Thorax 2004;59:643–5.
157. Tsang KW, Ooi GC, Ho PL. Diagnosis and pharmacotherapy of severe acute respiratory syndrome: what have we learnt? Eur Respir J 2004;24:1025–32.
158. Ong KC, Ng AW, Lee LS, et al. 1-year pulmonary function and health status in survivors of severe acute respiratory syndrome. Chest 2005;128:1393–400.
159. Xie L, Liu Y, Xiao Y, et al. Follow-up study on pulmonary function and lung radiographic changes in rehabilitating severe acute respiratory syndrome patients after discharge. Chest 2005;127:2119–24.
160. Tansey CM, Louie M, Loeb M, et al. One-year outcomes and health care utilization in survivors of severe acute respiratory syndrome. Arch Intern Med 2007;167:1312–20.
161. Chua SE, Cheung V, McAlonan GM, et al. Stress and psychological impact on SARS patients during the outbreak. Can J Psychiatry 2004;49:385–90.
162. Cheng SK, Wong CW, Tsang J, et al. Psychological distress and negative appraisals in survivors of severe acute respiratory syndrome (SARS). Psychol Med 2004;34:1187–95.
163. Lee DT, Wing YK, Leung HC, et al. Factors associated with psychosis among patients with severe acute respiratory syndrome: a case-control study. Clin Infect Dis 2004;39:1247–9.
164. Chen Z, Zhang L, Qin C, et al. Recombinant modified vaccinia virus Ankara expressing the spike glycoprotein of severe acute respiratory syndrome coronavirus induces protective neutralizing antibodies primarily targeting the receptor binding region. J Virol 2005;79:2678–88.
165. He Y, Li J, Heck S, et al. Antigenic and immunogenic characterization of recombinant baculovirus-expressed severe acute respiratory syndrome coronavirus spike protein: implication for vaccine design. J Virol 2006;80:5757–67.
166. Weingartl H, Czub M, Czub S, et al. Immunization with modified vaccinia virus Ankara-based recombinant vaccine against severe acute respiratory syndrome is associated with enhanced hepatitis in ferrets. J Virol 2004;78:12672–6.
167. Petersen NC, Boyle JF. Immunologic phenomena in the effusive form of feline infectious peritonitis. Am J Vet Res 1980;41:868–76.
168. Vennema H, de Groot RJ, Harbour DA, et al. Early death after feline infectious peritonitis virus challenge due to recombinant vaccinia virus immunization. J Virol 1990;64:1407–9.
169. Chan PK, Ip M, Ng KC, et al. Severe acute respiratory syndrome-associated coronavirus infection. Emerg Infect Dis 2003;9:1453–4.

Respiratory Infections Due to Drug-Resistant Bacteria

Jae-Hoon Song, MD, PhD[a,b,*], Doo Ryeon Chung, MD, PhD[a]

KEYWORDS

- Community-acquired pneumonia
- Hospital-acquired pneumonia • Antimicrobial resistance
- Epidemiology • Clinical impact • Treatment guidelines

Lower respiratory tract infections were ranked as the third leading cause of death worldwide in 2004.[1] The reported mortality of community-acquired pneumonia (CAP) ranges from less than 5% among outpatients to approximately 12% among all hospitalized patients with CAP, but is more than 30% among those admitted to the intensive care unit (ICU).[2] The crude mortality for hospital-acquired pneumonia (HAP) is reported to be 30% to 70%, and attributable mortality is estimated to be 33% to 50%.[3,4] Furthermore, increasing prevalence of antimicrobial resistance in major respiratory pathogens has become a serious threat to clinical medicine, with increased morbidity and mortality as a result of treatment failures. Antimicrobial resistance is a critical issue not only in CAP due to resistance in *Streptococcus pneumoniae* but also in HAP or ventilator-associated pneumonia (VAP) due to methicillin-resistant *Staphylococcus aureus* (MRSA) or resistant gram-negative bacilli. Emergence of antimicrobial resistance has also resulted in an additional economic burden of respiratory infections. Therefore, the recent increase in antimicrobial resistance in respiratory pathogens has resulted in a significant negative impact on clinical outcome of pneumonia and huge economic loss. This article reviews the current

[a] Division of Infectious Diseases, Samsung Medical Center, Sungkyunkwan University School of Medicine, 50 Ilwon-dong, Gangnam-gu, Seoul, 135-710, Korea
[b] Asia Pacific Foundation for Infectious Diseases (APFID), 50 Ilwon-dong, Gangnam-gu, Seoul, 135-710, Korea
* Corresponding author. Division of Infectious Diseases, Samsung Medical Center, Sungkyunkwan University School of Medicine, 50 Ilwon-dong, Gangnam-gu, Seoul, 135-710, Korea.
E-mail addresses: songjh@skku.edu, jhsong@ansorp.org

Infect Dis Clin N Am 24 (2010) 639–653
doi:10.1016/j.idc.2010.04.007
0891-5520/10/$ – see front matter © 2010 Elsevier Inc. All rights reserved.

id.theclinics.com

knowledge of respiratory infections caused by antibiotic-resistant pathogens, and treatment options of CAP and HAP.

CAP

Although the distribution of causative organisms of CAP differs by geographic regions, *S pneumoniae*, which accounts for 30% to 70% of cases requiring hospitalization,[5,6] has been the most frequent causal organism of CAP worldwide.[7–9] The incidence of *S aureus*, *Enterobacteriaceae*, and *Pseudomonas* spp in CAP was relatively higher in the United States compared with other regions. Some Asian countries also showed a higher frequency of occurrence of *Enterobacteriaceae* and *Pseudomonas* spp.[9]

CAP Due to Streptococcus pneumoniae

Major types of antimicrobial resistance in *S pneumoniae* include resistance to penicillin and β-lactam agents, macrolides, fluoroquinolones, and multidrug resistance.

S pneumoniae with penicillin resistance

According to the previous breakpoints, penicillin nonsusceptibility in *S pneumoniae* isolates (penicillin minimum inhibitory concentration [MIC] ≥0.12 mg/L) has been increasing worldwide and the prevalence reached 70% to 80% in some geographic regions.[10] However, clinical data suggest that in vitro penicillin resistance in *S pneumoniae* is not associated with increased mortality in nonmeningeal infections.[9,11–13] Because of this discrepancy, the Clinical and Laboratory Standards Institute (CLSI) has revised the MIC breakpoints for penicillin in nonmeningeal Isolates in 2008 (susceptible ≤2 mg/L, intermediate 4 mg/L, and resistant ≥8 mg/L).[14] According to the revised criteria, the prevalence of penicillin-resistant pneumococcal isolates in nonmeningeal infections is very low worldwide. For instance, in the United States, the prevalence of penicillin-resistant *S pneumoniae* (PRSP) decreased from 10.3% (MIC ≥2 mg/L) to 1.2% (MIC ≥8 mg/L).[15] In Asian countries that have reported the highest rates of penicillin resistance among pneumococci, the prevalence of PRSP also decreased from 29.4% to 4.0%.[10] Therefore, in vitro penicillin resistance is not a common problem in respiratory infections with these new breakpoints. Clinical impact of highly resistant strains with penicillin MIC ≥8 mg/L is yet to be evaluated.

S pneumoniae with macrolide resistance

In contrast to penicillin resistance, macrolide resistance in *S pneumoniae* remains a prominent and serious issue in the clinical practice worldwide. The prevalence of macrolide resistance has increased in diverse geographic regions across the world. In particular, Asian countries such as Korea, Japan, China, Taiwan, and Vietnam have shown the highest prevalence rates (>75%) of macrolide resistance[16] compared with the United States (29.4%) or Western Europe including France (57.6%), Italy (42.9%), and Belgium (32.1%) (**Fig. 1**).[17,18] Whereas *erm*B with high erythromycin MICs (>64 mg/L) is the most prevalent genotype for macrolide resistance in many European countries, South Africa, and Asian countries, *mef*(A) with lower level of erythromycin resistance (1–32 mg/L) is the most prevalent resistance genotype identified in the United States.[16–19] In Asian countries, South Africa, and the United States, the emergence and spread of multidrug-resistant pneumococcal clones such as Taiwan 19F, Spain 23F, or Taiwan 23F containing *erm*B and *mef*A have been reported.[20,21] The clinical significance of macrolide resistance among pneumococcal isolates is not well established. Although there have been reports on clinical or microbiological failures with macrolides in respiratory tract infections caused by macrolide-resistant isolates,[22–25] clinical data have shown an inconsistent relationship between

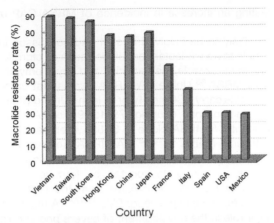

Fig. 1. Macrolide-resistant rates in *S pneumoniae* in different countries.[16–18]

in vitro macrolide resistance and clinical outcome.[26,27] However, a recent study showed that the low- and high-level macrolide resistance were important risk factors for macrolide failure of therapy for pneumococcal bacteremia.[28]

S pneumoniae with fluoroquinolone resistance

Fluoroquinolone resistance in *S pneumoniae* is relatively infrequent, but an increasing tendency is observed with increased use of fluoroquinolone.[29–31] Prior use of fluoroquinolones is an important risk factor for fluoroquinolone resistance. Nowadays the emergence of reduced susceptibility to respiratory fluoroquinolones such as levofloxacin is being increasingly reported.[32] The clinical impact of fluoroquinolone-resistant isolates in the treatment of pneumonia is still unclear, with several anecdotal reports on treatment failure with fluoroquinolones.

S pneumoniae with multidrug resistance

Multidrug resistance (MDR), which is defined as resistance to 3 or more antimicrobial classes, has been increasing in pneumococcal isolates especially from Asian countries. MDR in *S pneumoniae* usually involves resistance to β-lactams, macrolides, tetracycline, or trimethoprim/sulfamethoxazole, and rarely, fluoroquinolones.[33] MDR in pneumococci is increasing worldwide, and recent data from the Prospective Resistant Organism Tracking and Epidemiology for the Ketolide Telithromycin (PROTEKT) study indicate that about 40% of pneumococci display multidrug-resistant phenotypes.[34] The increase in MDR pneumococcal isolates has further limited the choice of empiric antimicrobial options.

CAP Due to Methicillin-Resistant Staphylococcus aureus (MRSA)

S aureus was an uncommon cause of CAP, accounting for 1% to 5% of all CAP cases and occurring mostly in patients with influenza.[35] However, a new variant of MRSA, containing SCC*mec* type IV, has recently emerged in the community as an important CAP pathogen. In a cohort study in United States hospitals from 2002 to 2003, MRSA accounted for 8.9% of CAP, 26.5% of HCAP, 22.9% of HAP, and 14.6% of VAP.[36] Although there have been increasing numbers of case reports, the true incidence of community-associated (CA)-MRSA pneumonia remains unknown. A recent systematic review showed that the estimated incidence of MRSA CAP was 0.51 to 0.64 cases per 100,000, suggesting an increase in incidence of MRSA CAP over the last few years.[37]

CA-MRSA is more likely to be involved in skin and soft-tissue infections, and is usually more susceptible to non–β-lactam antibiotics such as ciprofloxacin, clindamycin, trimethoprim-sulfamethoxazole, gentamicin, and erythromycin compared with hospital-acquired (HA)-MRSA.[38] Unlike HA-MRSA strains that carry SCC*mec* types I, II, or III, CA-MRSA strains carry SCC*mec* IV or V. In the United States, USA300 clone with ST8 is the most common clone, causing 97% to 99% of CA-MRSA infections.[39] In Europe, the predominant CA-MRSA clone is ST80, whereas ST30 is an important clone in Asia and Oceania (**Table 1**).[40–48] CA-MRSA isolates also showed a high percentage of Panton-Valentine leukocidin (PVL), an exotoxin that is able to cause tissue necrosis and destruction of leukocytes by forming pores in the cellular membrane. However, many CA-MRSA isolates from the United Kingdom, Korea, Japan, and Western Australia are negative for PVL.[43,47,49] A murine model suggested that PVL plays a major role in the development of severe pneumonia.[50]

CA-MRSA pneumonia generally affects young people. The median age of the patients is 21 years, and 59% of patients are younger than 35 years.[37] Influenza-like illness and documented influenza infection were reported in 41% to 57% and 21% to 38% of patients, respectively.[37,51] Tachypnea (92%), hemoptysis (29%), leukopenia (45%), and thrombocytopenia (68%) are common.[37] Multiorgan failure and acute respiratory distress syndrome developed in 44% and 23.5% of patients, respectively. Necrotizing pneumonia based on radiographic or autopsy findings was reported in 61% to 77% of CA-MRSA CAP cases.[37] Multiple lobes are usually affected, with scattered areas of cavitary consolidations, pleural effusion, or empyema.[37,52] In most cases, the median time from symptoms onset to death (8 days) or from admission to death (3 days) was very short.[37] Mortality in the individual case series ranged from 20% to 60%. CA-MRSA pneumonia is a fatal disease with about 15 times higher fatality than skin and soft-tissue infections caused by CA-MRSA.[53] CA-MRSA isolates have now spread into hospitals, causing various nosocomial infections including pneumonia.[51]

Treatment of CAP by Antibiotic-Resistant Pathogens

Recommendations of antimicrobial agents for CAP depend on the etiology of CAP, including the role of atypical pathogens, antibiotic resistance of major organisms, clinical relevance of antibiotic resistance, and other local issues such as antibiotic availability.[54–56] Antimicrobial resistance in major organisms causing CAP is an important

Table 1
Genotypic characteristics of CA-MRSA strains from different geographic regions

Region	Genotypic Characteristics		
	PVL	Sequence Type	SCC*mec* Type
North America[42]	+	ST8	IVa
UK[43]	–	ST1	IVa
Denmark[44]	+	ST80	IV
France[45]	+	ST80	IV
Taiwan[46]	+	ST59	V
Korea[47]	–	ST72	IVa
Australia[48]	+	ST1	IV

consideration for appropriate empiric antimicrobial therapy, which should be regularly updated based on appropriate surveillance studies. Penicillin resistance in S pneumoniae is not a major consideration for selecting antimicrobial options in the treatment of CAP because true penicillin resistance with MIC ≥8 mg/L is rare and lower-level resistance (MIC <8 mg/L) does not match with the clinical response to penicillin treatment. The United States guidelines recommend macrolides, doxycycline, respiratory fluoroquinolones, or the combination of a β-lactam and macrolide for treatment of outpatients with CAP.[54] In contrast, the British Thoracic Society guidelines recommend β-lactams, and atypical pathogens are not covered by an initial empiric regimen.[54] Macrolides have been widely used to empirically treat CAP because of their efficacy in treating typical pathogens such as S pneumoniae and atypical respiratory pathogens. However, given a global increase in macrolide resistance in S pneumoniae, especially in the Asian countries where high-level resistance to macrolides is widely prevalent, a single empiric use of macrolides is not recommended for treatment of CAP.[10,17] For the same reason, doxycycline may not be a good empiric choice for CAP in Asian countries or other areas with high prevalence of resistance. Empiric use of respiratory fluoroquinolones is recommended by the American Thoracic Society and the Infectious Diseases Society of America (ATS/IDSA) guidelines because of excellent clinical efficacy of these drugs against drug-resistant pneumococci and atypical pathogens. However, there are some concerns about the use of these agents as an empiric choice because they can induce the emergence of fluoroquinolone resistance in major respiratory pathogens as well as other bacterial organisms including Mycobacterium tuberculosis.

In the region where CA-MRSA is a concern, the initial empiric regimen should be effective against CA-MRSA although the most effective therapy has not been defined.[54] Although CA-MRSA is frequently susceptible to non–β-lactams including clindamycin, rifampin, fluoroquinolones, and trimethoprim/sulfamethoxazole, their efficacy in the treatment of CA-MRSA pneumonia has not been established. Experience in treatment of nosocomial pneumonia due to MRSA suggests that linezolid may be superior to vancomycin in the treatment of pneumonia. The effectiveness of new antimicrobial agents such as tigecycline or ceftobiprole in CA-MRSA pneumonia is yet to be evaluated. In the treatment of necrotizing pneumonia caused by CA-MRSA, which is associated with production of PVL and other toxins, the use of linezolid or addition of clindamycin to vancomycin may improve outcome.[35,54]

HAP

HAP and VAP are the most serious and fatal hospital-acquired infection. Early-onset HAP is defined as pneumonia occurring within the first 4 days of hospitalization, whereas late-onset HAP is defined as pneumonia occurring 5 days or more after hospitalization.[3] Late-onset VAP can be defined either by cases occurring 5 days or more after hospitalization[3] or by cases occurring 5 days or more after the initiation of mechanical ventilation in the British guidelines.[56] There are significant differences in the distribution of causative pathogens according to the geographic region and timing of onset. At present, S aureus, especially MRSA, has emerged as the most important pathogen causing HAP or VAP in many hospitals. Most frequent gram-negative organisms of HAP or VAP are Pseudomonas aeruginosa and Enterobactereiaceae (Klebsiella spp, Escherichia coli, Enterobacter spp) (Table 2).[3,36,57–59] In some Asian countries, nonfermenters such as Acinetobacter spp and P aeruginosa were reported as the most frequent causal organisms of HAP or VAP.[60]

Table 2
Major causative organisms of HAP or VAP

	NNIS (ICU)[57] (1992–1998) HAP + VAP (n = 9877)	USA[36] (2002–2003) HAP (n = 835)	USA[10] (2002–2003) VAP (n = 499)	EPIC (Europe)[58] (1992) HAP + VAP	Worldwide[59] (1989–2000) VAP (n = 2490)
Gram-positive (in %)					
S aureus	17.0	47.1	42.5	31.7	20.4
(MRSA/S aureus, %)	–	(48.6)	(34.4)	–	(55.7)
Streptococcus	–	13.9	7.0	–	8.0
S pneumoniae	1.6	3.1	5.8	–	4.1
Other gram-positive	9.3	8.1	8.6	10.6	1.4
Gram-negative (in %)					
Pseudomonas spp	15.6	18.4	21.2	29.8	24.4
Haemophilus spp	–	5.6	12.2	10.2	9.8
Klebsiella spp	7.0	7.1	8.4	8.0	2.2
Escherichia coli	4.4	4.7	6.4	6.8	3.4
Enterobacter spp	10.9	4.3	5.6	8.0	2.7
Proteus spp	–	–	–	–	3.1
Acinetobacter spp	2.9	2.0	3.0	10.0	7.9
Other gram-negative	32.3	3.7	6.2	–	7.0

Abbreviation: EPIC, European Prevalence of Infection in Intensive Care.

Early-onset HAP or VAP is often caused by organisms such as *S pneumoniae* or *Haemophilus influenzae*, whereas late-onset HAP or VAP is commonly caused by multidrug-resistant organisms including MRSA, *P aeruginosa*, or other gram-negative bacteria.

HAP Due to MRSA

Over the past 3 decades the percentage of respiratory infections in hospitals caused by MRSA has dramatically increased, and MRSA accounts for 20% to 40% of all HAP and VAP cases.[35] In many countries including United States and most Asian countries, more than 50% of *S aureus* isolates causing ICU infections are methicillin-resistant. Most of the MRSA strains causing HAP and VAP are typical nosocomial strains with SCC*mec* types I, II, or III, and CA-MRSA strains with SCC*mec* type IV or V have been introduced into the hospital recently.[61,62] Methicillin resistance in *S aureus* VAP may be associated with excess mortality, although this association may be probably because of confounders, such as the adequacy of the empiric treatment and severity of illness.[63] MRSA VAP also prolongs the duration of ICU hospitalization and increases overall health care cost.[64,65]

HAP Due to Pseudomonas aeruginosa

P aeruginosa is the second most common pathogen of HAP in the United States[66] and the most common pathogen in some Asian countries. Infections caused by *P aeruginosa* are frequently life threatening and often difficult to treat because of the intrinsic resistance of *P aeruginosa* to many antimicrobial agents. Data from United States showed that more than 20% of *P aeruginosa* isolates in ICU surveillance were resistant to ceftazidime or imipenem.[67] Increase in the prevalence of multidrug resistance to β-lactams, aminoglycosides, and fluoroquinolones is the greatest concern for *P aeruginosa* associated with HAP. Independent predictors for carbapenem resistance were prior receipt of mechanical ventilation and prior exposure to fluoroquinolones or carbapenems.[68] Risk factors for the presence of MDR *P aeruginosa* are 48 hours or more of hospital stay before ICU admission, prolonged ICU stay, longer duration of mechanical ventilation because of acute lung injury, taking antibiotics for longer duration, and long duration of indwelling central catheters.[69] Metallo-β-lactamases (MBL) production is an emerging mechanism in gram-negative bacilli, particularly in *P aeruginosa*. MBLs hydrolyze all β-lactam agents with the exception of aztreonam, including the carbapenems.[70] Because their genes are carried on highly mobile elements, they are easily disseminated between gram-negative bacilli. MBLs have been widely spreading into many countries including Europe, Asia, and Latin America.[71] Patients with MDR, colistin-susceptible *P aeruginosa* VAP are characterized by previous VAP episodes, prior broad-spectrum antimicrobial therapy for more than 10 days (particularly carbapenem), and delayed onset of VAP from the time of ICU admission.[72] The emergence of pandrug-resistant (PDR) *P aeruginosa* in Taiwan has been reported.[73] The prolonged combined use of carbapenems and colistin predisposed to VAP by PDR *P aeruginosa*. A prospective cohort study on HAP and VAP due to *P aeruginosa* revealed that the 30-day mortality was 37.3%.[71] In this study, patients with HAP or VAP by MBL-producing *P aeruginosa* showed higher mortality (57.1%) than those infected by non–MBL-producing strains (29.6%). Inappropriate antimicrobial therapy was an independent factor for the 30-day mortality period.

HAP Due to Acinetobacter spp

Acinetobacter spp has emerged as a significant nosocomial pathogen, especially in ICUs. HAP or VAP is the most common manifestation of nosocomial *Acinetobacter* infection, accounting for 6.9% of gram-negative pneumonia in the ICU in the NNIS (National Nosocomial Infections Surveillance System) study.[67] The important predisposing factors are mechanical ventilation, especially after prolonged intubation, type and duration of prior antibiotic therapy, underlying pulmonary disease and systemic comorbidities, longer length of ICU stay, aspiration, head injury, and neurosurgery.[74] *Acinetobacter* spp can develop resistance rapidly to different classes of antimicrobial agents, including β-lactams, aminoglycosides, fluoroquinolones, and tetracyclines.[75] Data from the NNIS System in the United States between 1986 and 2003 showed an increase in the prevalence of resistance to ceftazidime (24% to 67%), amikacin (3% to 20%), and imipenem (0% to 20%) in *Acinetobacter* spp[67] Recently, carbapenem resistance has been steadily increasing in *Acinetobacter* spp worldwide.[76,77] The major driving force for the emergence of carbapenem resistance is the heavy use of third-generation cephalosporins, aztreonam, and carbapenems.[78] Carbapenem-resistant *Acinetobacter* spp are disseminated within the hospital and between institutions. Multidrug resistance in *Acinetobacter* spp is associated with longer hospital stay in the ICU (odds ratio [OR] 2.1) or in the hospital (OR 2.5).[79] Emergence of carbapenem resistance and multidrug resistance has led to the revival of colistin in the clinical practice to treat *Acinetobacter* infection. However, colistin resistance in *Acinetobacter baumannii* isolates has already been reported. The prevalence rates of resistance to polymyxin B and colistin in a Korean hospital was 18.1% and 27.9%, respectively.[80] In addition, PDR strains that are resistant to all available antibiotics have emerged in some regions.[81,82]

Nosocomial *Acinetobacter* pneumonia is associated with high mortality rates that range from 35% to 70%, which is particularly high in patients with VAP.[83,84] A recent case-control study showed that VAP caused by *A baumannii* was not associated with an increase in the risk of death, although imipenem resistance was associated with higher mortality rates.[85] However, another study found that VAP caused by *Pseudomonas* and *Acinetobacter* had higher mortality rates compared with VAP caused by other etiologies.[86] Mortality of *Acinetobacter* pneumonia may be related to the extent of antimicrobial resistance, the effectiveness of empiric therapy, and the severity of illness. In one study, adequacy of empiric antibiotic therapy was a protective factor (OR 0.067) of in-hospital mortality, whereas sequential organ failure assessment (SOFA) score was the predictor of in-hospital mortality (OR 1.22).[84]

HAP Due to ESBL-producing Klebsiella pneumoniae

Enterobacteriaceae such as *K pneumoniae* are one of the most frequent causes of HAP, with nonfermenters including *P aeruginosa* and *A baumannii*. In a report from the United States, *Klebsiella* spp accounted for 7.1% of HAP and 8.4% of VAP.[36] *Klebsiella* spp are intrinsically resistant to ampicillin and other aminopenicillins, and resistance to the third- and fourth-generation cephalosporins has increased worldwide as a result of the spread of plasmid-mediated extended-spectrum β-lactamases (ESBLs). The proportion of ESBL production in *K pneumoniae* and the types of ESBLs vary by the region. The rate of ESBL production is highest among the *K pneumoniae* isolates collected in Latin America (44.0%), followed by the Asia/Pacific rim (22.4%), Europe (13.3%), and North America (7.5%).[87] In recent years, CTX-M type ESBLs have emerged as the predominant type of ESBL in many regions of the world.[88–90] Risk factors associated with ESBL-producing organisms are: increasing duration of hospital or ICU stay, greater severity of clinical status, insertion of various types of indwelling catheters, performance of certain types of invasive procedures or surgical interventions, receipt of renal replacement therapy, or mechanical ventilator support.[91] Because ESBL-producing *K pneumoniae* is emerging as important pathogens causing HAP or VAP, it is more likely to develop into inappropriate empiric antimicrobial agents that could be associated with high mortality. Recently, *K pneumoniae* carbapenemase (KPC)-producing *K pneumoniae* has increasingly been isolated in China, Israel, Greece, South America, and the United States, posing perhaps the most serious potential threat to antimicrobial treatment because of lack of effective antimicrobial agents.[92]

Treatment Issues for HAP Caused by Antibiotic-Resistant Pathogens

With increasing incidence of HAP caused by MDR pathogens, strategies for the management of HAP mainly focused on the evaluation of risk factors for MDR pathogens. Early-onset HAP or VAP is usually associated with lower risk for MDR pathogens, but late-onset HAP or VAP is associated with MDR pathogens that require broad-spectrum antibiotics.[3] Risk factors for MDR pathogens in HAP or VAP include antimicrobial therapy within the preceding 90 days, current hospitalization of 5 days or longer, high frequency of antibiotic resistance in the community or specific hospital units, admission from a health care–associated facility, and immunosuppressive disease or immunosuppressant therapy.[3] In the clinical setting with suspicion of MDR pathogens, antipseudomonal β-lactams such as carbapenem, ceftazidime, cefepime, or piperacillin/tazobactam have been recommended as initial empiric antibiotics in current guidelines.[3,93] Combination of β-lactams with fluoroquinolone or aminoglycoside is usually preferred to monotherapy in patients at risk for *P aeruginosa* to enhance the appropriateness of initial empiric therapy in most guidelines.[3,93] Theoretically, the use of combination therapy could minimize the emergence of resistance and increase likelihood of therapeutic success from antimicrobial synergy. The combination therapy in *P aeruginosa* pneumonia might reduce the likelihood of inappropriate treatment, especially if local resistant patterns or individual patient risk factors for resistant pathogens suggest the possibility of MDR organisms. However, clinical data has shown that the administration of a single effective antimicrobial agent provides a similar outcome to combination therapy, suggesting that switching to monotherapy once the susceptibility is documented could be a safe option.[94]

The increasing prevalence of ESBL-producing *Enterobacteriaceae* in HAP in many countries has led to increasing use of carbapenems. Because carbapenem-resistant gram-negative bacilli have been also increasing, colistin has reemerged as a promising drug for these MDR pathogens. However, there are no proven effective therapeutic options for HAP or VAP caused by colistin-resistant *K pneumoniae* and *A baumannii*. Initial empiric therapy with glycopeptides or linezolid against MRSA is usually not recommended unless local microbiology data suggest a high likelihood of MRSA infection, mainly because of concerns over the emergence of vancomycin-resistant *S aureus* or enterococci.

REFERENCES

1. World Health Organization. The global burden of disease: 2004 update. Switzerland: World Health Organization; 2008.
2. Fine MJ, Smith MA, Carson CA, et al. Prognosis and outcomes of patients with community-acquired pneumonia. A meta-analysis. JAMA 1996;275(2): 134–41.
3. American Thoracic Society, Infectious Diseases Society of America. Guidelines for the management of adults with hospital-acquired, ventilator-associated, and

healthcare-associated pneumonia. Am J Respir Crit Care Med 2005;171(4): 388–416.

4. Leu HS, Kaiser DL, Mori M, et al. Hospital-acquired pneumonia. Attributable mortality and morbidity. Am J Epidemiol 1989;129(6):1258–67.

5. Bartlett JG, Mundy LM. Community-acquired pneumonia. N Engl J Med 1995; 333(24):1618–24.

6. Ortqvist A, Hedlund J, Kalin M. Streptococcus pneumoniae: epidemiology, risk factors, and clinical features. Semin Respir Crit Care Med 2005;26(6):563–74.

7. Lim WS, Macfarlane JT, Boswell TC, et al. Study of community acquired pneumonia aetiology (SCAPA) in adults admitted to hospital: implications for management guidelines. Thorax 2001;56(4):296–301.

8. Almirall J, Boixeda R, Bolibar I, et al. Differences in the etiology of community-acquired pneumonia according to site of care: a population-based study. Respir Med 2007;101(10):2168–75.

9. Song JH, Oh WS, Kang CI, et al. Epidemiology and clinical outcomes of community-acquired pneumonia in adult patients in Asian countries: a prospective study by the Asian network for surveillance of resistant pathogens. Int J Antimicrob Agents 2008;31(2):107–14.

10. Song JH, Jung SI, Ko KS, et al. High prevalence of antimicrobial resistance among clinical Streptococcus pneumoniae isolates in Asia (an ANSORP study). Antimicrob Agents Chemother 2004;48(6):2101–7.

11. Pallares R, Linares J, Vadillo M, et al. Resistance to penicillin and cephalosporin and mortality from severe pneumococcal pneumonia in Barcelona, Spain. N Engl J Med 1995;333(8):474–80.

12. Klugman KP. Bacteriological evidence of antibiotic failure in pneumococcal lower respiratory tract infections. Eur Respir J Suppl 2002;36:3s–8s.

13. Yu VL, Baddour LM. Infection by drug-resistant Streptococcus pneumoniae is not linked to increased mortality. Clin Infect Dis 2004;39(7):1086–7.

14. Wikler MA, Clinical and Laboratory Standards Institute. Performance standards for antimicrobial susceptibility testing: eighteenth informational supplement. Wayne (PA): Clinical and Laboratory Standards Institute; 2008.

15. Centers for Disease Control and Prevention. Effects of new penicillin susceptibility breakpoints for Streptococcus pneumoniae—United States, 2006–2007. MMWR Morb Mortal Wkly Rep 2008;57(50):1353–5.

16. Song JH, Chang HH, Suh JY, et al. Macrolide resistance and genotypic characterization of Streptococcus pneumoniae in Asian countries: a study of the Asian network for surveillance of resistant pathogens (ANSORP). J Antimicrob Chemother 2004;53(3):457–63.

17. Doern GV, Richter SS, Miller A, et al. Antimicrobial resistance among Streptococcus pneumoniae in the United States: have we begun to turn the corner on resistance to certain antimicrobial classes? Clin Infect Dis 2005;41(2):139–48.

18. Felmingham D, Reinert RR, Hirakata Y, et al. Increasing prevalence of antimicrobial resistance among isolates of Streptococcus pneumoniae from the PROTEKT surveillance study, and comparative in vitro activity of the ketolide, telithromycin. J Antimicrob Chemother 2002;50(Suppl S1):25–37.

19. Kresken M, Henrichfreise B, Bagel S, et al. High prevalence of the ermB gene among erythromycin-resistant Streptococcus pneumoniae isolates in Germany during the winter of 2000-2001 and in vitro activity of telithromycin. Antimicrob Agents Chemother 2004;48(8):3193–5.

20. Klugman KP, Lonks JR. Hidden epidemic of macrolide-resistant pneumococci. Emerg Infect Dis 2005;11(6):802–7.

21. Ko KS, Song JH. Evolution of erythromycin-resistant *Streptococcus pneumoniae* from Asian countries that contains *erm*(B) and *mef*(A) genes. J Infect Dis 2004; 190(4):739–47.

22. Moreno S, Garcia-Leoni ME, Cercenado E, et al. Infections caused by erythromycin-resistant *Streptococcus pneumoniae*: incidence, risk factors, and response to therapy in a prospective study. Clin Infect Dis 1995;20(5):1195–200.

23. Lynch IJ, Martinez FJ. Clinical relevance of macrolide-resistant *Streptococcus pneumoniae* for community-acquired pneumonia. Clin Infect Dis 2002; 34(Suppl 1):S27–46.

24. Lonks JR, Garau J, Medeiros AA. Implications of antimicrobial resistance in the empirical treatment of community-acquired respiratory tract infections: the case of macrolides. J Antimicrob Chemother 2002;50(Suppl S2):87–92.

25. Musher DM, Dowell ME, Shortridge VD, et al. Emergence of macrolide resistance during treatment of pneumococcal pneumonia. N Engl J Med 2002;346(8):630–1.

26. Plouffe J, Schwartz DB, Kolokathis A, et al. Clinical efficacy of intravenous followed by oral azithromycin monotherapy in hospitalized patients with community-acquired pneumonia. The azithromycin intravenous clinical trials group. Antimicrob Agents Chemother 2000;44(7):1796–802.

27. Vergis EN, Indorf A, File TM Jr, et al. Azithromycin vs cefuroxime plus erythromycin for empirical treatment of community-acquired pneumonia in hospitalized patients: a prospective, randomized, multicenter trial. Arch Intern Med 2000; 160(9):1294–300.

28. Daneman N, McGeer A, Green K, et al. Macrolide resistance in bacteremic pneumococcal disease: implications for patient management. Clin Infect Dis 2006; 43(4):432–8.

29. Chen DK, McGeer A, de Azavedo JC, et al. Decreased susceptibility of *Streptococcus pneumoniae* to fluoroquinolones in Canada. Canadian bacterial surveillance network. N Engl J Med 1999;341(4):233–9.

30. Urban C, Rahman N, Zhao X, et al. Fluoroquinolone-resistant *Streptococcus pneumoniae* associated with levofloxacin therapy. J Infect Dis 2001;184(6): 794–8.

31. Bhavnani SM, Hammel JP, Jones RN, et al. Relationship between increased levofloxacin use and decreased susceptibility of *Streptococcus pneumoniae* in the United States. Diagn Microbiol Infect Dis 2005;51(1):31–7.

32. Davidson R, Cavalcanti R, Brunton JL, et al. Resistance to levofloxacin and failure of treatment of pneumococcal pneumonia. N Engl J Med 2002;346(10):747–50.

33. Draghi DC, Jones ME, Sahm DF, et al. Geographically-based evaluation of multidrug resistance trends among *Streptococcus pneumoniae* in the USA: findings of the fast surveillance initiative (2003–2004). Int J Antimicrob Agents 2006;28(6): 525–31.

34. Farrell DJ, Couturier C, Hryniewicz W. Distribution and antibacterial susceptibility of macrolide resistance genotypes in *Streptococcus pneumoniae*: PROTEKT year 5 (2003-2004). Int J Antimicrob Agents 2008;31(3):245–9.

35. Rubinstein E, Kollef MH, Nathwani D. Pneumonia caused by methicillin-resistant *Staphylococcus aureus*. Clin Infect Dis 2008;46(Suppl 5):S378–85.

36. Kollef MH, Shorr A, Tabak YP, et al. Epidemiology and outcomes of health-care-associated pneumonia: results from a large US database of culture-positive pneumonia. Chest 2005;128(6):3854–62.

37. Vardakas KZ, Matthaiou DK, Falagas ME. Incidence, characteristics and outcomes of patients with severe CA-MRSA pneumonia. Eur Respir J 2009;34: 1148–58.

38. Naimi TS, LeDell KH, Como-Sabetti K, et al. Comparison of community- and health care-associated methicillin-resistant *Staphylococcus aureus* infection. JAMA 2003;290(22):2976–84.

39. King MD, Humphrey BJ, Wang YF, et al. Emergence of community-acquired methicillin-resistant *Staphylococcus aureus* USA 300 clone as the predominant cause of skin and soft-tissue infections. Ann Intern Med 2006;144(5):309–17.

40. Larsen AR, Bocher S, Stegger M, et al. Epidemiology of European community-associated methicillin-resistant *Staphylococcus aureus* clonal complex 80 type IV strains isolated in Denmark from 1993 to 2004. J Clin Microbiol 2008;46(1): 62–8.

41. Tristan A, Bes M, Meugnier H, et al. Global distribution of Panton-Valentine Leukocidin-positive methicillin-resistant *Staphylococcus aureus*, 2006. Emerg Infect Dis 2007;13(4):594–600.

42. Fridkin SK, Hageman JC, Morrison M, et al. Methicillin-resistant *Staphylococcus aureus* disease in three communities. N Engl J Med 2005;352(14):1436–44.

43. Otter JA, Havill NL, Boyce JM, et al. Comparison of community-associated methicillin-resistant *Staphylococcus aureus* from teaching hospitals in London and the USA, 2004-2006: Where is USA300 in the UK? Eur J Clin Microbiol Infect Dis 2009;28(7):835–9.

44. Larsen AR, Stegger M, Bocher S, et al. Emergence and characterization of community-associated methicillin-resistant *Staphylococcus aureus* infections in Denmark, 1999 to 2006. J Clin Microbiol 2009;47(1):73–8.

45. Dauwalder O, Lina G, Durand G, et al. Epidemiology of invasive methicillin-resistant *Staphylococcus aureus* clones collected in France in 2006 and 2007. J Clin Microbiol 2008;46(10):3454–8.

46. Huang YC, Ho CF, Chen CJ, et al. Comparative molecular analysis of community-associated and healthcare-associated methicillin-resistant *Staphylococcus aureus* isolates from children in northern Taiwan. Clin Microbiol Infect 2008; 14(12):1167–72.

47. Kim ES, Song JS, Lee HJ, et al. A survey of community-associated methicillin-resistant *Staphylococcus aureus* in Korea. J Antimicrob Chemother 2007;60(5): 1108–14.

48. Nimmo GR, Coombs GW, Pearson JC, et al. Methicillin-resistant *Staphylococcus aureus* in the Australian community: an evolving epidemic. Med J Aust 2006; 184(8):384–8.

49. Hisata K, Kuwahara-Arai K, Yamanoto M, et al. Dissemination of methicillin-resistant staphylococci among healthy Japanese children. J Clin Microbiol 2005;43(7):3364–72.

50. Labandeira-Rey M, Couzon F, Boisset S, et al. *Staphylococcus aureus* Panton-Valentine Leukocidin causes necrotizing pneumonia. Science 2007;315(5815): 1130–3.

51. Hidron AI, Low CE, Honig EG, et al. Emergence of community-acquired methicillin-resistant *Staphylococcus aureus* strain USA300 as a cause of necrotising community-onset pneumonia. Lancet Infect Dis 2009;9(6):384–92.

52. Ebert MD, Sheth S, Fishman EK. Necrotizing pneumonia caused by community-acquired methicillin-resistant *Staphylococcus aureus*: an increasing cause of "Mayhem in the lung". Emerg Radiol 2009;16(2):159–62.

53. Moore CL, Hingwe A, Donabedian SM, et al. Comparative evaluation of epidemiology and outcomes of methicillin-resistant *Staphylococcus aureus* (MRSA) USA300 infections causing community- and healthcare-associated infections. Int J Antimicrob Agents 2009;34(2):148–55.

54. Mandell LA, Wunderink RG, Anzueto A, et al. Infectious Diseases Society of America/American Thoracic Society consensus guidelines on the management of community-acquired pneumonia in adults. Clin Infect Dis 2007;44(Suppl 2): S27–72.

55. Woodhead M, Blasi F, Ewig S, et al. Guidelines for the management of adult lower respiratory tract infections. Eur Respir J 2005;26(6):1138–80.

56. Masterton RG, Galloway A, French G, et al. Guidelines for the management of hospital-acquired pneumonia in the UK: report of the working party on hospital-acquired pneumonia of the British Society for Antimicrobial Chemotherapy. J Antimicrob Chemother 2008;62(1):5–34.

57. Richards MJ, Edwards JR, Culver DH, et al. Nosocomial infections in combined medical-surgical intensive care units in the United States. Infect Control Hosp Epidemiol 2000;21(8):510–5.

58. Vincent JL, Bihari DJ, Suter PM, et al. The prevalence of nosocomial infection in intensive care units in Europe. Results of the European prevalence of infection in intensive care (EPIC) study. Epic international advisory committee. JAMA 1995; 274(8):639–44.

59. Chastre J, Fagon JY. Ventilator-associated pneumonia. Am J Respir Crit Care Med 2002;165(7):867–903.

60. Chawla R. Epidemiology, etiology, and diagnosis of hospital-acquired pneumonia and ventilator-associated pneumonia in Asian countries. Am J Infect Control 2008;36(Suppl 4):S93–100.

61. Gonzalez BE, Rueda AM, Shelburne SA 3rd, et al. Community-associated strains of methicillin-resistant Staphylococcus aureus as the cause of healthcare-associated infection. Infect Control Hosp Epidemiol 2006;27(10):1051–6.

62. Patel M, Waites KB, Hoesley CJ, et al. Emergence of USA300 MRSA in a tertiary medical centre: implications for epidemiological studies. J Hosp Infect 2008; 68(3):208–13.

63. Athanassa Z, Siempos II, Falagas ME. Impact of methicillin resistance on mortality in Staphylococcus aureus VAP: a systematic review. Eur Respir J 2008;31(3):625–32.

64. Shorr AF, Combes A, Kollef MH, et al. Methicillin-resistant Staphylococcus aureus prolongs intensive care unit stay in ventilator-associated pneumonia, despite initially appropriate antibiotic therapy. Crit Care Med 2006;34(3):700–6.

65. Shorr AF, Tabak YP, Gupta V, et al. Morbidity and cost burden of methicillin-resistant Staphylococcus aureus in early onset ventilator-associated pneumonia. Crit Care 2006;10(3):R97.

66. El Solh AA, Alhajhusain A. Update on the treatment of Pseudomonas aeruginosa pneumonia. J Antimicrob Chemother 2009;64(2):229–38.

67. Gaynes R, Edwards JR, National Nosocomial Infections Surveillance System. Overview of nosocomial infections caused by gram-negative bacilli. Clin Infect Dis 2005;41(6):848–54.

68. Lodise TP Jr, Miller C, Patel N, et al. Identification of patients with Pseudomonas aeruginosa respiratory tract infections at greatest risk of infection with carbapenem-resistant isolates. Infect Control Hosp Epidemiol 2007;28(8): 959–65.

69. Parker CM, Kutsogiannis J, Muscedere J, et al. Ventilator-associated pneumonia caused by multidrug-resistant organisms or Pseudomonas aeruginosa: prevalence, incidence, risk factors, and outcomes. J Crit Care 2008;23(1):18–26.

70. Rossolini GM. Acquired metallo-beta-lactamases: an increasing clinical threat. Clin Infect Dis 2005;41(11):1557–8.

71. Zavascki AP, Barth AL, Fernandes JF, et al. Reappraisal of *Pseudomonas aeruginosa* hospital-acquired pneumonia mortality in the era of metallo-beta-lactamase-mediated multidrug resistance: a prospective observational study. Crit Care 2006;10(4):R114.

72. Rios FG, Luna CM, Maskin B, et al. Ventilator-associated pneumonia due to colistin susceptible-only microorganisms. Eur Respir J 2007;30(2):307–13.

73. Wang CY, Jerng JS, Chen KY, et al. Pandrug-resistant *Pseudomonas aeruginosa* among hospitalised patients: clinical features, risk-factors and outcomes. Clin Microbiol Infect 2006;12(1):63–8.

74. Kanafani ZA, Kara L, Hayek S, et al. Ventilator-associated pneumonia at a tertiary-care center in a developing country: incidence, microbiology, and susceptibility patterns of isolated microorganisms. Infect Control Hosp Epidemiol 2003; 24(11):864–9.

75. Naas T, Coignard B, Carbonne A, et al. VEB-1 extended-spectrum beta-lactamase-producing *Acinetobacter baumannii*, France. Emerg Infect Dis 2006; 12(8):1214–22.

76. Pournaras S, Markogiannakis A, Ikonomidis A, et al. Outbreak of multiple clones of imipenem-resistant *Acinetobacter baumannii* isolates expressing OXA-58 carbapenemase in an intensive care unit. J Antimicrob Chemother 2006;57(3):557–61.

77. Playford EG, Craig JC, Iredell JR. Carbapenem-resistant *Acinetobacter baumannii* in intensive care unit patients: risk factors for acquisition, infection and their consequences. J Hosp Infect 2007;65(3):204–11.

78. Manikal VM, Landman D, Saurina G, et al. Endemic carbapenem-resistant *Acinetobacter* species in Brooklyn, New York: citywide prevalence, interinstitutional spread, and relation to antibiotic usage. Clin Infect Dis 2000;31(1):101–6.

79. Sunenshine RH, Wright MO, Maragakis LL, et al. Multidrug-resistant *Acinetobacter* infection mortality rate and length of hospitalization. Emerg Infect Dis 2007;13(1):97–103.

80. Ko KS, Suh JY, Kwon KT, et al. High rates of resistance to colistin and polymyxin B in subgroups of *Acinetobacter baumannii* isolates from Korea. J Antimicrob Chemother 2007;60(5):1163–7.

81. Wang SH, Sheng WH, Chang YY, et al. Healthcare-associated outbreak due to pan-drug resistant *Acinetobacter baumannii* in a surgical intensive care unit. J Hosp Infect 2003;53(2):97–102.

82. Hsueh PR, Teng LJ, Chen CY, et al. Pandrug-resistant *Acinetobacter baumannii* causing nosocomial infections in a university hospital, Taiwan. Emerg Infect Dis 2002;8(8):827–32.

83. Fagon JY, Chastre J, Domart Y, et al. Mortality due to ventilator-associated pneumonia or colonization with *Pseudomonas* or *Acinetobacter* species: assessment by quantitative culture of samples obtained by a protected specimen brush. Clin Infect Dis 1996;23(3):538–42.

84. Garnacho-Montero J, Ortiz-Leyba C, Fernandez-Hinojosa E, et al. *Acinetobacter baumannii* ventilator-associated pneumonia: epidemiological and clinical findings. Intensive Care Med 2005;31(5):649–55.

85. Garnacho J, Sole-Violan J, Sa-Borges M, et al. Clinical impact of pneumonia caused by *Acinetobacter baumannii* in intubated patients: a matched cohort study. Crit Care Med 2003;31(10):2478–82.

86. Fagon JY, Chastre J, Domart Y, et al. Nosocomial pneumonia in patients receiving continuous mechanical ventilation. Prospective analysis of 52 episodes with use of a protected specimen brush and quantitative culture techniques. Am Rev Respir Dis 1989;139(4):877–84.

87. Reinert RR, Low DE, Rossi F, et al. Antimicrobial susceptibility among organisms from the Asia/Pacific Rim, Europe and Latin and North America collected as part of test and the in vitro activity of tigecycline. J Antimicrob Chemother 2007;60(5): 1018–29.
88. Hawkey PM. Prevalence and clonality of extended-spectrum beta-lactamases in Asia. Clin Microbiol Infect 2008;14(Suppl 1):159–65.
89. Canton R, Novais A, Valverde A, et al. Prevalence and spread of extended-spectrum beta-lactamase-producing Enterobacteriaceae in Europe. Clin Microbiol Infect 2008;14(Suppl 1):144–53.
90. Bush K. Extended-spectrum beta-lactamases in North America, 1987-2006. Clin Microbiol Infect 2008;14(Suppl 1):134–43.
91. Falagas ME, Karageorgopoulos DE. Extended-spectrum beta-lactamase-producing organisms. J Hosp Infect 2009;73:345–54.
92. Nordmann P, Cuzon G, Naas T. The real threat of *Klebsiella pneumoniae* carbapenemase-producing bacteria. Lancet Infect Dis 2009;9(4):228–36.
93. Song JH, Asian Hospital Acquired Pneumonia Working G. Treatment recommendations of hospital-acquired pneumonia in Asian countries: first consensus report by the Asian HAP working group. Am J Infect Control 2008;36(Suppl 4):S83–92.
94. Garnacho-Montero J, Sa-Borges M, Sole-Violan J, et al. Optimal management therapy for *Pseudomonas aeruginosa* ventilator-associated pneumonia: an observational, multicenter study comparing monotherapy with combination antibiotic therapy. Crit Care Med 2007;35(8):1888–95.

Occupation-Related Respiratory Infections Revisited

Daphne Ling, MPH[a], Dick Menzies, MD, MSc[b],*

KEYWORDS

- Tuberculosis • Nosocomial transmission • Infection control
- Occupational health

Tuberculosis (TB) is the best known, and most studied, occupational respiratory infectious disease. The wealth of published information regarding nosocomial transmission of TB can provide insight into the risks, mechanisms, and potential preventive measures for the nosocomial transmission of other airborne infections including severe acute respiratory syndrome (SARS), influenza, measles, varicella, and anthrax. The study of occupational TB is particularly informative because transmission can be monitored in 2 ways. The cumulative or periodic incidence of latent infection can be estimated using tests of immune reactions to TB antigens, such as the tuberculin skin test (TST).[1] Transmission that results in disease can be measured with a high degree of specificity using molecular epidemiologic tools such as restriction fragment length polymorphism (RFLP) analysis.[2]

Much of the information regarding risk, risk factors, and prevention of nosocomial transmission is derived from studies conducted in high-income countries.[3] There was considerable interest in this topic in the preantibiotic era, but this waned with the introduction of effective antibiotics.[4] However, the coincident advent of human immunodeficiency virus (HIV) infection and multidrug-resistant (MDR) TB resulted in several major outbreaks in high-income countries, particularly the United States. In a few of these outbreaks more than half of exposed patients became infected, developed disease, and died.[5] In the same hospitals a large number of health care workers were infected, although few developed disease and even fewer died.[5] These outbreaks led to renewed interest in the prevention of transmission of airborne respiratory infections. In the past decade attention has shifted to workers in low- and middle-income countries (LMIC), where risk of disease may be high.[3,6]

[a] Respiratory Epidemiology & Clinical Research Unit, Montreal Chest Institute, McGill University, 3650 St Urbain, Room K1.20, Montreal, QC H2X 2P4, Canada
[b] Respiratory Epidemiology & Clinical Research Unit, Montreal Chest Institute, McGill University, 3650 St Urbain, Room K1.24, Montreal, QC H2X 2P4, Canada
* Corresponding author.
E-mail address: dick.menzies@mcgill.ca

Infect Dis Clin N Am 24 (2010) 655–680
doi:10.1016/j.idc.2010.04.013
0891-5520/10/$ – see front matter © 2010 Elsevier Inc. All rights reserved.

id.theclinics.com

RISK AND RISK FACTORS FOR TB INFECTION AND DISEASE

Several narrative and systematic reviews have been published on the risk of TB infection and disease among health care workers in high-income[4,5] and LMIC.[3,6] Nosocomial TB transmission has also been reviewed in guidelines issued by authoritative agencies including the US Centers for Disease Control[7] and most recently the World Health Organization.[8]

Until recently prevalence and incidence of latent TB infection (LTBI) could be measured only with the TST. In the past decade interferon γ release assays (IGRA) have been increasingly used to measure LTBI prevalence.[9,10] However, few studies have measured incidence of TB infection through serial performance of IGRA. Although IGRA have significantly better specificity in bacille Calmette-Guérin (BCG)-vaccinated populations,[9,10] their ability to predict who will develop active TB is unclear. In addition, studies of serial IGRA testing have reported substantial rates of conversion and spontaneous reversion.[11,12] Until these issues are clarified the usefulness of IGRA for estimation of nosocomial transmission remains questionable, although this is an area of active research. Hence this review focuses on studies using TST to detect prevalent and incident LTBI.

As summarized in **Table 1** a large number of studies have estimated risk of TB infection or disease. Although the estimates are variable, there is consistent evidence that the prevalence and incidence of LTBI in health care workers is substantially higher than the general population, in all settings. In high-income countries the pooled risk of TB disease among workers is only twice that of the general population, whereas the risk of infection is 10 times higher. In low-income countries disease and infection are about 5-fold higher than the general population. The reason for the difference in relative risk between infection and disease in high-income countries may reflect the healthy worker effect[53] or may reflect overestimation of LTBI because of the nonspecificity of tuberculin skin testing in BCG-vaccinated populations.

Risk factors associated with TB infection and disease in all countries are summarized in **Table 2**. Despite the differences in levels of exposure, risk factors are similar. Most of these risk factors can be interpreted to indicate simply that infection and disease are proportionate to likelihood of exposure to patients with TB. It is self-evident that more years of work, in jobs that involve direct patient care, and in hospitals or units caring for more patients with TB, are more likely to result in TB infection and disease. One useful indicator is the number of patients with TB per worker,[3,5] because the same number of patients with TB inevitably creates greater probability of exposure if cared for by a small group of workers, than the per-worker exposure

Table 1
Summary of risk of TB in health care workers relative to general populations

	Studies (N)	Relative Risk	References
LTBI			
High-income countries	27	10.1	[13–38]
LMIC	9	5.8	[39–47]
Active TB disease			
High-income countries	12	2.0	[48–57]
LMIC	20 (222)	5.7	[58–79]

Data from World Health Organization, Stop TB Department. WHO policy on TB infection control in health-care facilities, congregate settings and households. Geneva (Switzerland): World Health Organization; 2009.

Table 2
Occupational risk factors for TB

General	Specific	LMIC References	High-income References
LTBI			
Exposure	Years of work	44,45,47,58,80–82	37
	TB admissions	—	37
	Known TB contact	43,58	18,37,83
Type of work	Health care/patient care	45,84	83,85
	Physicians	80,86	37,87
	Nurses	45,80,86	21,37,85,88
	Respiratory therapists	58	85
	Trainees	—	18
Location of work	Medical ward	58,81,89	21,88
	HIV ward/care	—	21
	Emergency	86	16
	Laboratory/pathology	86	88,90
	TB ward/clinic	—	18
TB disease			
Exposure	—	—	—
Type of work	Health care/patient care	—	49,50,53,56
	Physicians	63,68,72,73	51,53,55
	Nurses	61,63,67,68,70–73	52,53,55
	Respiratory therapists	—	52
	Trainees	—	54
Location of work	Medical ward	58,70,72,91	—
	TB ward/clinic	58,59,62,66,70,72	—
	HIV ward/clinic	—	—
	Emergency	58,70	—
	Laboratory/pathology	58,63	—

risk in a larger hospital. Other risk factors relate to increased chance of exposure to undiagnosed patients; these include work in emergency departments, or HIV services (the latter because of the atypical clinical manifestations of TB in HIV-coinfected patients). The third category of risk factor relates to specific activities that increase patients' contagiousness. For example, respiratory therapists,[52,92] and pathology workers[2,90,93] have been consistently identified as high-risk workers, because certain of their tasks can result in aerosolization of TB bacilli (eg, intubation,[94,95] sputum induction,[96,97] bronchoscopy,[98] or autopsy[99,100]).

These epidemiologic observations have improved our understanding of nosocomial transmission, and guided the development of infection control recommendations. The consistent observation that risk is proportional to the number of patients with TB per worker has resulted in risk-stratified recommendations: large hospitals with few patients with TB are required to implement fewer measures to prevent nosocomial TB transmission than hospitals with more TB cases. The knowledge that workers in high-incidence countries have 5 times greater risk of infection and disease than the general population has led to the realization that TB is the most common and serious occupational illness in these countries. This finding has stimulated concerted efforts to raise awareness, not least among the workers themselves, many of whom have a stoic and fatalistic approach to occupational TB. This finding also resulted in development of guidelines for TB control in resource poor settings,[101] which have been updated recently.[8]

The identification of high-risk professionals such as respiratory therapists or pathology workers led to the realization that certain tasks were high-risk activities, such as bronchoscopy or autopsy. This finding in turn led to specific infection-control measures for these activities. The identification of increased risk associated with work in emergency departments resulted in administrative measures in these departments to improve triage and separation of patients suspected of TB.

INTERVENTIONS TO PREVENT NOSOCOMIAL TB TRANSMISSION

Interventions to prevent nosocomial TB transmission are generally divided into 3 broad categories: administrative, personal, and engineering.[7] These categories are often referred to as a hierarchy of control measures. Administrative controls are institutional policies that have the general aim of reducing the time between arrival of a patient at a health care facility and their placement in respiratory isolation, definitive diagnosis, and initiation of effective treatment. These controls include rapid triage of patients suspected of active TB, rapid performance of chest radiographs or other screening tests, expeditious processing of sputum samples for acid-fast bacillus (AFB) smear and culture, and more rapid separation of patients with TB (usually in isolation rooms). Personal controls are measures directed at individual workers. These measures include use of personal respirators (masks) and screening for, and treatment of, latent or active TB. Engineering controls are environmental measures that act to reduce the likelihood of workers' exposure to viable airborne TB bacilli. These controls include ventilation to remove and/or dilute airborne bacilli, and to ensure correct direction of flow of contaminated air, and ultraviolet germicidal irradiation (UVGI), which kills airborne bacilli.

As shown in **Table 3**, several studies have examined the effect on indicators of nosocomial transmission when multiple interventions were applied simultaneously. Harries and colleagues[65] implemented a program in 40 facilities in Malawi to train workers to triage, and separate patients with TB, and to enhance natural ventilation. These efforts resulted in a modest decline in overall TB incidence, which was not statistically significant. However, compliance with these measures was suboptimal. In Thailand, 1202 health care workers had serial tuberculin testing before and after administrative, personal, and engineering measures were instituted in one provincial referral hospital. Incidence of LTBI declined substantially but incidence of disease increased.[47] However, the increase in disease may have been a result of a concomitant increase in HIV prevalence, and because the number of patients with TB almost doubled at the same time. In 2 Brazilian hospitals incidence of TST conversion was 8 per 1000 person-months following implementation of the full hierarchy of administrative, personal, and engineering controls, compared with 16 per 1000 person-months in 2 other hospitals without any TB infection-control measures.[45]

Delays in institution of adequate isolation, or diagnosis and institution of effective therapy, have been consistently identified as important factors in almost all reports of nosocomial TB outbreaks.[5] The importance of administrative measures has been identified in a modeling study,[107] but the epidemiologic evidence of the effectiveness of these measures is limited, because, as shown in **Table 4**, few studies have implemented these measures alone. In one Italian hospital, the occurrence of new MDR disease among patients was eliminated after implementation of administrative measures alone.[108] In a US hospital TST conversion was reduced 80% by administrative measures alone.[109] In the Malawi study most of the changes were administrative; these had minimal effect, but as noted earlier, compliance with the measures was poor.[65] In 2 US hospitals administrative measures were introduced first, and interim tuberculin testing was performed before implementation of the rest of the infection control measures. In both hospitals incidence of TST conversion decreased significantly after the implementation of the administrative measures.[110,111] Administrative controls are the cheapest and simplest measures to implement, and all evidence suggests that they are effective and important. Hence, implementation of administrative control measures should be the first priority in all health care facilities.

Personal respirators or masks were the subject of considerable confusion in the early 1990s. Infection control and occupational health practitioners, regulatory agencies, and researchers struggled with conflicting recommendations and confusing terminology regarding personal respirators. In 1994 a single standard was recommended: that personal respirators (masks) should filter at least 95% of particles of 1 μm or larger, with less than 10% face seal air leak.[112] Respirators meeting these standards are referred to as N-95. Given that TB bacilli are 3 to 5 μm in length, these masks should filter at least 95% of TB bacilli out of the air inhaled by health care workers. Modeling studies have concluded that personal respirators should work well.[113] On the other hand, there is no epidemiologic evidence of their effectiveness. No studies have been published in which only personal respirators were implemented. Some modeling studies have found that the effect of personal respirators is modest if they are used in a setting with proper engineering control measures.[114] Fit testing of personal respirators is particularly controversial because studies have shown that the results of fit testing are not reliable or reproducible.[115,116] Nevertheless, most regulatory authorities and most health care institutions insist on fit testing because in theory a better-fitting personal respirator should provide more protection than one that allows some leakage.

Virtually all TB transmission occurs indoors. The risk of TB transmission outdoors is considered virtually nil, because of the bactericidal effect of sunlight as well as the rapid dispersion and dilution of airborne bacilli.[117] Ventilation can reduce the risk of indoor transmission by removal and dilution of airborne TB bacilli.[118] As shown in **Fig. 1**, the concentration of any airborne particles, including TB bacilli, can be reduced effectively with greater air exchange rates. However, the incremental gains diminish as air exchange rates are progressively increased, and the energy costs and construction/capital costs to achieve these higher air exchange rates increase considerably.[119] Natural ventilation, through open windows and doors, can achieve high air exchange rates,[120] but the direction of airflow within the building is unpredictable, as it is largely determined by outdoor temperature and wind direction.[85,121] This situation means that contaminated air from a TB patient's room can move to other occupied areas including staff rooms and other patient rooms. Natural ventilation also has limitations when outdoor temperatures are very high or very low.

When properly designed and installed, mechanical ventilation can control direction of airflow and achieve adequate outdoor air exchange rates. However, the initial capital costs for mechanical ventilation systems are high, as are the operating costs. The latter reflect the need for trained personnel to operate mechanical ventilation systems constantly, and to inspect and maintain them regularly. Energy costs of mechanical ventilation can be substantial in very cold or very hot climates,[119] particularly if high outdoor air exchange rates are mandated.

The effect of ventilation alone has been examined in only 3 studies, summarized in **Table 5**. In a Canadian study of 1274 workers in 17 hospitals, nurses and respiratory therapists who worked on units with ventilation of less than 2 air changes per hour in general patient rooms and wards (ie, nonisolation rooms) had a 3.8 times higher risk of tuberculin conversion than those who worked on units with better ventilation in general wards.[92] Air exchange rates in respiratory isolation rooms were not associated with

Table 3
Effect of administrative, personal, and engineering control measures applied concurrently on nosocomial transmission of TB

LMIC

Author, Year Country Facilities Year of intervention	Preventive Strategy Used			Epidemiologic Measure in Absence of Preventive Measure	Epidemiologic Measure in Presence of Preventive Measure	Effect
	Administrative	Personal	Engineering			
Harries 2002,[65] Malawi 40 TB care facilities (1998)	(1) Priority to patients with chronic cough in OPD (2) Rapid sputum collection, transport and reporting (3) Visitors kept to a minimum (4) CXR at quiet times of the day (5) Patients with TB spend more day time outdoors when possible	(1) Proper cough hygiene (2) Mask worn by patients with TB when undergoing surgical procedures	(1) Increased natural ventilation (2) Windows left open most of the time	Incidence of TB disease before prevention (1996) Clin officer 7407 Pt attd 5014 Wd attd 3543 TB officer 3030 Nurses 2835 Overall 3707	Incidence of TB disease after prevention (1999) Clin officer 3603 Pt attd 4348 Wd attd 3954 TB officer 1785 Nurses 2060 Overall 3222	Incidence of TB disease declined after preventive measures used. Statistically NS
Yanai 2003,[47] Thailand Provincial referral hospital (1997–98)	(1) Early suspicion of TB (2) Early sputum collection and reporting (3) Early initiation of TB treatment (4) Isolation of patients with TB (5) One-stop OPD TB service	(1) N95 mask use by HCWs (2) HEPA filter in laboratory areas	(1) TB isolation room in wards (2) Maximizing ventilation in wards (3) Class II safety cabinets in laboratory (4) UVGI system in laboratory	Incidence of TB disease control measures (1995–1997) All HCWs 179.21 Annual incidence of LTBI before control measures (1995–97) 9.3% (3.3%–15.3%)	Incidence of TB disease after control measures (1999) All HCWs 252.68 Annual incidence of LTBI after control measures (1999) 2.2% (0%–5.1%)	Increase in TB disease Statistically NS Decrease in LTBI rates Statistically significant
Roth 2005,[45] Brazil, 2 hospitals with, and 2 without control measures (1998)	(1) Rapid diagnosis and treatment of Patients with TB (2) Isolation of patients with TB in private rooms	(1) N95 mask use by HCWs (2) HEPA filter in laboratory areas	(1) Negative pressure rooms[a] (one hospital) (2) Class II biosafety cabinets in laboratory areas	Incidence of LTBI in 2 hospitals without control measures (1998–99) 16 per 1000 person-months	Incidence of LTBI in 2 hospitals with control measures (1998–99) 8 per 1000 person-months	Difference in LTBI rates Statistically significant

High-Income Countries

Author, Year Country	Workers Facilities Year of Intervention	TST Baseline Conversion Definition	Infection Control Strategy Used			Outcomes		
			Administrative	Personal	Engineering	Measure	Before	After
Wenger 1990[102] United States	All HCW 1 hospital 1991	1-Step $T_1<10$, $T_2 \geq 10$ mm TST ≥ 10 mm and ↑6+ mm	↑Isolation ↑Speed for AFB Sputum induction in respiratory isolation rooms	TST every 4 mo Sub-μm masks Dust-mist masks	Auto door closers Negative pressure isolation rooms	Conv/tested ARI	7/25 28%	3/17 18%
Maloney 1991[103] United States	All HCW 1 hospital 1991	1-Step $T_1<10$, $T_2 \geq 10$ mm	↑Isolation ↑Treatment ↑Speed for AFB	Molded surgical masks	Window exhaust fans	Conv/tested ARI	26/840 3.1%	22/727 3.0%
Fella 1991[104] United States	All HCW 1 hospital 1991–1993	1-Step $T_1<10$, $T_2 \geq 10$ mm	↑Isolation	Better mask (dust-mist)	Window exhaust fans Upper air UV light	Conv/tested ARI	30/145 21%	51/1007 5.1%
Bangsberg 1992[105] United States	Residents 1 hospital 1992	1-Step $T_1<10$, $T_2 \geq 10$ mm and ↑6+ mm	↑Isolation	Respiratory masks	Negative pressure rooms in ER+OPD Upper-air UV lights	Conv/tested ARI	11/90 5.4%	1/90 0.7%
Blumberg 1992[106] United States	All HCW 1 hospital 1991–1992	1-Step $T_1<10$, $T_2 \geq 10$ mm	↑Respiratory isolation	TST every 6 months Sub-μm masks	Window exhaust fans	Conv/tested ARI	118/3579 3.3%	185/17618 1.1%
Boudreau 1997[18] United States	All HCW 1 hospital 1989–1992	1-Step $T_1<10$, $T_2 \geq 10$ mm	Drug therapy improved ↑Isolation procedures Worker education	Better masks	Sputum induction booth UV lights	ARI in HCW	6.9%	1.9%
Blumberg 1998[17] United States	Residents 1 hospital 1992–1997	1-Step $T_1<10$, $T_2 \geq 10$ mm	Isolation procedures TB infection control nurse	Better masks TST of HCWs	50 respiratory isolation rooms	ARI in HCW	6%	1.1%
Louther 1997[26] United States	All HCW 1 hospital 1991–1994	1-Step $T_1<10$, $T_2 \geq 10$ mm and ↑10+ mm	↑Isolation	Better masks	↑Ventilation	ARI in HCW	7.2%	4.8%

Abbreviations: ARI, annual risk of infection; Clin officer, clinical officer; Conv, conversions; CXR, chest radiograph; ER, emergency room; HCW, health care worker; HEPA, high-efficiency particulate air; NS, nonsignificant; OPD, outpatient department; Pt attd, patient attendant; Wd attd, ward attendant.
a Single rooms, R6 air changes per hour, negative pressure or inward airflow, automatic door closing.

Table 4
Effect of administrative measures (triage and separation of patients with TB) (studies in which effect of administrative measures only were studied)

Author (References)	Country	Year of Intervention	Effect Measured in	Outcome Measure	Before	After
Moro[108]	Italy	1993	Patients	New MDR disease	26/90	0/44
Jarvis[109]	United States	1995	HCWs	TST conversion	14.6%	2.9%

Abbreviation: HCW, health care worker.

workers' tuberculin conversion rates.[92] In the same study laboratory workers had greater rates of tuberculin conversions if they worked in laboratories or autopsy suites with lower ventilation levels.[90] A single study has reported on TST conversion rates before and after improvements in ventilation only.[16] In the emergency department of a US hospital, 4 respiratory isolation rooms were created, recirculation of air was eliminated, and laminar airflow introduced. Following these measures tuberculin conversion declined substantially among staff in the emergency department and in other departments (possibly because of reduced recirculation of air from the emergency departments to these other departments).[16]

UVGI is an older technology that was evaluated extensively in the preantibiotic era. With the advent of effective antibiotic therapy, UVGI fell into disuse (along with most aspects of TB infection control). UVGI also fell into disrepute because of concerns regarding skin cancer. These concerns were completely unfounded because the type of ultraviolet irradiation generated by the lamps (UV-C) does not penetrate the skin and so cannot cause mutagenesis in the skin.[117,122] Direct exposure to UVGI can cause skin rash (similar to sunburn) and keratoconjunctivitis (similar to snow blindness). Outbreaks of both conditions have been reported, and all have been mild and self-limited.[122] In every instance these outbreaks were caused by errors in the installation, or operation of the lamps.[122]

Modern lamps are designed to minimize risk of direct exposure. Usually these are installed above eye level in rooms with reflectors so that only the upper air in the

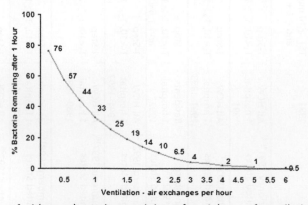

Fig. 1. Percent of airborne bacteria remaining after 1 hour of ventilation at different exchange rates.

Table 5
Effect of ventilation on nosocomial TB transmission (studies in which effect of ventilation alone was studied)

Author (References)	Country	Year of Intervention	Ventilation	Outcome Measure	Effect Measured in		N	Outcomes	
					Type			Lower Ventilation	Higher Ventilation
Menzies[90,92]	Canada	1996–98	Mechanical	Relative risk of cumulative TST conversion	Nurses, respiratory therapists		1270	3.8	1.0
					Laboratory workers		120	1.3	1.0
Behrman[16]	United States	1993–96	4 respiratory isolation rooms	TST conversion per 6 months	Emergency department staff		88	10.5%	0
			Nonrecirculating air laminar airflow		Other departments		3000	5.0%	1.2%

room is irradiated. Occasionally such lamps have caused eye irritation as a result of reflected UV light from glossy ceilings.[122] This reflection can be eliminated by use of low-gloss ceiling paint or louvered lamps so that the UV light is emitted only in a narrow beam in the upper air. Effectiveness of UVGI is summarized in **Table 6**. Effect of UVGI installation on TST conversion among hospital workers has been reported in 4 studies. In all 4, the incidence of tuberculin conversion declined substantially, but this may have been a result of other interventions, because UVGI was one of several interventions introduced at the same time. Two studies have irradiated upper air in rooms of patients with TB with UVGI; the air exhausted from these rooms was fed through an animal enclosure. In both studies, animals exposed to air from rooms with UV irradiation had substantially reduced incidence of TB infection and disease.[123,124,128] In vitro studies have also shown the high potency of UVGI in reducing the number of viable airborne BCG,[129] or viable mycobacterial cultures in solid media. Despite solid animal evidence of efficacy and clear evidence that it is safe for humans, authoritative agencies remain reluctant to endorse use of UVGI. As summarized in **Table 7**, UVGI has many advantages compared with mechanical ventilation in terms of proven effectiveness, low initial and recurrent costs, as well as proven safety, yet authoritative agencies continue to recommend it only as an adjunct measure.

SARS

The SARS epidemic from November 2002 until July 2003 provided many important observations regarding determinants and prevention of nosocomial transmission. Interest in infection control with SARS was high because no effective vaccine or treatment was available at the time of the epidemic, and a high proportion of all SARS cases occurred as a result of nosocomial transmission. Ultimately the epidemic subsided following strict enforcement of control measures within health care facilities and in the community. Hence, this epidemic provides many important lessons that are applicable for prevention of nosocomial transmission of TB and influenza.

Several features of SARS were unusual. First, the incubation period was longer than typical for influenza or other respiratory tract viral infections (4–6 days instead of 1–2 days; see **Table 8**) and the course of the illness was slower.[147] Of particular relevance for nosocomial transmission, in most patients the viral load and viral shedding increased to a peak about 10 to 12 days after the onset of symptoms, following which there was a slow decline.[146,147] Because patients typically sought medical care and were hospitalized after a few days of symptoms they became progressively more contagious after their arrival in health care facilities. This situation may have accounted for the disproportionate share of transmission that occurred within health care facilities; it was estimated that 78% of all cases in Singapore, among patients and health care workers, resulted from nosocomial transmission.[150] Overall, health care workers accounted for 21% of all cases,[132] although in most countries they account for only 2% to 3% of the adult population. A rough estimate is that the risk of disease in health care workers was approximately 10-fold higher than the general population. A similar estimate can be derived from Hong Kong, where there was more extensive community transmission, yet the rates in health care workers were more than 10 times higher than the community rates in the worst affected areas.[141]

This situation is similar to TB in high-income countries; community transmission is rare, and patients are often hospitalized when they present with symptoms. After admission, contagiousness and transmission often increase, because the diagnosis is missed or delayed by days to weeks.[156]

Table 6
Effect of improved UVGI only on nosocomial TB transmission

Author (References)	Country	Year of Intervention	Intervention Measured in Type	N	Outcomes	Before UVGI	After UVGI	Reduction (%)
Studies of HCWs[a]								
Bourdeau[18]	United States	1989–91	All HCWs		TST conv/y	21%	5.1%	76
Fella[104]	United States	1991	All HCWs	1000	TST conv/y	6.9%	1.9%	72
Bangsberg[105]	United States	1991–92	Trainees (residents)	90	TST conv/y	5.4%	0.7%	87
Yanai[b],[47]	Thailand	1997–98	All HCWs	1202	TST conv/y	9.3%	2.2%	76
Studies of laboratory animals								
Riley[123]	United States	1957	Guinea pigs	ns	BCG infection	100%	0	100
Escombe[124]	Peru	2008	Guinea pigs	150	MTB infection	106	29	72
					MTB disease	26	11	60
Studies of microbes								
Ray[125]	United States	1957	Culture plates		Viable MTB	150–350	15–30	90
Riley[126]	United States	1976	Airborne BCG		BCG killing	9	1	90
Xu[127]	United States	2003	Airborne BCG		Viable airborne BCG	5.7×10^4	3.2×10^3	96

Abbreviations: conv, conversions; HCW, health care worker; MTB, *Mycobacterium tuberculosis.*
[a] All 4 studies in health care workers involved multiple interventions applied concurrently. Hence, the reduction seen may have been caused by other interventions (partially or entirely).
[b] UVGI applied in laboratory areas only. In this study there was no reduction in incidence of disease.

Table 7
Comparison of engineering control measures: ventilation versus UVGI (a gap between evidence and recommendations?)

Parameters	Mechanical Ventilation	UVGI
Maximum air exchange rate[a]	12–15	20–25
Effectiveness		
Proved	—	—
In workers	Partially	Partially
In animals	No	Yes
In vitro	No	Yes
Safety		
In theory	Yes	Yes
Shown in workers	No	Yes
Costs		
Initial capital costs	Very high	Moderate
Recurrent costs	—	—
Maintenance	High	Low
Energy	Moderate-High	Low
Personnel (operation)	Moderate	None
Personnel (inspection)	Low	Low
Recommendations (reference)		
United States[7]	Primary mode	Adjunct measure
Canada[130]	Primary mode	Use when recommended ventilation cannot be achieved
WHO[8]	Primary mode	Use when recommended ventilation cannot be achieved

[a] Maximum outdoor air exchange rate that can reasonably be achieved in occupied spaces, yet maintain noise, draft, and temperature within human comfort range. For UVGI this refers to the removal of viable airborne organisms that would be achieved with equivalent levels of ventilation.

Another feature of the SARS epidemic was that a few patients were identified as more contagious than others, so-called superspreaders of the epidemic (SSEs).[137,152,157] One of these persons transmitted SARS to several others on the same floor in a hotel,[141] and another to more than 50 others living in the same apartment complex but different buildings.[137] Neither patient had any direct contact with these secondary cases, supporting the possibility of airborne spread. Reasons for this contagiousness were not identified, but again there is a close parallel with TB. In several studies, the contagiousness of patients with TB has varied widely.[123,158,159] Although contagiousness is generally correlated with extent of pulmonary disease, it is substantially increased if there is laryngeal involvement.[123,159] One can only speculate why the phenomenon of SARS superspreaders occurred, but it seems these few patients were efficient generators of infectious aerosols.

Delayed diagnosis was common to all outbreaks of SARS, as with TB. Triage and separation of patients proved important in containing SARS epidemic, as shown in **Table 9**, another parallel with TB. Other administrative measures, particularly

Table 8
Key epidemiologic and clinical features of influenza A (including H$_1$N$_1$) and SARS

Features	Influenza A Values (References)	SARS Values (References)
Incubation	1.4 days[131]	4.6–6.4 days[132,133]
Transmission		
Mode	Primary droplet[134] Possible contact Possible airborne[134,136] —	Primary droplet[132] Fecal-oral[135] Possible contact[135] Possible airborne[137,138]
Asymptomatic	Minimal[139]	None[140,141]
Increased by	Intubation —	Intubation[142–144] NIPPV[a,144,145]
Infectiousness (new infections per case)	1.8–20.0	2.4–2.7[146,147]
Duration of contagiousness	3 days[b,131]	10–20 days[146,147]
Nosocomial transmission		
Outbreaks shown	Yes[139,148,149]	All reports
% Nosocomial	Unknown–low[148,149]	78% in Singapore[150]
Transmission to HCWs		
Estimated risk of infection	No estimates	1%–3% per h[143,151]
HCW as % of all cases	No estimates	21%[132]
Incidence		
Total global cases	401, 276 (H$_1$N$_1$ as of September 25, 2009)[c]	8098 (as of July 2003)[132]
Severity (% admitted to ICU)	3.8% (Quebec)	19%–34%[132,141,152]
Mortality (overall)	1.1%[153]	9.6%[132]
age <60 y	—	2.9%–7.0%[141,143]
age >60 y	—	53%–55%[141,143]
HCWs (all ages)	—	2%[141]

Abbreviations: HCW, health care worker; ICU, intensive care unit; NIPPV, nasal intermittent positive pressure ventilation.

[a] Noninvasive positive pressure ventilation such as continuous positive airway pressure or bilevel positive airway pressure.

[b] Contagiousness estimate for nonimmunocompromised adult. Duration is longer if immunocompromised,[154] severely ill[155] or young infant.[154]

[c] US estimates were that more than 1 million cases had occurred in the United States alone by September 12, 2009.[153]

isolation of symptomatic health care workers, limited the health care workers as a source of nosocomial transmission, an important message for influenza control (see later discussion). Personal protective measures seemed the most important in containing the spread of SARS. In almost all situations in which full protective measures were implemented, there was no further nosocomial transmission.[135,145] In an analysis of workers who became infected with SARS despite using full personal protective equipment, lapses or breaches in infection-control procedures were found that could explain every apparent failure.[142] In one ward in a Hong Kong hospital, more than 20 patients were placed on noninvasive positive ventilation, a significant

Table 9
Evidence of importance and effectiveness of infection control measures for influenza and SARS

Influence Control Measures	Influenza Studies Showing Benefit, N (References)	SARS Studies Showing Benefit, N (References)
Administrative		
Triage/separation of patients	2[154,160]	2[135,150]
Reduce crowding	1[136]	1[144]
Screen/furlough sick workers	2[154,161]	2[144,150]
Personal		
Vaccination of health care worker	3[162–164]	No vaccine available
Knowledge/training in infection control	—	1[165]
Hand washing	—	2[144,166]
Masks: surgical or N-95	1[167],[a]	2[151,166] [b,c]
Compliance with all measures	—	3[142,165,166]
Engineering		
UVGI	1[168]	—
Ventilation (risk factor, not intervention)	2[136,169]	1 (Ha 2004)
Full hierarchy of measures	1[160]	2[143,150]
Most important measure	Vaccination	Infection control

[a] Loeb 2009[167]: Randomized controlled trial of surgical versus N-95 masks: no difference in sero-conversion of workers.
[b] Seto 2003[166]: paper masks were not effective; surgical and N-95 were not different.
[c] Loeb 2004[151]: N-95 masks were better than surgical masks, which were better than no masks.

risk factor for aerosolization of infectious particles.[144,145] All workers on this ward were required to be meticulous in their infection-control procedures and use of personal protective equipment; despite the intense exposure, none became infected with SARS.

One controversial issue with regard to personal protective measures remains the type of respiratory protection, or masks. In one survey, nonuse of masks was clearly associated with increased risk of SARS,[165] whereas in another use of either surgical or N-95 masks was protective, although use of paper masks was not.[166] In a Toronto study, use of N-95 masks was associated with greater protection than use of surgical masks, and both type of masks were associated with greater protection than no mask use.[151] Need for N-95 masks depends on the mode of transmission. If transmission is solely by droplet, then face shields, eye protection, and surgical masks are adequate. However, if transmission is airborne, than N-95 masks should be used. As reviewed earlier, there is evidence that airborne transmission of SARS occurred, at least from the superspreaders[137,152] or during aerosol-generating activities such as intubation or suctioning.[142–144,151] Given that superspreaders are identified only in retrospect, it may be more prudent for workers to wear N-95 masks at all times.

Ventilation of occupied indoor spaces is important for diluting and removing airborne contaminants. This practice can help prevent nosocomial transmission of airborne pathogens. As reviewed earlier there is some evidence that SARS could be transmitted by the airborne route; this was the most plausible explanation for the community outbreak.[138] The ward in which nasal intermittent positive pressure ventilation was used achieved high air exchange rates with exhaust fans, which may have helped prevent nosocomial transmission. The efficacy of UVGI was not studied with SARS.

INFLUENZA

There is less information regarding the determinants, and effective prevention, of nosocomial transmission. This situation reflects the availability, for more than 20 years, of an effective vaccine. Also, influenza is typically less severe, with lower case fatality rates than SARS. Influenza also has a shorter incubation period, so that patients are more quickly contagious during the symptomatic phase than with SARS. Hence, there is greater community transmission, making it difficult to identify and study nosocomial influenza transmission. The new pandemic of H_1N_1, which spread rapidly through air travel,[170] and caused millions of cases,[153] before a vaccine became available, underscores the importance of understanding the determinants of nosocomial transmission of influenza, to implement effective infection control.

The effect of nosocomial transmission of influenza is difficult to estimate but there have been well-documented outbreaks in nursing homes, intensive care units, and general medical facilities.[149] Attack rates in these outbreaks ranged from 11% to 59% overall, and from 8% to 63% in exposed health care workers.[149] Mortality among patients ranged from 0% to 66%, with highest mortality among elderly nursing home residents[140,171] and very young infants.[149] Individuals with other immunocompromising conditions are also highly susceptible. An additional problem created by nosocomial influenza transmission is the large number of health care workers who may become ill and unable to work.[163] Their absenteeism may create significant problems in delivery of care, at a time when they are needed most.

As with SARS and TB, delayed diagnosis of cases is a common feature of nosocomial influenza outbreaks.[149] In these outbreaks, health care workers were the most commonly identified source cases,[149] as well as frequently playing a major role in spreading the infection from patient to patient.[148,171] Two studies have reported that screening workers to identify those with influenza and send them home was an effective measure to prevent nosocomial outbreaks.[154]

Little attention has been given to the importance of personal protective equipment such as gowns, gloves, and masks in practice and in guidelines for prevention and management of influenza.[172,173] This situation is because vaccination of health care workers has been shown to reduce or prevent nosocomial transmission.[148,155,163] In one randomized trial, vaccinating health care workers reduced mortality among elderly people in nursing homes.[162] Treatment of influenza with antivirals is effective for individual benefit, but the effect of antiviral therapy on community or nosocomial transmission has not been studied.

The role of airborne transmission of influenza in nosocomial outbreaks is controversial, because the evidence is limited. As reviewed elsewhere,[134,148] there is convincing animal and in vitro evidence that airborne transmission of influenza can occur. There is also evidence from a limited number of outbreaks that supports the role of airborne transmission.[136] As with SARS and TB, a few individuals may be extremely contagious and contribute to airborne transmission, or particularly contagious during aerosol-generating procedures such as intubation or noninvasive ventilation. Given this uncertainty, it seems prudent for nonvaccinated workers to use N-95 masks, particularly during high-risk procedures or with very ill patients.

There is limited evidence, from an older study, that upper-air UVGI is effective in reducing influenza transmission rates.[168] Upper-air UVGI was also shown to be effective in reducing measles transmission among schoolchildren.[174]

SUMMARY

1. The risk of TB infection in health care workers is 5 to 10 times greater than that in the general population, and risk of disease is 2 to 5 times higher. Risk factors for TB infection and disease are mostly associated with greater risk of exposure to patients with TB, particularly undiagnosed patients. Some risk factors relate to specific work activities that can cause aerosolization of TB bacilli.

2. The simplest, cheapest, and quickest interventions to implement, with proven effectiveness, are the administrative measures of triage and separation of patients. These measures should be a part of all TB infection-control programs in all health care facilities.

3. There is little direct evidence for the effectiveness of N-95 personal respirators for protection against occupational TB. Nevertheless, on theoretic grounds alone, their use is supported.

4. There are sound theoretic reasons why air exchange (ventilation) should help reduce nosocomial TB transmission. There is evidence from several observational studies and one interventional study that higher levels of ventilation reduce risk of TB transmission. Natural ventilation can achieve high air exchange rates and should be effective as well as feasible in health facilities in LMIC. However, resultant airflow patterns within buildings are unpredictable, so natural ventilation may result in inadvertent exposure of workers or other patients.

5. UVGI is grossly underused. This is a low-cost, simple, and safe technology. All available evidence suggests that it should be safe and highly effective in reducing nosocomial TB transmission.

6. There are few epidemiologic studies on the effectiveness of infection control measures, alone or in combination, and their effect on reducing nosocomial TB transmission.

7. For the prevention of nosocomial transmission of influenza, the most important action is vaccination of health care workers. However, if an effective vaccine is not available, then other infection-control measures become of paramount importance. For TB, SARS, and influenza, delayed diagnosis (or delayed institution of an effective treatment, if available) is the most common and important factor in nosocomial transmission. Hence, the most important measures are to promptly identify patients with these illnesses and separate them from other patients and from susceptible health care workers.

8. Personal protective equipment including gowns, masks, and gloves is important to prevent transmission by droplet. This is a major mechanism of transmission for SARS and influenza, so should be the major method of protection for health care workers and prevention of spread by health care workers from one patient to another.

9. However, there is clear evidence that airborne transmission of influenza and SARS can occur. Transmission is most likely during performance of procedures that

cause aerosolization of infectious droplets, or with severely ill patients. Therefore, N-95 personal respirators, which should be more effective in preventing acquisition of airborne infections, should be used by workers caring for severely ill patients, or workers performing aerosol-generating procedures. In addition, these patients should be cared for, and procedures performed, in rooms with adequate ventilation and/or upper-air UVGI, as these environmental measures can further reduce the risk of airborne transmission.

REFERENCES

1. Menzies D, Doherty TM. Diagnosis of latent tuberculosis infection. In: Raviglione MC, editor. Reichman and Hershfield's tuberculosis, a comprehensive international approach. New York: Informa Healthcare USA; 2006. p. 215–63.
2. Harrington JM, Shannon HS. Incidence of tuberculosis, hepatitis, brucellosis, and shigellosis in British medical laboratory workers. Br Med J 1976;1:759–62.
3. Joshi R, Reingold A, Menzies D, et al. Tuberculosis among healthcare workers in low and middle income countries: a systematic review. PLoS Med 2006;3(12): c494.
4. Sepkowitz K. Tuberculosis and the health care worker: a historical perspective. Ann Intern Med 1994;120:71–9.
5. Menzies RI, Fanning A, Yuan L. Tuberculosis among health care workers. N Engl J Med 1995;332:92–8.
6. Menzies D, Joshi R, Pai M. Risk of tuberculosis infection and disease associated with work in health care settings. Int J Tuberc Lung Dis 2007;11(6):593–605.
7. Centers for Diease Control. Guidelines for preventing the transmission of *Mycobacterium tuberculosis* in health-care settings, 2005. MMWR Recomm Rep 2005;54(RR–17):1–141.
8. World Health Organization, Stop TB Department. WHO policy on TB infection control in health-care facilities, congregate settings and households. Geneva (Switzerland): World Health Organization; 2009.
9. Menzies D, Pai M, Comstock GW. New tests for diagnosis of latent tuebrculosis infection - areas of uncertainty and recommendations for research. Ann Intern Med 2007;146(5):340–54.
10. Pai M, Zwerling A, Menzies D. Systematic review: T-cell based assays for the diagnosis of latent tuberculosis infection–an update. Ann Intern Med 2008; 149(177):184.
11. Pai M, Joshi R, Dogra S, et al. T-cell assay conversions and reversions among household contacts of tuberculosis patients in rural India. Int J Tuberc Lung Dis 2009;13(1):84–92.
12. Pai M, Joshi R, Dogra S, et al. Serial testing of health care workers for tuberculosis using interferon-gamma assay. Am J Respir Crit Care Med 2006;174(3): 349–55.
13. Adal KA, Anglim AM, Palumbo CL, et al. Preventing nosocomial tuberculosis with HEPA respirators: a cost-effectiveness analysis. N Engl J Med 1994; 331(3):169–73.
14. Aitken ML, Anderson KM, Albert RK. Is the tuberculosis screening program of hospital employees still required? Am Rev Respir Dis 1987;136:805–7.
15. Baussano I, Bugiani M, Caros ELA, et al. Risk of tuberculin conversion among healthcare workers and the adoption of preventive measures. Occup Environ Med 2007;64(3):161–6.

16. Behrman AJ, Shofer FS. Tuberculosis exposure and control in an urban emergency department. Ann Emerg Med 1998;31(3):370–5.
17. Blumberg HM, Sotir M, Erwin M, et al. Risk of house staff tuberculin skin test conversion in an area with a high incidence of tuberculosis. Clin Infect Dis 1998;27:826–33.
18. Bourdreau AY, Baron SL, Steenland NK, et al. Occupational risk of *Mycobacterium tuberculosis* infection in hospital workers. Am J Ind Med 1997;32:528–34.
19. Chan CC, Tabak JI. Risk of tuberculous infection among house staff in an urban teaching hospital. South Med J 1985;78:1061–4.
20. Christie CD, Constantinou P, Marx ML, et al. Low risk for tuberculosis in a regional pediatric hospital: nine-year study of community rates and the mandatory employee tuberculin skin-test program. Infect Control Hosp Epidemiol 1998;19:168–74.
21. Dooley SW, Villarino ME, Lawrence M, et al. Nosocomial transmission of tuberculosis in a hospital unit for HIV-infected patients. JAMA 1992;267(19):2632–4.
22. Fraser VJ, Kilo CM, Bailey TC, et al. Screening of physicians for tuberculosis. Infect Control Hosp Epidemiol 1994;15(2):95–100.
23. Lainez RM, Consul M, Olona M, et al. Tuberculous infection in nursing students: prevalence and conversion during a 3-year follow-up. Med Clin 1999;113(18): 685–9.
24. Larsen NM, Biddle CL, Sotir MJ, et al. Risk of tuberculin skin test conversion among health care workers: occupational versus community exposure and infection. Clin Infect Dis 2002;35(7):796–801.
25. LoBue PA, Catanzaro A. Effectiveness of a nosocomial tuberculosis control program at an urban teaching hospital. Chest 1998;113(5):1184–9.
26. Louther J, Riviera P, Feldman J, et al. Risk of tuberculin conversion according to occupation among health care workers at a New York City hospital. Am J Respir Crit Care Med 1997;156:201–5.
27. Manusov EG, Bradshaw RD, Fogarty JP. Tuberculosis screening in medical students. Fam Med 1996;28(9):645–9.
28. Menzies D, Fanning A, Yuan L, et al. The Canadian Collaborative Group in Nosocomial Transmission of Tuberculosis. Tuberculosis in health care workers: a multicentre Canadian prevalence survey: preliminary results. Int J Tuberc Lung Dis 1998;2(9):S98–102.
29. Plitt SS, Soskolne CL, Fanning EA, et al. Prevalence and determinants of tuberculin reactivity among physicians in Edmonton, Canada: 1996–1997. Int J Epidemiol 2001;30(5):1022–8.
30. Price LE, Rutala WA, Samsa GP. Tuberculosis in hospital personnel. Infect Control 1987;8:97–101.
31. Ramirez JA, Anderson P, Herp S, et al. Increased rate of tuberculin skin test conversion among workers at a university hospital. Infect Control Hosp Epidemiol 1992;13(10):579–81.
32. Ruben FL, Norden CW, Schuster N. Analysis of a community hospital employee tuberculosis screening program 31 months after its inception. Am Rev Respir Dis 1977;115:23–8.
33. Rullan JV, Herrera D, Cano R, et al. Nosocomial transmission of multidrug-resistant *Mycobacterium tuberculosis* in Spain. Emerg Infect Dis 1996;2(2): 125–9.
34. Stuart RL, Bennett NJ, Forbes AB, et al. Assessing the risk of tuberculosis infection among healthcare workers: the Melbourne Mantoux Study. Melbourne Mantoux Study Group. Med J Aust 2001;174(11):569–73.

35. Bailey TC, Fraser VJ, Spitznagel EL, et al. Risk factors for a positive tuberculin skin test among employees of an urban, midwestern teaching hospital. Ann Intern Med 1995;122:580–5.

36. Vogeler DM, Burke JP. Tuberculosis screening for hospital employees: a five-year experience in a large community hospital. Am Rev Respir Dis 1978;117: 227–32.

37. Zahnow K, Matts JP, Hillman D, et al. Rates of tuberculosis infection in health-care workers providing services to HIV-infected populations. Terry Beirn Community Programs for Clinical Research on AIDS. Infect Control Hosp Epidemiol 1998;19(11):829–35.

38. Zarzuela-Ramirez M, Cordoba-Dona JA, Perea-Milla E, et al. Factors associated with tuberculin conversion among staff at a university-affiliated hospital. Infect Control Hosp Epidemiol 1999;20(9):589–90.

39. Bonifacio N, Saito M, Gilman RH, et al. High risk for tuberculosis in hospital physicians, Peru. Emerg Infect Dis 2002;8(7):747–8.

40. Corbett EL, Muzangwa J, Chaka K, et al. Nursing and community rates of Mycobacterium tuberculosis infection among students in Harare, Zimbabwe. Clin Infect Dis 2007;44(3):317–23.

41. Hohmuth BA, Yamanjia JC, Dayal AS, et al. Latent tuberculosis: risks to health care students at a hospital in Lima, Peru. Int J Tuberc Lung Dis 2006;10(10): 1146–51.

42. Lopes LK, Teles SA, Souza AC, et al. Tuberculosis risk among nursing professionals from Central Brazil. Am J Infect Contr 2008;36(2):148–51.

43. Maciel EL, Viana MC, Zeitoune RC, et al. Prevalence and incidence of Mycobacterium tuberculosis infection in nursing students in Vitoria, Espirito Santo. Rev Soc Bras Med Trop 2005;38(6):469–72.

44. Pai M, Gokhale K, Joshi R, et al. Mycobacterium tuberculosis infection in health care workers in rural India – comparison of a whole-blood interferon gamma assay with tuberculin skin testing. JAMA 2005;293(22):2746–55.

45. Roth VR, Garrett DO, Laserson KF, et al. A multicenter evaluation of tuberculin skin test positivity and conversion among health care workers in Brazilian hospitals. Int J Tuberc Lung Dis 2005;9:1335–42.

46. Silva VM, Cunha AJ, Oliveira JR, et al. Medical students at risk of nosocomial transmission of Mycobacterium tuberculosis. Int J Tuberc Lung Dis 2000;4(5): 420–6.

47. Yanai H, Limpakarnjanarat K, Uthaivoravit W, et al. Risk of Mycobacterium tuberculosis infection and disease among health care workers, Chiang Rai, Thailand. Int J Tuberc Lung Dis 2003;7(1):36–45.

48. Center for Disease Control. Proportionate mortality from pulmonary tuberculosis associated with occupations–28 states, 1979–1990. MMWR Morb Mortal Wkly Rep 1995;44(1):14–9.

49. Diel R, Seidler A, Nienhaus A, et al. Occupational risk of tuberculosis transmission in a low incidence area. Respir Res 2005;6(1):35.

50. Driver CR, Stricof RL, Granville K, et al. Tuberculosis in health care workers during declining tuberculosis incidence in New York State. Am J Infect Contr 2005;33(9):519–26.

51. Hill A, Burge A, Skinner C. Tuberculosis in National Health Service hospital staff in the west Midlands region of England, 1992–5. Thorax 1997;52(11):994–7.

52. McKenna MT, Hutton M, Cauthen G, et al. The association between occupation and tuberculosis. A population-based survey. Am J Respir Crit Care Med 1996; 154:587–93.

53. Meredith S, Watson JM, Citron KM, et al. Are healthcare workers in England and Wales at increased risk of tuberculosis? BMJ 1996;313(7056):522–5.

54. Pleszewski B, FitzGerald JM. Tuberculosis among health care workers in British Columbia. Int J Tuberc Lung Dis 1998;2(11):898–903.

55. Raitio M, Helenius H, Tala E. Is the risk of occupational tuberculosis higher for young health care workers? Int J Tuberc Lung Dis 2003;7(6):556–62.

56. Sepkowitz KA, Friedman CR, Hafner A, et al. Tuberculosis among urban health care workers: a study using restriction fragment length polymorphism typing. Clin Infect Dis 1995;21:1098–102.

57. van DH, Gerritsen JJ, van SD, et al. A molecular epidemiological approach to studying the transmission of tuberculosis in Amsterdam. Clin Infect Dis 1997; 25(5):1071–7.

58. Alonso-Echanove J, Granich RM, Laszlo A, et al. Occupational transmission of Mycobacterium tuberculosis to health care workers in a university hospital in Lima, Peru. Clin Infect Dis 2001;33(5):589–96.

59. Babus V. Tuberculosis morbidity risk in medical nurses in specialized institutions for the treatment of lung diseases in Zagreb. Int J Tuberc Lung Dis 1997;1(3): 254–8.

60. Balt E, Durrheim DN, Weyer K. Nosocomial transmission of tuberculosis to health care workers in Mpumalanga [8]. S Afr Med J 1998;88(11):1363–6.

61. Cuhadaroglu C, Erelel M, Tabak L, et al. Increased risk of tuberculosis in health care workers: a retrospective survey at a teaching hospital in Istanbul, Turkey. BMC Infect Dis 2002;2:14.

62. Dimitrova B, Hutchings A, Atun R, et al. Increased risk of tuberculosis among health care workers in Samara Oblast, Russia: analysis of notification data. Int J Tuberc Lung Dis 2005;9(1):43–8.

63. Eyob G, Gebeyhu M, Goshu S, et al. Increase in tuberculosis incidence among the staff working at the Tuberculosis Demonstration and Training Centre in Addis Ababa, Ethiopia: a retrospective cohort study (1989–1998). Int J Tuberc Lung Dis 2002;6(1):85–8.

64. Gopinath KG, Siddique S, Kirubakaran H, et al. Tuberculosis among healthcare workers in a tertiary-care hospital in South India. J Hosp Infect 2004;57(4): 339–42.

65. Harries AD, Hargreaves NJ, Gausi F, et al. Preventing tuberculosis among health workers in Malawi. Bull World Health Organ 2002;80(7):526–31.

66. Harries AD, Kamenya A, Namarika D, et al. Delays in diagnosis and treatment of smear-positive tuberculosis and the incidence of tuberculosis in hospital nurses in Blantyre, Malawi. Trans R Soc Trop Med Hyg 1997;91(1):15–7.

67. Harries AD, Nyirenda TE, Banerjee A, et al. Tuberculosis in health care workers in Malawi. Trans R Soc Trop Med Hyg 1999;93(1):32–5.

68. Hosoglu S, Tanrikulu AC, Dagli C, et al. Tuberculosis among health care workers in a short working period. Am J Infect Contr 2005;33(1):23–6.

69. Jelip J, Mathew GG, Yusin Y, et al. Risk factors of tuberculosis among health care workers in Sabah, Malaysia. Tuberculosis 2004;84(1–2):19–23.

70. Jiamjarasrangsi W, Hirunsuthikul N, Kamolratanakul P. Tuberculosis among health care workers at King Chulalongkorn Memorial Hospital, 1988–2002. Int J Tuberc Lung Dis 2005;9(11):1253–8.

71. Kanyerere HS, Salaniponi FM. Tuberculosis in health care workers in a central hospital in Malawi. Int J Tuberc Lung Dis 2003;7(5):489–92.

72. Kilinc O, Ucan ES, Cakan MD, et al. Risk of tuberculosis among healthcare workers: can tuberculosis be considered as an occupational disease? Respir Med 2002;96(7):506–10.

73. Kruuner A, Danilovitsh M, Pehme L, et al. Tuberculosis as an occupational hazard for health care workers in Estonia. Int J Tuberc Lung Dis 2001;5(2): 170–6.

74. Laniado-Laborin R, Cabrales-Vargas N. Tuberculosis in healthcare workers at a general hospital in Mexico. Infect Control Hosp Epidemiol 2006;27(5):449–52.

75. Naidoo S, Mahommed A. Knowledge, attitudes, behaviour and prevalence of TB infection among dentists in the western Cape. SADJ 2002;57(11):476–8.

76. Rao KG, Aggarwal AM, Behera D. Tuberculosis among physicians in training. Int J Tuberc Lung Dis 2004;8(11):1392–4.

77. Skodric V, Savic B, Jovanovic M, et al. Occupational risk of tuberculosis among health care workers at the Institute for Pulmonary Diseases of Serbia. Int J Tuberc Lung Dis 2000;4(9):827–31.

78. Sotgiu G, Arbore AS, Cojocariu V, et al. High risk of tuberculosis in health care workers in Romania. Int J Tuberc Lung Dis 2008;12(6):606–11.

79. Wilkinson D, Gilks CF. Increasing frequency of tuberculosis among staff in a South African district hospital: impact of the HIV epidemic on the supply side of health care. Trans R Soc Trop Med Hyg 1998;92(5):500–2.

80. Do AN, Limpakarnjarat K, Uthaivoravit W, et al. Increased risk of *Mycobacterium tuberculosis* infection related to the occupational exposures of health care workers in Chiang Rai, Thailand. Int J Tuberc Lung Dis 1999;3(5):377–81.

81. Kassim S, Zuber P, Wiktor SZ, et al. Tuberculin skin testing to assess the occupational risk of *Mycobacterium tuberculosis* infection among health care workers in Abidjan, Cote d'Ivoire. Int J Tuberc Lung Dis 2000;4(4):321–6.

82. Orrett FA. Prevalence of tuberculin skin test reactivity among health care workers at a teaching hospital in Trinidad. Clin Microbiol Infect 2000;6(1):45–8.

83. Liss GM, Khan R, Koven E, et al. Tuberculosis infection among staff at a Canadian community hospital. Infect Control Hosp Epidemiol 1996;17(1):29–35.

84. Keskiner R, Ergonul O, Demiroglu Z, et al. Risk of tuberculous infection among healthcare workers in a tertiary-care hospital in Ankara, Turkey. Infect Control Hosp Epidemiol 2004;25(12):1067–71.

85. Schwartzman K, Loo V, Pasztor J, et al. Tuberculosis infection among health care workers in Montreal. Am J Respir Crit Care Med 1996;154:1006–12.

86. Garcia-Garcia ML, Jimenez-Corona A, Jimenez-Corona ME, et al. Factors associated with tuberculin reactivity in two general hospitals in Mexico. Infect Control Hosp Epidemiol 2001;22(2):88–93.

87. Warren DK, Foley KM, Polish LB, et al. Tuberculin skin testing of physicians at a midwestern teaching hospital: a 6-year prospective study. Clin Infect Dis 2001;32(9):1331–7.

88. Berman J, Levin ML, Orr ST, et al. Tuberculosis risk of hospital employees: analysis of a five-year tuberculin skin testing program. Am J Public Health 1981;71: 1217–22.

89. Kayanja HK, Debanne S, King C, et al. Tuberculosis infection among health care workers in Kampala, Uganda. Int J Tuberc Lung Dis 2005;9(6):686–8.

90. Menzies D, Fanning A, Yuan L, et al. Factors associated with tuberculin conversion in Canadian microbiology and pathology workers. Am J Respir Crit Care Med 2003;167(4):599–602.

91. Harries AD, Maher D, Nunn P. Practical and affordable measures for the protection of health care workers from tuberculosis in low-income countries. Bull World Health Organ 1997;75(5):477–89.

92. Menzies RI, Fanning A, Yuan L, et al. Hospital ventilation and risk of tuberculous infection in Canadian Health Care Workers. Ann Intern Med 2000;133(10): 779–89.

93. Sugita M, Tsutsumi Y, Suchi M, et al. Pulmonary tuberculosis: an occupational hazard for pathologists and pathology technicians in Japan. Acta Pathol Jpn 1990;40:116–27.

94. Ehrenkranz NJ, Kicklighter JL. Tuberculosis outbreak in a general hospital: evidence for airborne spread of infection. Ann Intern Med 1972;77:377–82.

95. Haley CE, McDonald RC, Rossi L, et al. Tuberculosis epidemic among hospital personnel. Infect Control Hosp Epidemiol 1989;10:204–10.

96. Calder RA, Duclos P, Wilder MH, et al. Mycobacterium tuberculosis: transmission in a health clinic. Bull Int Union Tuberc Lung Dis 1991;66:103–6.

97. Menzies D, Adhikari N, Arieta M, et al. Efficacy of environmental measures in reducing potentially infectious bioaerosols during sputum induction. Infect Control Hosp Epidemiol 2003;24(7):483–9.

98. Catanzaro A. Nosocomial tuberculosis. Am Rev Respir Dis 1982;125:559–62.

99. Kantor HS, Poblete R, Pusateri SL. Nosocomial transmission of tuberculosis from unsuspected disease. Am J Med 1988;84:833–8.

100. Lundgren R, Norrman E, Asberg I. Tuberculosis infection transmitted at autopsy. Tubercle 1987;68:147–50.

101. International Union Against Tuberculosis and Lung Disease, World Health Organization. Control of tuberculosis transmission in health care settings. Tuberc Lung Dis 1994;75:94–5.

102. Wenger PN, Otten J, Breeden A, et al. Control of nosocomial transmission of multidrug-resistant Mycobacterium tuberculosis among healthcare workers and HIV-infected patients. Lancet 1995;345:235–40.

103. Maloney SA, Pearson ML, Gordon MT, et al. Efficacy of control measures in preventing nosocomial transmission of multidrug-resistant tuberculosis to patients and health care workers. Ann Intern Med 1995;122:90–5.

104. Fella P, Rivera P, Hale M, et al. Dramatic decrease in tuberculin skin test conversion rate among employees at a hospital in New York City. Am J Infect Contr 1995;23:352–6.

105. Bangsberg DR, Crowley K, Moss A, et al. Reduction in tuberculin skin-test conversions among medical house staff associated with improved tuberculosis infection control practices. Infect Control Hosp Epidemiol 1997;18:566–70.

106. Blumberg HM, Watkins DL, Jeffrey PA-C, et al. Preventing the nosocomial transmission of tuberculosis. Ann Intern Med 1995;122:658–63.

107. Nicas M. Assessing the relative importance of the components of an occupational tuberculosis control program. J Occup Environ Med 1998;40(7):648–54.

108. Moro ML, Errante I, Infuso A, et al. Effectiveness of infection control measures in controlling a nosocomial outbreak of multidrug-resistant tuberculosis among HIV patients in Italy. Int J Tuberc Lung Dis 2000;4(1):61–8.

109. Jarvis WR. Nosocomial transmission of multidrug-resistant Mycobacterium tuberculosis. Am J Infect Contr 1995;23(2):146–51.

110. Otten J, Chen J, Cleary T. Successful control of an outbreak of multi-drug resistant tuberculosis in an urban teaching hospital [abstract 51D]. World Congress on Tuberculosis; 1992.

111. Stroud LA, Tokars JI, Grieco MH, et al. Evaluation of infection control measures in preventing the nosocomial transmission of multidrug-resistant *Mycobacterium tuberculosis* in a New York City hospital. Infect Control Hosp Epidemiol 1995; 16(3):141–7.

112. Centers for Disease Control and Prevention. Recommendations and Reports. Guidelines for preventing the transmission of mycobacterium tuberculosis in health-care facilities. MMWR Recomm Rep 1994;43(RR13):1–132.

113. Nicas M. Respiratory protection and the risk of mycobacterium tuberculosis infection. Am J Ind Med 1995;27:317–33.

114. Fennelly KP, Nardell EA. The relative efficacy of respirators and room ventilation in preventing occupational tuberculosis. Infect Control Hosp Epidemiol 1998; 19(10):754–9.

115. Coffey CC, Lawrence RB, Campbell DL, et al. Fitting characteristics of eighteen N95 filtering-facepiece respirators. J Occup Environ Hyg 2004;1(4):262–71.

116. Lee MC, Joffe M, Long R, et al. Qualitative fit testing does not ensure health care worker protection. Can J Infect Dis Med Microbiol 2005;16(2):172.

117. Nardell EA. Fans, filters, or rays? Pros and cons of the current environmental tuberculosis control technologies. Infect Control Hosp Epidemiol 1993;14: 681–5.

118. Nardell EA, Keegan J, Cheney SA, et al. Airborne infection: theoretical limits of protection achievable by building ventilation. Am Rev Respir Dis 1991;144(2): 302–6.

119. Nardell EA. Environmental infection control of tuberculosis. Semin Respir Infect 2003;18(4):307–19.

120. Escombe AR, Oeser CC, Gilman RH, et al. Natural ventilation for the prevention of airborne contagion. PLoS Med 2007;4(2):e68.

121. Menzies RI, Schwartzman K, Loo V, et al. Measuring ventilation of patient care areas in hospitals: description of a new protocol. Am J Respir Crit Care Med 1995;152:1992–9.

122. Nardell EA, Bugher SJ, Brickner PW, et al. Safety of upper-room ultraviolet germicidal air disinfection for room occupants: results from the Tuberculosis Ultraviolet Shelter Study. Public Health Rep 2008;123(1):52–60.

123. Riley RL, Mills CC, O'Grady FO, et al. Infectiousness of air from a tuberculosis ward: ultraviolet irradiation of infected air – comparative infectiousness of different patients. Am Rev Respir Dis 1962;85:511–25.

124. Escombe AR, Moore DAJ, Gilman RH, et al. Upper-room ultraviolet light and negative air ionization to prevent tuberculosis transmission. PLoS Med 2009; 6(3):e1000043.

125. Ray KC, Johnson BH. An evaluation of ultraviolet lamps in a dental clinic (tuberculosis hospital). Dent Items Interest 1951;73:521–9.

126. Riley RL, Knight M, Middlebrook G. Ultraviolet susceptibilty of BCG and virulent tubercule baccilli. Am Rev Respir Dis 1976;113:413–8.

127. Xu P, Peccia J, Fabian P, et al. Efficacy of ultraviolet germicidal irradiation of upper-room air in inactivating airborne bacterial spores and mycobacteria in full-scale studies. Atmos Environ 2003;37:405–19.

128. Riley RL, Nardell EA. Controlling transmission of tuberculosis in health care facilities: ventilation, filtration, and ultraviolet air disinfection. In: Tomasik KM, editor. Plant, technology, safety management series. 1st edition. Oakbrook Terrace (IL): Joint Commission Accreditation of Healthcare Organizations; 1993. p. 25–31.

129. Riley RL, Nardell EA. Clearing the air: the theory and application of ultraviolet air disinfection. Am Rev Respir Dis 1989;139:1286–94.

130. Long R. Canadian tuberculosis standards 6th edition - 2007. Ottawa (Canada): Canadian Lung Association and Public Health Agency of Canada; 2007.

131. Lessler J, Reich NG, Brookmeyer R, et al. Incubation periods of acute respiratory viral infections: a systematic review. Lancet Infect Dis 2009;9:291–300.

132. Chan-Yeung M, Ooi GC, Hui DS, et al. Severe acute respiratory syndrome. Int J Tuberc Lung Dis 2003;7(12):1117–30.

133. Donnelly CA, Chani AC, Leung GM, et al. Epidemiological determinants of spread of causal agent of severe acute respiratory syndrome in Hong Kong. Lancet 2003;361:1761–6.

134. Brankston G, Gitterman L, Hirji Z, et al. Transmission of influenza A in human beings. Lancet Infect Dis 2007;7:257–65.

135. Ho AS, Sung J, Chan-Yeung M. An outbreak of severe acute respiratory syndrome among hospital workers in a community hospital in Hong Kong. Ann Intern Med 2003;139:564–7.

136. Moser MR, Bender TR, Margolis HS, et al. An outbreak of influenza aboard a commercial airliner. Am J Epidemiol 1979;110(1):1–6.

137. Li Y, Yu I, Xu P, et al. Predicting super spreading events during the 2003 severe acute respiratory syndrome epidemics in Hong Kong and Singapore. Am J Epidemiol 2004;160:719–28.

138. Yu I, Li Y, Wong T, et al. Evidence of airborne transmission of the severe acute respiratory syndrome virus. N Engl J Med 2004;350:1731–8.

139. Patrozou E, Mermel LA. Does influenza transmission occur from asymptomatic infection or prior to symptom onset? Public Health Rep 2009;124(2):193–6.

140. Gamage B, Moore D, Copes R, et al. Protecting health care workers from SARS and other respiratory pathogens: a review of the infection control literature. Am J Infect Contr 2005;33:114–21.

141. Leung GM, Hedley AJ, Ho LM, et al. The epidemiology of severe acute respiratory syndrome in the 2003 Hong Kong epidemic: an analysis of all 1755 patients. Ann Intern Med 2004;141:662–73.

142. Ofner-Agostini M, Gravel D, McDonald LC, et al. Cluster of cases of severe acute respiratory syndrome among Toronto healthcare workers after implementation of infection control precautions: a case series. Infect Control Hosp Epidemiol 2006;27(5):473–8.

143. Varia M, Wilson S, Sarwal S, et al. Investigation of a nosocomial outbreak of severe acute respiratory syndrome (SARS) in Toronto, Canada. CMAJ 2003; 169(4):285.

144. Yu IT, Xie ZH, Tsoi KK, et al. Why did outbreaks of severe acute respiratory syndrome occur in some hospital wards but not in others? Clin Infect Dis 2007;44(8):1017–25.

145. Dwosh AH, Hong H, Austgarden D, et al. Identification and containment of an outbreak of SARS in a community hospital. CMAJ 2003;168(11):1415.

146. Cheng P, Wong DA, Tong L, et al. Viral shedding patterns of coronavirus in patients with probable severe acute respiratory syndrome. Lancet 2004; 363(9422):1699–700.

147. Peiris JSM, Chu CM, Cheng VCC, et al. Clinical progression and viral load in a community outbreak of coronavirus-associated SARS pneumonia: a prospective study. Lancet 2003;361:1767–72.

148. Bridges CB, Kuehnert J, Hall CB. Transmission of influenza: implications for control in health care settings. Clin Infect Dis 2003;37(8):1094.

149. Voirin N, Barret B, Metzger MH, et al. Hospital-acquired influenza: a synthesis using the Outbreak Reports and Intervention Studies of Nosocomial Infection (ORION) statement. J Hosp Infect 2009;71:1–14.

150. Tan CC. SARS in Singapore – key lessons from an epidemic. Ann Acad Med Singap 2006;35:345–9.

151. Loeb M, McGreer A, Henry B, et al. SARS among critical care nurses, Toronto. Emerg Infect Dis 2004;10(2):251–5.

152. Chan P, Tang J, Hui D. SARS: clinical presentation, transmission, pathogenesis and treatment options. Clin Sci 2006;110:193–204.

153. Center for Disease Control. Update: influenza activity – United States, April–August 2009. MMWR Morb Mortal Wkly Rep 2009;58(36):1009–12.

154. Salgado SD, Farr BM, Hall KK, et al. Influenza in the acute hospital setting. Lancet Infect Dis 2002;2(3):145–55.

155. Sandrock C, Stollenwerk N. Acute febrile respiratory illness in the ICU: reducing disease transmission. Chest 2008;133:1221–31.

156. Greenaway C, Menzies D, Fanning A, et al. Delay in diagnosis among hospitalized patients with active tuberculosis–predictors and outcomes. Am J Respir Crit Care Med 2002;165(7):927–33.

157. Riley S, Fraser C, Donnelly CA, et al. Transmission dynamics of the etiological agent of SARS in Hong Kong: impact of public health interventions. Science 2003;300(5627):1961.

158. Escombe AR, Moore DA, Gilman RH, et al. The infectiousness of tuberculosis patients coinfected with HIV. PLoS Med 2008;5(9):e188.

159. Riley RL, Mills CC, Nyka W, et al. Aerial dissemination of pulmonary tuberculosis: a two year study of contagion in a tuberculosis ward. Am J Hyg 1050; 70:185–96.

160. Munoz F, Campbell J, Atmar R, et al. Influenza A virus outbreak in a neonatal intensive care unit. Pediatr Infect Dis J 1999;18(9):811–5.

161. Low JGH, Wilder-Smith A. Infectious respiratory illnesses and their impact on healthcare workers: a review. Ann Acad Med Singap 2005;34:105–10.

162. Carman WF, Elder AG, Wallce LA, et al. Effects of influenza vaccination of health-care workers on mortality of elderly people in long-term care: a randomised controlled trial. Lancet 2000;355:93–7.

163. Maltezou HC. Nosocomial influenza: new concepts and practice. Curr Opin Infect Dis 2008;21:337–43.

164. Pachucki CT, Pappas SA, Fuller GF, et al. Influenza A among hospital personnel and patients. Implications for recognition, prevention, and control. Arch Intern Med 1989;149(1):77–80.

165. Lau JT, Fung KS, Wong TW, et al. SARS transmission among hospital workers in Hong Kong. Emerg Infect Dis 2004;10(2):280–6.

166. Seto WH, Tsang D, Yung RWH, et al. Effectiveness of precautions against droplets and contact in prevention of nosocomial transmission of severe acute respiratory syndrome (SARS). Lancet 2003;361:1519.

167. Loeb M, Dafoe N, Mahony J, et al. Surgical mask vs N95 respirator for preventing influenza among health care workers. JAMA 2009;302(17):1865–71.

168. McLean RL. The effect of ultraviolet radiation upon the transmission of epidemic influenza in long-term hospital patients. Am Rev Respir Dis 1961;83:36–8.

169. Drinka PJ, Krause P, Schilling M, et al. Clinical investigation: reporting of an outbreak: nursing home architecture and Influenza-A attack rates. J Am Geriatr Soc 1996;44(8):910–3.

170. Khan K, Arino J, Hu W, et al. Spread of novel influenza A (H1N1) virus via global airline transportation. N Engl J Med 2009;361(2):212.

171. Morens DM, Rash VM. Lessons from a nursing home outbreak of influenza A. Infect Control Hosp Epidemiol 1995;16:275–80.

172. Committee on Infectious Diseases. Infection prevention and control in pediatric ambulatory settings. Pediatrics 2007;120:650.

173. Uhnoo I, Linde A, Pauksens K, et al. Treatment and prevention of influenza: Swedish recommendations. Scand J Infect Dis 2003;35(1):3–11.

174. Wells WF. Airborne contagion and air hygiene. Cambridge (MA): Harvard University Press; 1955.

Pulmonary Infectious Complications of Tumor Necrosis Factor Blockade

Robert S. Wallis, MD, FIDSA[a,b,c,*], Neil W. Schluger, MD[d]

KEYWORDS

- Tumor necrosis factor • Infection • Tuberculosis • Granuloma
- Etanercept • Infliximab • Adalimumab • Mechanism of action

In the decade since tumor necrosis factor-alpha (TNF α) antagonists were first approved for clinical use, they have proven invaluable for the treatment of chronic inflammation. Currently licensed TNF blockers fall into two classes, monoclonal antibody and soluble receptor. Although they are equally effective in rheumatoid arthritis (RA) and psoriasis, important differences have emerged with regard to efficacy in granulomatous inflammation and risks of granulomatous infections, particularly tuberculosis (TB). This article focuses on recent studies that inform prevention and management of infections in this susceptible patient population.

TNF ANTAGONISTS

Four monoclonal anti-TNF antibodies are presently in clinical use: infliximab, adalimumab, golimumab, and certolizumab pegol (**Fig. 1**). Infliximab is comprised of human immunoglobulin G1 (IgG1) constant regions and murine variable regions, whereas adalimumab and golimumab have both human IgG1 constant and variable regions. Certolizumab pegol is a pegylated, humanized Fab' fragment. Infliximab, adalimumab, and golimumab are approved for treatment of RA, psoriatic arthritis, and ankylosing spondylitis. Infliximab, adalimumab, and certolizumab are approved for treatment of Crohn disease (CD).[1,2] Infliximab also is approved for ulcerative colitis, and may be

Dr Wallis has served as a consultant for Wyeth and Amgen, and is presently employed by Pfizer.
[a] Pfizer, 50 Pequot Avenue, B3149, New London, CT 06320, USA
[b] Department of Medicine, UMDNJ-New Jersey School of Medicine, Newark, NJ, USA
[c] Department of Medicine, Case School of Medicine, Cleveland, OH, USA
[d] Division of Pulmonary, Allergy, and Critical Care Medicine, Department of Medicine, Epidemiology and Environmental Health Sciences, Columbia University College of Physicians and Surgeons, PH-8 East, Room 101, 630 West 168th Street, New York, NY 10032, USA
* Corresponding author. Pfizer, 50 Pequot Avenue, B3149, New London, CT 06320.
E-mail address: rswallis@gmail.com

Infect Dis Clin N Am 24 (2010) 681–692
doi:10.1016/j.idc.2010.04.010
0891-5520/10/$ – see front matter © 2010 Elsevier Inc. All rights reserved.

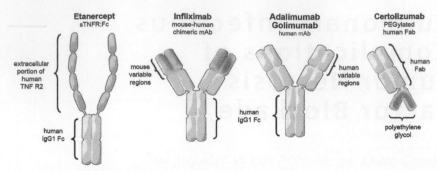

Fig. 1. Structures of the tumor necrosis factor (TNF) antagonists. *Adapted from* Wallis RS. Tumor necrosis factor antagonists: structure, function, and tuberculosis risks. Lancet Infect Dis 2008;8(10):602; with permission.

effective in sarcoidosis.[3–5] Certolizumab appears to also be effective for RA.[6–8] Infliximab is administered by intravenous infusion, producing peak blood concentrations of 80 μg/mL.[9] Adalimumab, certolizumab, and golimumab are administered by subcutaneous injection. Peak blood concentrations of 10 μg/mL have been reported for adalimumab, 90 μg/mL for certolizumab, and 2.5 μg/mL for golimumab.[10–13]

Etanercept is the only soluble TNF receptor presently in clinical use. It is comprised of two extracellular domains of human TNF-R2 fused to the Fc fragment of human IgG1. It binds both TNF and lymphotoxin. Etanercept is approved for the treatment of RA, psoriatic arthritis, psoriasis, juvenile RA, and ankylosing spondylitis.[14] Etanercept is not effective against granulomatous inflammatory conditions such as CD or sarcoidosis.[15,16] It is administered by subcutaneous injection, usually once or twice weekly, producing blood concentrations of 1 to 2.4 μg/mL.[14]

GRANULOMATOUS INFECTIONS

Clinical studies of the impact of TNF antagonists on granulomatous infections face several challenges. These infections are relatively uncommon in the United States and European Union. Rates vary substantially by country, and may be influenced by underlying medical conditions. Studies in southern Europe and East Asia appear to indicate that RA, for example, increases TB risk aside from that due to anti-TNF treatment.[17–19] Granulomatous infections that do not require public health notification may be greatly under-reported. Their natural histories may be complicated by long periods of clinical latency. Tests for latent *Mycobacterium tuberculosis* infection (LTBI) may be falsely positive in persons in whom the infection has been eradicated by chemotherapy or host immunity.[20] They may be falsely negative in persons with RA, either because of the underlying disease or its treatment.[21] No tests presently exist for diagnosis of latent granulomatous infections other than TB.

These challenges notwithstanding, several adequately powered studies have examined the differential impact of TNF blockers on granulomatous infections including TB, and have reached rather similar conclusions. In 2004, the authors and colleagues published a study of granulomatous infections associated with infliximab or etanercept reported to the US Food and Drug Administration (FDA) adverse event reporting system from January 1998 through September 2002.[22] The report was corrected shortly thereafter to remove European TB cases.[23] Compared to etanercept, infliximab was associated with significantly greater risks (two- to sevenfold) of TB, coccidioidomycosis and histoplasmosis, shorter time to TB onset (17 vs 48 weeks), and a higher proportion of TB cases with disseminated or extrapulmonary disease (25% vs 10%). The findings with regard to coccidioidomycosis were confirmed by a retrospective study conducted in the southwestern United States, which found a fivefold higher rate due to infliximab than other antirheumatic drugs ($P<.01$).[24]

A large prospective study of TB using the French research axed on tolerance of bio-therapies (RATIO) registry identified 69 cases in patients treated with TNF blockers over 3 years.[25] The sex- and age-adjusted TB incidence rate was 1.17 per 1000 patient–years, 12.2 times that of the general population. Nearly all of the excess risk was due to infliximab (standardized incidence ratio [SIR] = 18.6, 95% confidence interval [CI] =1 3.4 to 25.8) and adalimumab (SIR=29.3, 95% CI = 20.2 to 42.4) rather than etanercept (SIR = 1.8, 95% CI = 0.7 to 4.3). A similar conclusion was reached by a Portuguese biologics registry study of 13 TB cases that found the TB risk of TNF anti-bodies 6.4-fold greater than etanercept.[26] These studies indicate that adalimumab and infliximab share a high risk of reactivating LTBI despite very different pharmacokinetics.

An additional study, by Brassard and colleagues,[27] used prescriptions for isoniazid in a large pharmaceutical claims database to identify TB cases occurring in patients with a diagnosis of RA. TB rates in the entire RA cohort were greater than five times expected, and only a small additional risk was attributable to anti-TNF treatment. It appears likely that study findings were influenced by the misclassification of LTBI as active TB.[28,29]

The twin observations of increased risk and shorter time to onset provide important clues as to the etiology of tuberculosis caused by TNF antibody, as early clustering of excess cases is consistent with reactivation. In contrast, TB caused by progression of new infection occurs at random over time. A study by the one of the authors (RSW) systematically examined these issues using hidden Markov modeling, which describes transitions among clinical states.[30] The study revealed that greater than 20% of latent TB infections are reactivated each month by infliximab, 12.1-fold greater than etanercept ($P<.001$). The analysis also revealed, however, that both drugs caused a high proportion of new infections to progress directly to active disease. The findings were consistent with the reported effects of soluble murine TNF receptor (mTNFRII:mFc) and anti-mTNF antibody in acutely and chronically TB-infected mice.[31]

A recent survey of infectious disease physicians in the United States revealed that disease due to non-tuberculous mycobacteria (NTM) may surpass TB in patients treated with biologic therapies, in part because of increased awareness and screening for LTBI.[32] TNF antibodies and soluble receptor appear to pose equal risks of NTM infections.[23,32] This may reflect a reduced role for latency and reactivation in NTM pathogenesis compared with TB.[33]

VIRAL INFECTIONS

A recent study by Strangfeld and colleagues[34] used the rheumatoid arthritis observation of biologic therapy registry to examine the impact of TNF blockers on herpes zoster. The study identified 86 episodes in 5040 patients. After adjusting for age, RA severity, and glucocorticoid use, a small but significantly increased risk was observed for treatment with the monoclonal antibodies (hazard ratio [HR], 1.82 [95% CI, 1.05 to 3.15]) but not for etanercept (HR, 1.36 [95% CI, 0.73 to 2.55]). The risks posed by TNF antibodies were greater when the analysis was restricted to ophthalmic and multider-matomal disease, or when a within-subjects analysis was conducted in patients who had been treated with multiple agents.

Reactivation of hepatitis B infection also has been attributed to anti-TNF therapy, although this literature is limited to individual case reports of patients treated with infliximab or adalimumab.[35–40] A small retrospective study suggests hepatitis B virus (HBV) reactivation may be prevented by concurrent antiviral therapy.[41] In contrast, hepatitis C infection appears relatively unaffected by TNF blockers of either class.[42,43]

STRUCTURE–FUNCTION RELATIONSHIP

The differences in biologic activity and infection risks of the two classes of TNF blockers have been attributed to their molecular structures.[44] Most research in this area has focused on the ability of anti-TNF antibodies to cross-link transmembrane TNF and thereby induce apoptosis in TNF-expressing T cells. This activity can be demonstrated in vitro using reporter cell constructs, and in vivo, in cells infiltrating the gut of CD patients.[45–50] Other studies have examined complement-mediated lysis of TNF-expressing T cells. A recent study by Bruns and colleagues,[51] for example, found that the number of circulating effector memory CD8 T cells was reduced by infliximab treatment.

Experience with the Fab' TNF antibody fragment certolizumab pegol call into question the significance of these observations, however. With only one TNF binding region and without Fc, certolizumab can neither cross-link tmTNF nor activate complement. Nonetheless, two phase 3 placebo-controlled trials of certolizumab in RA (RA prevention of structural damage 1 and 2) reported TB rates of 8.5 and 12.5 cases per 1000 patient–years of certolizumab exposure, with no cases in controls.[6,8,52] Certolizumab is also highly effective as therapy for CD.[7,53] These findings indicate that despite its structural differences, certolizumab shares with other TNF antibodies efficacy against granulomatous inflammation and efficiency in reactivating LTBI. Other properties, such as binding avidity and inhibition of cell activation, therefore must be more important than induction of cell death in this regard.[54–56]

LTBI DIAGNOSIS AND TREATMENT

Strategies to reduce TB risk caused by TNF blockade emphasize detection and treatment of LTBI. Although the largest experience for LTBI diagnosis exists for the tuberculin skin test (TST), its specificity is reduced by antigens shared by M bovis bacilli Calmette-Guerin, and other NTM. BCG vaccine is administered in infancy in over 100 countries. It is not administered in the United States because of concerns that it interferes with the TST. TST reactions due to BCG vaccine, however, decline rapidly in adults and infants.[57,58] Large reactions in adults are therefore unlikely to be caused solely by vaccination in infancy.

The specificity of testing for LTBI can be improved by the use of the antigens ESAT-6 and CFP-10, encoded by genes absent from all BCG vaccine strains.[59] T cell responses to these antigens are detected by in vitro assays as the release of interferon (IFN)g (interferon gamma release assay [IGRA]), either by enzyme-linked immunosorbent assay (ELISA) or ELISPOT. Some studies have reported reduced sensitivity of testing with ESAT-6 and CFP-10 compared with PPD,[60] although others have not.[61] Studies in India and Peru indicate that most TST reactivity in regions of high TB prevalence is indeed due to M tuberculosis infection rather than merely BCG vaccine sensitization.[61,62] However, no studies have reported outcomes when IGRA testing is used rather than TST to identify persons with LTBI prior to starting anti-TNF therapy, nor have any studies compared IGRA with boosted (two-step) TST.

TST responses are reduced in RA.[21,63,64] TST sensitivity may be increased by repeated testing 7 to 10 days after a negative test (boosting), at the cost of reduced specificity.[65,66] The sensitivity of screening can be improved further by chest radiography to identify regional scarring and hilar lymphadenopathy. The effectiveness of screening using a boosted (two-step) TST has been documented by the Spanish base de datos de productos biológicos de la sociedad española de reumatología (BIOBA-DASER) registry, initiated in 2000. Thirty-two cases of TB were reported among the first 1648 patients treated with infliximab, a rate 23 times the general population. Beginning in 2002, recommendations were implemented requiring patients to be screened by chest radiography and two-step TST using a 5 mm threshold. Persons with evidence of LTBI were required to receive at least the first of 9 months treatment with isoniazid before initiating anti-TNF therapy. TB rates in infliximab-treated patients declined by 74%.[67] Isoniazid was well tolerated. Elevated transaminases were reported in 7 of 324 isoniazid-treated patients, with no deaths or hospitalizations.

Boosted TST appears critical for successful LTBI detection in RA. A follow-up study by the BIOBADASER group found that the probability of developing TB after starting a TNF blocker was more than sevenfold greater if recommendations were not explicitly followed.[68] Lack of boosted testing was the main failure in complying with recommendations. This is consistent with the experience in the French RATIO registry, in which only a single TST was used. Of the 69 TB cases in the RATIO study, 45 had undergone TST screening, and 30 had been found negative (<5 mm).[25] No TB cases occurred in patients who had been prescribed and were compliant with appropriate LTBI treatment, indicating the failure was one of diagnosis rather than therapy.

Significant discussion has taken place regarding the management of persons with evidence of latent TB infection and planned treatment with TNF-antagonists. Some have advocated completing a course of isoniazid prior to beginning anti-TNF therapy, while others have suggested that the two treatments can be given concurrently. It is certainly true that the effectiveness of isoniazid treatment of LTBI decreases as its duration is reduced. Studies in the 1970s indicated that although a 52-week regimen was 75% effective, 24- and 12-week regimens were only 65% and 21% effective, respectively.[69,70] This has led some to suggest that the safest approach is to complete a course of isoniazid (INH) prior to initiating treatment with TNF blockade. Direct and indirect evidence, however, suggest that therapy can be, at least in large measure, concurrent. Several controlled trials of treatment of LTBI in people with human immunodeficiency virus (HIV) were carried out in the preantiretroviral era, and in these studies, reactivation of latent infection while on INH did not occur.[71-74] This suggests that even in the presence of significant immunocompromise, INH is sufficient to prevent progression to active TB. More directly, the Spanish experience cited previously also indicates that concurrent TNF blockade does not interfere with LTBI treatment, and that eradication of LTBI prior to starting TNF blockade is not required, but merely that preventive treatment has been initiated.

In other patient populations, larger TST or IFNg responses indicate higher TB risk.[75,76] The significance of large reactions in this population is not yet known. Patients being switched from etanercept to antibody should be tested and treated for LTBI if they have not been tested previously. Periodic retesting should be considered for patients who may have acquired LTBI since their first screening.[77] Treatment of LTBI will not prevent subsequent tuberculosis due to new infection. Alternative strategies, such as life-long preventive therapy, may be required when TNF-blockers are used in TB-endemic regions.

MANAGEMENT OF INCIDENT TB CASES

Many questions remain regarding optimal management of patients who develop TB due to TNF blockade. Although the RATIO database describes two TB patients who were continued on anti-TNF therapy without apparent ill effect, most guidelines recommend halting anti-TNF therapy until a response to anti-TB therapy is evident. However, these recommendations place patients at risk of disease exacerbation due to recovery of TNF-dependent inflammation. Such cases, termed paradoxical reactions (PR), are marked by worsening inflammation despite microbiologic improvement. They are most likely to occur in patients who develop disseminated or extrapulmonary TB due to treatment with anti-TNF antibody, and in whom that treatment is stopped.[26,78–81] The most common case definition for this syndrome requires an initial clinical response prior to subsequent deterioration. However, this definition may fail to identify cases caused by withdrawal of the short-acting TNF antibodies adalimumab and certolizumab, in which progressive exacerbation may occur without initial improvement. The syndrome is therefore likely under-recognized.

Two cases have been recently reported in which TNF antibodies were used to treat life-threatening TB PR. In one, a South African RA patient developed extensive bilateral lower lobe TB 8 months into treatment with adalimumab.[82] Adalimumab was withdrawn and standard TB therapy started. Culture and molecular testing revealed fully susceptible *M tuberculosis* at diagnosis that was appropriately cleared by treatment. Nonetheless, signs and symptoms worsened during the following 3 weeks, ultimately requiring ventilatory support and lung biopsy. Improvement did not occur until adalimumab was resumed at the dose for initial treatment of CD (**Fig. 2**). A contributing role of corticosteroid cannot be excluded in this case. However, other studies of prednisolone given in substantially greater doses in TB have not shown comparable levels of effectiveness.[83] This may be due to induction of hepatic enzymes by rifampin, which reduces methylprednisolone exposure and effect by 66%.[84] In the second case, infliximab was successfully used to treat an intractable paradoxical reaction of the central nervous system (CNS) in a patient with multiple tuberculomas that had failed to respond to high-dose corticosteroids.[85] In a third case, not yet published, adalimumab was used to treat recurrent immune reconstitution inflammatory syndrome (IRIS) in

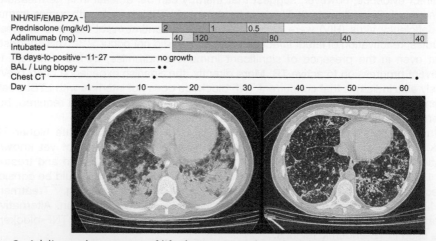

Fig. 2. Adalimumab treatment of life-threatening tuberculosis (TB). Day 1 indicates start of anti-TB therapy. Clearance of viable mycobacteria during the first 2 weeks of chemotherapy was accompanied by progressive clinical exacerbation attributed to withdrawal of the TNF antibody adalimumab. Clinical improvement was delayed until after day 20, when the patient received the full adalimumab dose recommended for initial treatment Crohn disease (160 mg). *Adapted from* Wallis RS, van Vuuren C, Potgieter S. Adalimumab treatment of life-threatening tuberculosis. Clin Infect Dis 2009;48(10):1430; with permission.

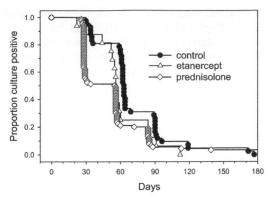

Fig. 3. Effects of etanercept (25 mg twice weekly) and high-dose methylprednisolone (2.75 mg/kg/d) on sputum culture conversion in pulmonary tuberculosis. *Reprinted from* Wallis RS. Reconsidering adjuvant immunotherapy for tuberculosis. Clin Infect Dis 2005;41(2):204; with permission.

a patient with acquired immunodeficiency syndrome and CNS cryptococcoma5674.[86] All three cases were remarkable for the rapidity of the radiographic and clinical responses to anti-TNF therapy. Further studies are warranted to confirm these observations.

Earlier resumption of anti-TNF therapy generally has not been recommended because of the concern that this might interfere with TB treatment. However, in none of these cases was the microbiologic response to therapy compromised. Indeed, two prospective controlled studies in patients with newly diagnosed pulmonary TB have indicated that TNF inhibition accelerates, rather than compromises, tissue sterilization (**Fig. 3**).[83,87] This may be due to enhanced penetration of TB drugs into granulomas, or enhanced drug bactericidal activity against metabolically active bacilli.[88,89] Further research is needed to investigate the potential role of anti-TNF antibody to accelerate and shorten TB chemotherapy.

REFERENCES

1. Humira prescribing information. Available at: http://www.rxabbott.com/pdf/humira.pdf. Accessed May 24, 2010.
2. Infliximab (Remicade) prescribing information. Available at: http://www.remicade.com/remicade/assets/HCP_PPI.pdf. Accessed May 24, 2010.
3. Baughman RP, Drent M, Kavuru M, et al. Infliximab therapy in patients with chronic sarcoidosis and pulmonary involvement. Am J Respir Crit Care Med 2006;174(7):795–802.
4. Rossman MD, Newman LS, Baughman RP, et al. A double-blinded, randomized, placebo-controlled trial of infliximab in subjects with active pulmonary sarcoidosis. Sarcoidosis Vasc Diffuse Lung Dis 2006;23(3):201–8.
5. Saleh S, Ghodsian S, Yakimova V, et al. Effectiveness of infliximab in treating selected patients with sarcoidosis. Respir Med 2006;100(11):2053–9.
6. Keystone E, Heijde D, Mason D Jr, et al. Certolizumab pegol plus methotrexate is significantly more effective than placebo plus methotrexate in active rheumatoid arthritis: findings of a fifty-two-week, phase III, multicenter, randomized, double-blind, placebo-controlled, parallel-group study. Arthritis Rheum 2008;58(11):3319–29.

7. Sandborn WJ, Feagan BG, Stoinov S, et al. Certolizumab pegol for the treatment of Crohn's disease. N Engl J Med 2007;357(3):228–38.

8. Smolen J, Brezezicki J, Mason D, et al. Efficacy and safety of certolizumab pegol in combination with methotrexate (MTX) in patients with active rheumatoid arthritis despite MTX therapy: results from the RAPID 2 study. Ann Rheum Dis 2007;66(Suppl 2):187.

9. St Clair EW, Wagner CL, Fasanmade AA, et al. The relationship of serum inflixi- mab concentrations to clinical improvement in rheumatoid arthritis: results from ATTRACT, a multicenter, randomized, double-blind, placebo-controlled trial. Arthritis Rheum 2002;46(6):1451–9.

10. Simponi (golimumab) prescribing information. Available at: http://www.simponi. com/simponi/Prescribing-Information/Prescribing-Information.pdf. Accessed May 24, 2010.

11. Nestorov I. Clinical pharmacokinetics of TNF antagonists: how do they differ? Semin Arthritis Rheum 2005;34:12–8.

12. Ucb. Cimzia prescribing information. Available at: http://www.cimzia.com/pdf/ Prescribing_Information.pdf. Accessed May 24, 2010.

13. Winter TA, Wright J, Ghosh S, et al. Intravenous CDP870, a PEGylated Fab' frag- ment of a humanized antitumour necrosis factor antibody, in patients with moderate-to-severe Crohn disease: an exploratory study. Aliment Pharmacol Ther 2004;20(11-12):1337–46.

14. Enbrel prescribing information. Agmen and Wyeth Pharmaceuticals, Thousand Oaks (CA); Madison (NJ). Available at: http://www.enbrel.com/prescribing-information.jsp. Accessed May 24, 2010.

15. Sandborn WJ, Hanauer SB, Katz S, et al. Etanercept for active Crohn's disease: a randomized, double-blind, placebo-controlled trial. Gastroenterology 2001; 121(5):1088–94.

16. Utz JP, Limper AH, Kalra S, et al. Etanercept for the treatment of stage II and III progressive pulmonary sarcoidosis. Chest 2003;124(1):177–85.

17. Carmona L, Hernandez-Garcia C, Vadillo C, et al. Increased risk of tuberculosis in patients with rheumatoid arthritis. J Rheumatol 2003;30(7):1436–9.

18. Seong SS, Choi CB, Woo JH, et al. Incidence of tuberculosis in Korean patients with rheumatoid arthritis (RA): effects of RA itself and of tumor necrosis factor blockers. J Rheumatol 2007;34(4):706–11.

19. Yamada T, Nakajima A, Inoue E, et al. Increased risk of tuberculosis in patients with rheumatoid arthritis in Japan. Ann Rheum Dis 2006;65(12):1661–3.

20. Nardell EA, Wallis RS. Here today–gone tomorrow: the case for transient acute tuberculosis infection. Am J Respir Crit Care Med 2006;174(7):734–5.

21. Coaccioli S, Di Cato L, Marioli D, et al. Impaired cutaneous cell-mediated immunity in newly diagnosed rheumatoid arthritis. Panminerva Med 2000; 42(4):263–6.

22. Wallis RS, Broder MS, Wong JY, et al. Granulomatous infectious diseases asso- ciated with TNF antagonists. Clin Infect Dis 2004;38(9):1261–5.

23. Wallis RS, Broder MS, Wong JY, et al. Granulomatous infections due to tumor necrosis factor blockade: correction. Clin Infect Dis 2004;39:1254–6.

24. Bergstrom L, Yocum DE, Ampel NM, et al. Increased risk of coccidioidomy- cosis in patients treated with TNF antagonists. Arthritis Rheum 2004;50(6): 1959–66.

25. Tubach F, Salmon D, Ravaud P, et al. Risk of tuberculosis is higher with antitumor necrosis factor monoclonal antibody therapy than with soluble tumor necrosis

factor receptor therapy: the three-year prospective French research axed on tolerance of biotherapies registry. Arthritis Rheum 2009;60(7):1884–94.

26. Fonseca JE, Canhao H, Silva C, et al. [Tuberculosis in rheumatic patients treated with tumour necrosis factor alpha antagonists: the Portuguese experience]. Acta Reumatol Port 2006;31(3):247–53 [in Portuguese].

27. Brassard P, Kezouh A, Suissa S. Antirheumatic drugs and the risk of tuberculosis. Clin Infect Dis 2006;43(6):717–22.

28. Mines D, Novelli L. Antirheumatic drugs and the risk of tuberculosis. Clin Infect Dis 2007;44(4):619–20.

29. Subramanyan GS, Yokoe DS, Sharnprapai S, et al. Using automated pharmacy records to assess the management of tuberculosis. Emerg Infect Dis 1999; 5(6):788–91.

30. Wallis RS. Mathematical modeling of the cause of tuberculosis during tumor necrosis factor blockade. Arthritis Rheum 2008;58(4):947–52.

31. Plessner HL, Lin PL, Kohno T, et al. Neutralization of tumor necrosis factor (TNF) by antibody but not TNF receptor fusion molecule exacerbates chronic murine tuberculosis. J Infect Dis 2007;195(11):1643–50.

32. Winthrop KL, Yamashita S, Beekmann SE, et al. Mycobacterial and other serious infections in patients receiving antitumor necrosis factor and other newly approved biologic therapies: case finding through the Emerging Infections Network. Clin Infect Dis 2008;46(11):1738–40.

33. Wallis RS. Mycobacterial disease attributable to tumor necrosis factor-alpha blockers. Clin Infect Dis 2008;47(12):1603–5.

34. Strangfeld A, Listing J, Herzer P, et al. Risk of herpes zoster in patients with rheumatoid arthritis treated with anti–TNF-α agents. JAMA 2009;301(7):737–44.

35. Esteve M, Saro C, Gonzalez-Huix F, et al. Chronic hepatitis B reactivation following Infliximab therapy in Crohn's disease patients: need for primary prophylaxis. Gut 2004;53(9):1363–5.

36. Michel M, Duvoux C, Hezode C, et al. Fulminant hepatitis after infliximab in a patient with hepatitis B virus treated for an adult onset still's disease. J Rheumatol 2003;30(7):1624–5.

37. Ostuni P, Botsios C, Punzi L, et al. Hepatitis B reactivation in a chronic hepatitis B surface antigen carrier with rheumatoid arthritis treated with infliximab and low dose methotrexate. Ann Rheum Dis 2003;62(7):686–7.

38. Sakellariou GT, Chatzigiannis I. Long-term anti-TNFalpha therapy for ankylosing spondylitis in two patients with chronic HBV infection. Clin Rheumatol 2007; 26(6):950–2.

39. Ueno Y, Tanaka S, Shimamoto M, et al. Infliximab therapy for Crohn's disease in a patient with chronic hepatitis B. Dig Dis Sci 2005;50(1):163–6.

40. Wendling D, Auge B, Bettinger D, et al. Reactivation of a latent precore mutant hepatitis B virus related chronic hepatitis during infliximab treatment for severe spondyloarthropathy. Ann Rheum Dis 2005;64(5):788–9.

41. Roux CH, Brocq O, Breuil V, et al. Safety of anti-TNF-alpha therapy in rheumatoid arthritis and spondylarthropathies with concurrent B or C chronic hepatitis. Rheumatology (Oxford) 2006;45(10):1294–7.

42. Ferri C, Ferraccioli G, Ferrari D, et al. Safety of antitumor necrosis factor-alpha therapy in patients with rheumatoid arthritis and chronic hepatitis C virus infection. J Rheumatol 2008;35(10):1944–9.

43. Oniankitan O, Duvoux C, Challine D, et al. Infliximab therapy for rheumatic diseases in patients with chronic hepatitis B or C. J Rheumatol 2004;31(1):107–9.

44. Wallis RS. Tumor necrosis factor antagonists: structure, function, and tuberculosis risks. Lancet Infect Dis 2008;8(10):601–11.
45. Di Sabatino A, Ciccocioppo R, Cinque B, et al. Defective mucosal T cell death is sustainably reverted by infliximab in a caspase-dependent pathway in Crohn's disease. Gut 2004;53(1):70–7.
46. Kirchner S, Holler E, Haffner S, et al. Effect of different tumor necrosis factor (TNF) reactive agents on reverse signaling of membrane integrated TNF in monocytes. Cytokine 2004;28(2):67–74.
47. Shen C, Assche GV, Colpaert S, et al. Adalimumab induces apoptosis of human monocytes: a comparative study with infliximab and etanercept. Aliment Pharmacol Ther 2005;21(3):251–8.
48. ten Hove T, van Montfrans C, Peppelenbosch MP, et al. Infliximab treatment induces apoptosis of lamina propria T lymphocytes in Crohn's disease. Gut 2002;50(2):206–11.
49. Van den Brande JM, Braat H, van den Brink GR, et al. Infliximab but not etanercept induces apoptosis in lamina propria T lymphocytes from patients with Crohn's disease. Gastroenterology 2003;124(7):1774–85.
50. Van den Brande JM, Koehler TC, Zelinkova Z, et al. Prediction of antitumour necrosis factor clinical efficacy by real-time visualisation of apoptosis in patients with Crohn's disease. Gut 2007;56(4):509–17.
51. Bruns H, Meinken C, Schauenberg P, et al. Anti-TNF immunotherapy reduces CD8+ T cell-mediated antimicrobial activity against Mycobacterium tuberculosis in humans. J Clin Invest 2009;119(5):1167–77.
52. Keystone EC. Certolizumab. Presented at the Annual European Congress of Rheumatology. Barcelona (Spain), June 13–16, 2007.
53. Nesbitt A, Fossati G, Bergin M, et al. Mechanism of action of certolizumab pegol (CDP870): in vitro comparison with other anti-tumor necrosis factor alpha agents. Inflamm Bowel Dis 2007;13(11):1323–32.
54. Bourne T, Fossati G, Nesbitt A. A PEGylated Fab' fragment against tumor necrosis factor for the treatment of Crohn disease: exploring a new mechanism of action. BioDrugs 2008;22(5):331–7.
55. Saliu O, Sofer C, Stein DS, et al. Tumor necrosis factor blockers: differential effects on mycobacterial immunity. J Infect Dis 2006;194:486–92.
56. Scallon B, Cai A, Solowski N, et al. Binding and functional comparisons of two types of tumor necrosis factor antagonists. J Pharmacol Exp Ther 2002;301(2):418–26.
57. Brewer MA, Edwards KM, Palmer PS, et al. Bacille Calmette-Guerin immunization in normal healthy adults. J Infect Dis 1994;170:476–9.
58. Mudido PM, Guwatudde D, Nakakeeto MK, et al. The effect of bacille Calmette-Guerin vaccination at birth on tuberculin skin test reactivity in Ugandan children. Int J Tuberc Lung Dis 1999;3(10):891–5.
59. Behr MA, Wilson MA, Gill WP, et al. Comparative genomics of BCG vaccines by whole-genome DNA microarray. Science 1999;284(5419):1520–3.
60. Brock I, Weldingh K, Leyten EM, et al. Specific T cell epitopes for immunoassay-based diagnosis of Mycobacterium tuberculosis infection. J Clin Microbiol 2004;42(6):2379–87.
61. Ponce de Leon D, cevedo-Vasquez E, Alvizuri S, et al. Comparison of an interferon-gamma assay with tuberculin skin testing for detection of tuberculosis (TB) infection in patients with rheumatoid arthritis in a TB-endemic population. J Rheumatol 2008;35(5):776–81.

62. Lalvani A, Nagvenkar P, Udwadia Z, et al. Enumeration of T cells specific for RD1-encoded antigens suggests a high prevalence of latent *Mycobacterium tuberculosis* infection in healthy urban Indians. J Infect Dis 2001;183(3):469–77.
63. Paimela L, Johansson-Stephansson EA, Koskimies S, et al. Depressed cutaneous cell-mediated immunity in early rheumatoid arthritis. Clin Exp Rheumatol 1990;8(5):433–7.
64. Ponce de Leon D, cevedo-Vasquez E, Sanchez-Torres A, et al. Attenuated response to purified protein derivative in patients with rheumatoid arthritis: study in a population with a high prevalence of tuberculosis. Ann Rheum Dis 2005; 64(9):1360–1.
65. Richards NM, Nelson KE, Batt MD, et al. Tuberculin test conversion during repeated skin testing, associated with sensitivity to nontuberculous mycobacteria. Am Rev Respir Dis 1979;120(1):59–65.
66. Thompson NJ, Glassroth JL, Snider DEJ, et al. The booster phenomenon in serial tuberculin testing. Am Rev Respir Dis 1979;119(4):587–97.
67. Carmona L, Gomez-Reino JJ, Rodriguez-Valverde V, et al. Effectiveness of recommendations to prevent reactivation of latent tuberculosis infection in patients treated with tumor necrosis factor antagonists. Arthritis Rheum 2005; 52(6):1766–72.
68. Gomez-Reino JJ, Carmona L, Angel DM. Risk of tuberculosis in patients treated with tumor necrosis factor antagonists due to incomplete prevention of reactivation of latent infection. Arthritis Rheum 2007;57(5):756–61.
69. Comstock GW, Baum C, Snider DE Jr. Isoniazid prophylaxis among Alaskan Eskimos: a final report of the Bethel isoniazid studies. Am Rev Respir Dis 1979; 119(5):827–30.
70. IUAT Committee on Prophylaxis. Efficacy of various durations of isoniazid preventive therapy for tuberculosis: five years of follow-up in the IUAT trial. International Union Against Tuberculosis Committee on Prophylaxis. Bull World Health Organ 1982;60(4):555–64.
71. Gordin FM, Matts JP, Miller C, et al. A controlled trial of isoniazid in persons with anergy and human immunodeficiency virus infection who are at high risk for tuberculosis. Terry Beirn Community Programs for Clinical Research on AIDS. N Engl J Med 1997;337(5):315–20.
72. Hawken M, Nunn P, Gathua S, et al. Increased recurrence of tuberculosis in HIV-1-infected patients in Kenya. Lancet 1993;342(8867):332–7.
73. Pape JW, Jean SS, Ho JL, et al. Effect of isoniazid prophylaxis on incidence of active tuberculosis and progression of HIV infection. Lancet 1993;342(8866): 268–72.
74. Whalen CC, Johnson JL, Okwera A, et al. A trial of three regimens to prevent tuberculosis in Ugandan adults infected with the human immunodeficiency virus. Uganda-Case Western Reserve University Research Collaboration. N Engl J Med 1997;337(12):801–8.
75. Edwards LB, Acquaviva FA, Livesay VT. Identification of tuberculous infected: dual tests and density of reaction. Am Rev Respir Dis 1973;108:1334–9.
76. Higuchi K, Harada N, Fukazawa K, et al. Relationship between whole-blood interferon-gamma responses and the risk of active tuberculosis. Tuberculosis (Edinb) 2008;88(3):244–8.
77. Cooray DV, Moran R, Khanna D, et al. Screening, rescreening and treatment of ppd positivity in patients on anti-TNF-α therapy. Arthritis Rheum 2008;58: S546–7.

78. Arend SM, Leyten EM, Franken WP, et al. A patient with de novo tuberculosis during antitumor necrosis factor-alpha therapy illustrating diagnostic pitfalls and paradoxical response to treatment. Clin Infect Dis 2007;45(11):1470–5.

79. Belknap R, Reves R, Burman W. Immune reconstitution to *Mycobacterium tuberculosis* after discontinuing infliximab. Int J Tuberc Lung Dis 2005;9(9):1057–8.

80. Garcia-Vidal C, Rodriguez FS, Martinez LJ, et al. Paradoxical response to antituberculous therapy in infliximab-treated patients with disseminated tuberculosis. Clin Infect Dis 2005;40(5):756–9.

81. Strady C, Brochot P, Ainine K, et al. Tuberculosis during treatment by TNFalpha-inhibitors. Presse Med 2006;35:1765–72.

82. Wallis RS, van Vuuren C, Potgieter S. Adalimumab treatment of life-threatening tuberculosis. Clin Infect Dis 2009;48(10):1429–32.

83. Mayanja-Kizza H, Jones-Lopez EC, Okwera A, et al. Immunoadjuvant therapy for HIV-associated tuberculosis with prednisolone: a phase II clinical trial in Uganda. J Infect Dis 2005;191(6):856–65.

84. McAllister WA, Thompson PJ, Al-Habet SM, et al. Rifampicin reduces effectiveness and bioavailability of prednisolone. Br Med J (Clin Res Ed) 1983; 286(6369):923–5.

85. Blackmore TK, Manning L, Taylor W, et al. Therapeutic use of infliximab in tuberculosis to control severe paradoxical reaction involving the brain, lung, and lymph nodes. Clin Infect Dis 2008;47(10):e79–82.

86. Sitapati AM, Kao CL, Cachay ER, et al. Treatment of HIV-related inflammatory cerebral cryptococcoma using adalimumab. Clin Infect Dis 2010;50(2):e7–10.

87. Wallis RS, Kyambadde P, Johnson JL, et al. A study of the safety, immunology, virology, and microbiology of adjunctive etanercept in HIV-1-associated tuberculosis. AIDS 2004;18(2):257–64.

88. Karakousis PC, Yoshimatsu T, Lamichhane G, et al. Dormancy phenotype displayed by extracellular *Mycobacterium tuberculosis* within artificial granulomas in mice. J Exp Med 2004;200(5):647–57.

89. Wallis RS. Reconsidering adjuvant immunotherapy for tuberculosis. Clin Infect Dis 2005;41(2):201–8.

The Convergence of the Global Smoking, COPD, Tuberculosis, HIV, and Respiratory Infection Epidemics

Richard N. van Zyl-Smit, MBChB, MRCP(UK)[a],*, Laurence Brunet, BSc[b],
Madhukar Pai, MD, PhD[b], Wing-Wai Yew, MBBS, FRCP(Edinb), FCCP[c]

KEYWORDS

• Tuberculosis • Smoking • HIV • Influenza • COPD
• Pneumonia • Epidemics

History appears to be repeating itself. This time, however, it might have a sting in its tail. At the end of the 19th century a vaguely familiar picture was developing, with consequences for global respiratory health. Tobacco smoking was widespread and increasing after the invention of the cigarette-rolling machine in 1881.[1] The discovery of *Mycobacterium tuberculosis* by Robert Koch 1 year later in 1882 occurred during a time that tuberculosis (TB) was rampant across many parts of the world.

By the turn of the 20th century, tobacco consumption had increased to approximately 50 billion cigarettes per year[1] at a time that TB mortality was declining in Europe most likely because of improved nutrition and social circumstances. A potential association between smoking and TB was suggested by Webb[2] in 1918. During the same year, the "Mother of all pandemics,"[3] the 1918 Spanish flu, killed nearly 50 million people worldwide.[3,4]

R.V.Z.S. is supported by a Discovery Foundation fellowship and by the Fogarty International Clinical Research Scholars/Fellows Support Center National Institutes of Health grant R24TW007988. M.P. is supported by grants from the Canadian Institutes of Health Research (CIHR) and European Commission (TBSusgent; EU FP-7).
[a] Lung Infection and Immunity Unit, Division of Pulmonology and UCT Lung Institute, Department of Medicine, University of Cape Town, Groote Schuur Hospital, Cape Town 7935, South Africa
[b] Department of Epidemiology, Biostatistics & Occupational Health, McGill University, 1020 Pine Avenue West, Montreal, Quebec H3A 1A2, Canada
[c] Tuberculosis and Chest Unit, Grantham Hospital, 125 Wong Chuk Hang Road, Hong Kong, China
* Corresponding author.
E-mail address: rvzs@iafrica.com

Infect Dis Clin N Am 24 (2010) 693–703
doi:10.1016/j.idc.2010.04.012
0891-5520/10/$ – see front matter © 2010 Elsevier Inc. All rights reserved.

id.theclinics.com

Nearly 100 years later, smoking rates are at an all time high with more than 6319 billion cigarettes consumed per year.[1] Faced with declining markets in the north, the tobacco industry is moving south, where smoking is on the increase, especially in countries such as China and India. TB remains uncontrolled in the developing world with increasing rates of multi-, extensively, and pan-drug–resistant tuberculosis. HIV has added a new face to respiratory disease with increased rates of TB and pneumonia and in addition we are facing the looming possibility of a highly virulent H5N1 "avian" influenza pandemic, with the novel strain of H1N1 "swine" flu recently added to the mix.

In this overview, we build on our previous reviews[5,6] and consider the predisposing effects of tobacco smoking, and the potential interactions of tuberculosis, HIV, chronic obstructive pulmonary disease (COPD), influenza, and other respiratory infection epidemics (**Fig. 1**).

METHODOLOGY AND SEARCH STRATEGY

We searched PubMed for peer-reviewed literature over the past 3 decades with a focus on studies that reported data on the associations among tuberculosis, smoking, HIV, influenza, pneumonia, and COPD. No language restrictions were imposed, although only English language studies were eventually included. In addition, we identified 3 systematic reviews[7–9] on the association between tobacco and TB, 1 systematic review on the association between tobacco and HIV,[10] and several narrative reviews[5,6,11–17] on the association between tobacco and all the conditions of interest. The reference lists of these reviews were also used to supplement the search. In addition, we identified a comprehensive report entitled "A WHO/The Union monograph on TB and tobacco control: joining efforts to control two related global epidemics"[18]; this was used as an additional resource to supplement our searches. Key words included tuberculosis, HIV, COPD, pneumonia, influenza, and tobacco smoking.

SMOKING AND PULMONARY IMMUNITY AND DISEASE

Current estimates of tobacco smoking rates are 49% for men and 8% for women in low- and middle-income countries, and 37% for men and 21% for women in high-income countries.[7] Tobacco is the single most preventable cause of death in the world today. It kills more than 5 million people per year, with more than 80% of those deaths occurring in the developing world.[19] There are a multitude of effects of tobacco smoke

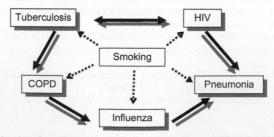

Fig. 1. The central role of smoking in pulmonary infections, HIV, and COPD, and the interactions of several of the individual diseases. The dashed lines indicate increased risk of disease associated with tobacco smoking. The solid line indicates increased risk associated with other diseases.

on the immune system, predisposing individuals to respiratory infections.[15–17] These effects have been summarized in **Fig. 2**. Briefly, smoking affects circulating immune cells and mucosal surface defenses (mucus, cilia), as well as local innate immune cell functions (macrophages, neutrophils). The associations with tobacco smoking have been well described for several of the diseases depicted in **Fig. 1**.

SMOKING AND TB

The association between tobacco smoke and tuberculosis was suggested many years ago.[2] Evidence of the impact of tobacco smoking on TB infection has been confounded by its almost universal association with poverty, overcrowding, and alcohol usage. Similar pathologic mechanisms induced by malnutrition, alcohol abuse, and smoking may indeed all predispose an individual to TB. There are now 3 comprehensive independent systematic reviews and meta-analyses that have synthesized the evidence for the association between TB and tobacco smoking.[7–9]

The association of smoking and TB has been analyzed for 3 outcomes: TB infection (defined by a positive tuberculin skin test), active TB disease, and death attributable to TB. **Table 1** provides the outcome-specific pooled relative risk estimates from the 3 independent meta-analyses.

It is evident from these meta-analyses that smoking approximately doubles the risk of each outcome, namely TB infection (relative risk [RR] ~1.5), active TB disease (RR ~2.0), and TB mortality (RR ~2.0). The evidence is strong for TB disease, but relatively weaker for TB infection. Because of the widespread nature of tobacco smoking, the population attributable risk (PAR%) is likely to be high. For example, if the relative risk for TB disease is estimated at 1.5, and population exposure to tobacco smoke is 30%, the PAR% will be approximately 15%. In other words, 15% of the TB cases in the world each year may be attributable to tobacco exposure.[4]

Since the publication of these meta-analyses, newer studies have been published, and these studies confirm the association between smoking and TB. In a large case-control study from India, Jha and colleagues[20] reported excess TB deaths among smokers, as compared with nonsmokers, among both women (RR, 3.0; 99% confidence interval [CI], 2.4 to 3.9) and men (RR, 2.3; 99% CI, 2.1 to 2.6). A subsequent large case-control study from India[21] reported that those who both smoked cigarettes and drank alcohol had considerably higher active TB incidence rates than those who did neither (TB incidence RR 3.5).

Similar results were also obtained in Taiwan and China. In a prospective cohort study from Taiwan, Lin and colleagues[22] reported that current smoking was associated with an increased risk of active TB (adjusted odds ratio [OR], 1.94; 95% confidence interval, 1.01–3.73). In a case-control study from 2 rural areas of China, Wang and Shen[23] reported an adjusted OR of 1.93 (95% CI: 1.51–2.48) for smoking and TB disease. Thus, these studies from India, Taiwan, and China added further support to the already strong evidence from the meta-analyses.

A cohort study in Brazil looked at the association between smoking and a fourth outcome, TB relapse. They reported that smoking was independently associated with relapse of TB, as defined by the requirement for re-treatment within 3 to 5 years after successful completion of TB treatment. After adjusting for socioeconomic variables and alcohol, the OR for relapse was 2.53 (95% CI, 1.23–5.21).[24]

Last, Lin and colleagues[25] did a mathematical modeling study, where they modeled future COPD and lung cancer mortality and TB incidence, taking into account the accumulation of hazardous effects of risk factors on COPD and lung cancer over time, and dependency of the risk of TB infection on the prevalence of disease. Their

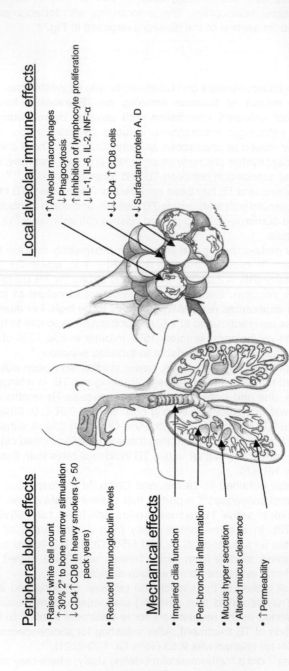

Local alveolar immune effects

- ↑Alveolar macrophages
- ↓ Phagocytosis
- ↑Inhibition of lymphocyte proliferation
- ↓IL-1, IL-6, IL-2, INF-α
- ↓↓ CD4 ↑CD8 cells
- ↓Surfactant protein A, D

Peripheral blood effects

- Raised white cell count
  ↑ 30% 2° to bone marrow stimulation
- ↓CD4↑CD8 In heavy smokers (> 50 pack years)
- Reduced Immunoglobulin levels

Mechanical effects

- Impaired cilia function
- Peri-bronchial inflammation
- Mucus hyper secretion
- Altered mucus clearance
- ↑ Permeability

Fig. 2. Overview of the systemic and local effects of tobacco smoke on the immune system and pulmonary defense mechanisms against infection.

Table 1			
The association between smoking and the relative risk of latent tuberculosis infection, progression to active disease, and mortality from active TB			
		Meta-analyses: Pooled Relative Risks (95% Confidence Interval)	
		Slama et al 2007[6]	Lin et al 2007[7]	Bates et al 2007[8]
TB outcome	TB infection	~1.8 (1.5–2.1)	1.7–2.2 (1.5–2.8)	~1.7 (1.5–2.0)
	TB disease	~2.3 (1.8–3.0)	~2.0 (1.6–2.6)	~2.3 (2.0–2.8)
	TB mortality	~2.2 (1.3–3.7)	~2.0 (1.1–3.5)	~2.1 (1.4–3.4)

Data from van Zyl-Smit RN, Pai M, Yew WW, et al. Global lung health: the colliding epidemics of tuberculosis, tobacco smoking, HIV and COPD. Eur Respir J 2010;35:27–33.

model suggested that complete cessation of smoking and solid-fuel use by 2033 could avoid 26 million deaths from COPD and 6.3 million deaths from lung cancer. Smoking cessation would also reduce the projected annual TB incidence in 2033 by 14% to 52% if 80% directly observed treatment short-course (DOTS) coverage is sustained. Based on these results, they concluded that reducing smoking and solid-fuel use can substantially lower predictions of COPD and lung cancer burden and would contribute to effective TB control in China.

SMOKING AND PNEUMONIA

Pneumonia occurs more frequently in individuals with impaired immunity. This is evident in the elderly and alcoholic individuals, and those who are malnourished, HIV-infected, and those with underlying COPD.[26] In addition, tobacco smoking appears to be an independent risk factor for pneumonia.[27,28] It is evident from several studies that smoking is a particularly important risk factor for streptococcal pneumonia (OR 1.88 to 4.1).[29,30] Passive smokers and importantly children also have an increased risk of infection, OR 2.5 (95% CI 1.2–5.1) and 1.88 (95% CI 1.04–3.39), respectively.[29,31] Severe pneumococcal disease is more frequently seen in smokers,[29,32] which may be partially explained by enhanced pneumococcal epithelial adherence caused by tobacco smoking.[33]

Although the frequency of pneumonia caused by other organisms is low, there is also strong evidence for increased risks of *Legionella* (OR 3.48; 95% CI 2.09–5.79),[34] *Mycoplasma* (OR 5.6; 95% CI, 1.5–20.4),[35] and *Haemophilus influenzae*[36] infection. In HIV-infected individuals, the already increased risk of community-acquired pneumonia is compounded by the increased risk associated with smoking[37–42] with an apparent dose response association.[39] In addition, the risks of other infection such as pneumocystis jiroveci pneumonia (PCP) are also increased by smoking (discussed in the following section).[40,43]

SMOKING AND INFLUENZA

With the prospect of an avian influenza epidemic ever increasing,[3] multiple measures will be required to control the epidemics. Although not recognized as a risk factor in the 1918 pandemic (data not collected),[2,3] there is substantial evidence in both mouse and human models for a negative effect of smoking on influenza.[44–48] The risk of infection is increased in smokers (OR 1.4–2.4),[46,47] as well as likelihood for severe disease and complications (OR 4.3; 95% CI 1.1–16.1).[49] In addition to predisposing individuals to infection, the efficacy of influenza vaccines is reduced in smokers.[50–52]

The predisposing risk factors for localized influenza outbreaks have been studied. An influenza A/USSR/90/77(H1N1) outbreak in Israeli military recruits in 1979 found a relative risk of 1.44 (95% CI; 1.03–2.01).[48] In a 1986 influenza A/Taiwan/1/86(H1N1) outbreak at a Florida naval air base, the seasonal trivalent vaccination offered no protection and smokers had a nonsignificant trend to increased infection (OR 1.4; 95% CI 0.9–2.2; $p = .27$).[53] There are little data on the current H1N1 epidemics and their potential association with tobacco smoking. Several recent observational studies have not reported on the smoking status of patients.[54–57] It is likely, however, given the extent of the global pandemic, that the association with tobacco smoking will become evident as the number of reported cases increases.

SMOKING AND HIV

Although both tobacco smoking and HIV infection may be associated through their common associations with poverty and high-risk behavior, tobacco smoking appears to be an independent and important risk factor for contracting HIV.[58–61] Other studies have demonstrated higher viral loads[62] and rate of progression of HIV infection to AIDS in smokers,[63,64] but this association has not been observed in all studies.[65–68]

Smoking further raises the extremely high risk of contracting TB in HIV-positive persons[43] in addition to increased susceptibility of community-acquired bacterial pneumonia.[37–40] HIV-infected smokers also have higher respiratory symptoms and risk of mortality (hazard ratio 1.99; 95% CI 1.03–3.86) when compared with nonsmokers.[41]

Several studies have examined the risk of other opportunistic infection such as PCP with conflicting results. Some have shown significantly increased risk but this has not been confirmed by others.[38–40,66]

Tobacco smoking and HIV are associated with an accelerated form of obstructive pulmonary disease.[69–73] If this form of COPD is phenotypically similar to that seen with HIV uninfected smokers, the risk of influenza and pneumonia may be further magnified.

SMOKING AND COPD

Although the focus of this article is primarily on the convergence of respiratory infections, HIV, and tobacco smoking, the importance of COPD in the interactions needs to be stressed. The causal link between smoking and COPD is well described and the multitude of consequences well known.[74] There is now a growing recognition of the importance of non-smoking causes for COPD.[75] There are several studies examining respiratory infections (particularly TB) as a cause of COPD.[76–80] The long-term effect on pulmonary function and response to treatment is not well documented,[75] although the increased susceptibility to other respiratory infections, particularly influenza and pneumonia are likely to be similar.

CONVERGENCE OF TB, HIV, COPD, PNEUMONIA, AND INFLUENZA

Tobacco smoking is undoubtedly at the center of convergence of the epidemics we are currently facing (not discounting the role of alcohol, malnutrition, poverty, indoor biomass fuel exposure, and outdoor air pollution).

As smoking increases the risk of TB and COPD, the long-term damage to pulmonary structures and respiratory function further increases the risk of bacterial pneumonia and influenza. Similarly, the increased susceptibility to influenza seen in smokers will magnify the risk of superadded bacterial pneumonia following severe influenza. The multitude of infections associated with HIV infection, particularly TB and pneumonia, are likely to be exacerbated by smoking, especially if the accelerated form of COPD further impairs pulmonary immunity to infection.

Even without the effect of tobacco smoke, the interactions of HIV, influenza, TB, and pneumonia compound the health on the individuals suffering from them as well as society in general. The interactions summarized in **Fig. 1** are likely to be far more complex and wide ranging. This is no more evident than what is being seen in many parts of the developing world where in addition to high smoking rates, malnutrition, overcrowding, and indoor biomass fuel usage, HIV is driving the TB epidemic. The net outcome, in several parts of the world (mainly low-income countries), is that these epidemics are simultaneously converging.

These high-burden, low-income countries are least likely to be able to put measures in place to effectively combat the spread of a worldwide influenza epidemic. The already overburdened TB control programs are struggling to cope with increasing HIV-positive subjects as well as complicated and expensive treatment regimes for multidrug-resistant and extremely drug-resistant TB. Whether local and national government structures are able to effectively improve service delivery, drug supplies, and infection control measures remains to be seen. The H1N1 epidemic clearly showed the inability of weak health care systems to launch any concerted, evidence-based programs to manage clinical cases and prevent transmission.

It is clear that smoking cessation and respiratory infection control are likely to be the cornerstone to halting the convergent epidemics. In addition, effective treatment strategies will be required to treat those who contract community-acquired pneumonia, tuberculosis, influenza, or HIV. The management of multiple infections with potentially interacting drug therapies, the need for quarantine, and rational allocation of critical care services will further challenge the most advanced health care services let alone those in under-resourced areas.

SUMMARY

At the beginning of the 21st century, the globe is facing an economic crisis in addition to the convergence of several potentially devastating infection epidemics. The emergence of H1N1 is adding to the burden on health care delivery systems, and is already diverting precious human and laboratory resources. This was clearly evident in countries such as Mexico and India. The final number of people who will succumb to TB, HIV, and influenza will depend on the combined efforts of governments, health agencies, and nongovernmental bodies. Interventional strategies will need to target preventive strategies as well as locally sustainable treatment options.

Karl Marx said, "History repeats itself—first as a tragedy, second as a farce." It remains to be seen if we have learned sufficiently over the past hundred years to effectively combat the looming epidemics or whether we are doomed to see history repeat itself.

REFERENCES

1. Mackay J, Eriksen M. The tobacco atlas. 2nd edition. Hong Kong (China): World Health Organisation; 2006.
2. Webb GB. The effect of the inhalation of cigarette smoke on the lungs. A clinical study. Am Rev Tuberc 1918;2(1):25–7.
3. Taubenberger JK, Morens DM. 1918 influenza: the mother of all pandemics. Emerg Infect Dis 2006;12(1):15–22.
4. Morens DM, Fauci AS. The 1918 influenza pandemic: insights for the 21st century. J Infect Dis 2007;195(7):1018–28.

5. Pai M, Mohan A, Dheda K, et al. Lethal interaction: the colliding epidemics of tobacco and tuberculosis. Expert Rev Anti Infect Ther 2007;5(3):385–91.
6. van Zyl-Smit RN, Pai M, Yew WW, et al. Global lung health: the colliding epidemics of tuberculosis, tobacco smoking, HIV and COPD. Eur Respir J 2010;35:27–33.
7. Slama K, Chiang CY, Enarson DA, et al. Tobacco and tuberculosis: a qualitative systematic review and meta-analysis. Int J Tuberc Lung Dis 2007;11(10):1049–61.
8. Lin HH, Ezzati M, Murray M. Tobacco smoke, indoor air pollution and tuberculosis: a systematic review and meta-analysis. PLoS Med 2007;4(1):e20.
9. Bates MN, Khalakdina A, Pai M, et al. Risk of tuberculosis from exposure to tobacco smoke: a systematic review and meta-analysis. Arch Intern Med 2007; 167(4):335–42.
10. Furber AS, Maheswaran R, Newell JN, et al. Is smoking tobacco an independent risk factor for HIV infection and progression to AIDS? A systemic review. Sex Transm Infect 2007;83(1):41–6.
11. Baris E, Ezzati M. Should interventions to reduce respirable pollutants be linked to tuberculosis control programmes? BMJ 2004;329(7474):1090–3.
12. Chiang CY, Slama K, Enarson DA. Associations between tobacco and tuberculosis. Int J Tuberc Lung Dis 2007;11(3):258–62.
13. Davies PD, Yew WW, Ganguly D, et al. Smoking and tuberculosis: the epidemiological association and immunopathogenesis. Trans R Soc Trop Med Hyg 2006; 100(4):291–8.
14. Maurya V, Vijayan VK, Shah A. Smoking and tuberculosis: an association overlooked. Int J Tuberc Lung Dis 2002;6(11):942–51.
15. Arcavi L, Benowitz NL. Cigarette smoking and infection. Arch Intern Med 2004; 164(20):2206–16.
16. Sopori M. Effects of cigarette smoke on the immune system. Nat Rev Immunol 2002;2(5):372–7.
17. Stampfli MR, Anderson GP. How cigarette smoke skews immune responses to promote infection, lung disease and cancer. Nat Rev Immunol 2009;9(5):377–84.
18. World Health Organisation. A WHO/The Union monograph on TB and tobacco control: joining forces to control two related global epidemics [WHO/HTM/TB/2007.390]. Geneva (Switzerland): World Health Organization; 2007.
19. WHO. WHO report on the global tobacco epidemic, 2008. The MPOWER package. Geneva (Switzerland): World Health Organisation; 2008.
20. Jha P, Jacob B, Gajalakshmi V, et al. A nationally representative case-control study of smoking and death in India. N Engl J Med 2008;358(11):1137–47.
21. Gajalakshmi V, Peto R. Smoking, drinking and incident tuberculosis in rural India: population-based case-control study. Int J Epidemiol 2009;38(4):1018–25.
22. Lin HH, Ezzati M, Chang HY, et al. Association between tobacco smoking and active tuberculosis in Taiwan: prospective cohort study. Am J Respir Crit Care Med 2009;180(5):475–80.
23. Wang J, Shen H. Review of cigarette smoking and tuberculosis in China: intervention is needed for smoking cessation among tuberculosis patients. BMC Public Health 2009;9:292.
24. d'Arc Lyra Batista J, de Fatima Pessoa Militao de Albuquerque M, de Alencar Ximenes RA, et al. Smoking increases the risk of relapse after successful tuberculosis treatment. Int J Epidemiol 2008;37(4):841–51.
25. Lin HH, Murray M, Cohen T, et al. Effects of smoking and solid-fuel use on COPD, lung cancer, and tuberculosis in China: a time-based, multiple risk factor, modelling study. Lancet 2008;372(9648):1473–83.

26. Feldman C, Anderson R. New insights into pneumococcal disease. Respirology 2009;14(2):167–79.
27. Farr BM, Woodhead MA, Macfarlane JT, et al. Risk factors for community-acquired pneumonia diagnosed by general practitioners in the community. Respir Med 2000;94(5):422–7.
28. Farr BM, Bartlett CL, Wadsworth J, et al. Risk factors for community-acquired pneumonia diagnosed upon hospital admission. British Thoracic Society Pneumonia Study Group. Respir Med 2000;94(10):954–63.
29. Nuorti JP, Butler JC, Farley MM, et al. Cigarette smoking and invasive pneumococcal disease. Active Bacterial Core Surveillance Team. N Engl J Med 2000; 342(10):681–9.
30. Almirall J, Gonzalez CA, Balanzo X, et al. Proportion of community-acquired pneumonia cases attributable to tobacco smoking. Chest 1999;116(2):375–9.
31. O'Dempsey TJ, McArdle TF, Morris J, et al. A study of risk factors for pneumococcal disease among children in a rural area of West Africa. Int J Epidemiol 1996;25(4):885–93.
32. Pastor P, Medley F, Murphy TV. Invasive pneumococcal disease in Dallas County, Texas: results from population-based surveillance in 1995. Clin Infect Dis 1998; 26(3):590–5.
33. Raman AS, Swinburne AJ, Fedullo AJ. Pneumococcal adherence to the buccal epithelial cells of cigarette smokers. Chest 1983;83(1):23–7.
34. Doebbeling BN, Wenzel RP. The epidemiology of Legionella pneumophila infections. Semin Respir Infect 1987;2(4):206–21.
35. Klement E, Talkington DF, Wasserzug O, et al. Identification of risk factors for infection in an outbreak of Mycoplasma pneumoniae respiratory tract disease. Clin Infect Dis 2006;43(10):1239–45.
36. Kofteridis D, Samonis G, Mantadakis E, et al. Lower respiratory tract infections caused by Haemophilus influenzae: clinical features and predictors of outcome. Med Sci Monit 2009;15(4):CR135–9.
37. Kohli R, Lo Y, Homel P, et al. Bacterial pneumonia, HIV therapy, and disease progression among HIV-infected women in the HIV epidemiologic research (HER) study. Clin Infect Dis 2006;43(1):90–8.
38. Burns DN, Hillman D, Neaton JD, et al. Cigarette smoking, bacterial pneumonia, and other clinical outcomes in HIV-1 infection. Terry Beirn Community Programs for Clinical Research on AIDS. J Acquir Immune Defic Syndr Hum Retrovirol 1996; 13(4):374–83.
39. Conley LJ, Bush TJ, Buchbinder SP, et al. The association between cigarette smoking and selected HIV-related medical conditions. AIDS 1996;10(10): 1121–6.
40. Miguez-Burbano MJ, Ashkin D, Rodriguez A, et al. Increased risk of Pneumocystis carinii and community-acquired pneumonia with tobacco use in HIV disease. Int J Infect Dis 2005;9(4):208–17.
41. Crothers K, Griffith TA, McGinnis KA, et al. The impact of cigarette smoking on mortality, quality of life, and comorbid illness among HIV-positive veterans. J Gen Intern Med 2005;20(12):1142–5.
42. Hirschtick RE, Glassroth J, Jordan MC, et al. Bacterial pneumonia in persons infected with the Human Immunodeficiency Virus. Pulmonary Complications of HIV Infection Study Group. N Engl J Med 1995;333(13):845–51.
43. Miguez-Burbano MJ, Burbano X, Ashkin D, et al. Impact of tobacco use on the development of opportunistic respiratory infections in HIV seropositive patients on antiretroviral therapy. Addict Biol 2003;8(1):39–43.

44. Gualano RC, Hansen MJ, Vlahos R, et al. Cigarette smoke worsens lung inflammation and impairs resolution of influenza infection in mice. Respir Res 2008;9:53.
45. Robbins CS, Bauer CM, Vujicic N, et al. Cigarette smoke impacts immune inflammatory responses to influenza in mice. Am J Respir Crit Care Med 2006;174(12): 1342–51.
46. Finklea JF, Sandifer SH, Smith DD. Cigarette smoking and epidemic influenza. Am J Epidemiol 1969;90(5):390–9.
47. Kark JD, Lebiush M, Rannon L. Cigarette smoking as a risk factor for epidemic a(H1N1) influenza in young men. N Engl J Med 1982;307(17):1042–6.
48. Kark JD, Lebiush M. Smoking and epidemic influenza-like illness in female military recruits: a brief survey. Am J Public Health 1981;71(5):530–2.
49. Hanshaoworakul W, Simmerman JM, Narueponjirakul U, et al. Severe human influenza infections in Thailand: oseltamivir treatment and risk factors for fatal outcome. PLoS One 2009;4(6):e6051.
50. Cruijff M, Thijs C, Govaert T, et al. The effect of smoking on influenza, influenza vaccination efficacy and on the antibody response to influenza vaccination. Vaccine 1999;17(5):426–32.
51. Pearson WS, Dube SR, Ford ES, et al. Influenza and pneumococcal vaccination rates among smokers: data from the 2006 Behavioral Risk Factor Surveillance System. Prev Med 2009;48(2):180–3.
52. Finklea JF, Hasselblad V, Riggan WB, et al. Cigarette smoking and hemagglutination inhibition response to influenza after natural disease and immunization. Am Rev Respir Dis 1971;104(3):368–76.
53. Klontz KC, Hynes NA, Gunn RA, et al. An outbreak of influenza A/Taiwan/1/86 (H1N1) infections at a naval base and its association with airplane travel. Am J Epidemiol 1989;129(2):341–8.
54. Dawood FS, Jain S, Finelli L, et al. Emergence of a novel swine-origin influenza A (H1N1) virus in humans. N Engl J Med 2009;360(25):2605–15.
55. Fraser C, Donnelly CA, Cauchemez S, et al. Pandemic potential of a strain of influenza A (H1N1): early findings. Science 2009;324(5934):1557–61.
56. Cutler J, Schleihauf E, Hatchette TF, et al. Investigation of the first cases of human-to-human infection with the new swine-origin influenza A (H1N1) virus in Canada. CMAJ 2009;181(3–4):159–63.
57. Perez-Padilla R, de la Rosa-Zamboni D, Ponce de Leon S, et al. Pneumonia and respiratory failure from swine-origin influenza A (H1N1) in Mexico. N Engl J Med 2009;361(7):680–9.
58. Boulos R, Halsey NA, Holt E, et al. HIV-1 in Haitian women 1982–1988. The Cite Soleil/JHU AIDS Project Team. J Acquir Immune Defic Syndr 1990;3(7):721–8.
59. Halsey NA, Coberly JS, Holt E, et al. Sexual behavior, smoking, and HIV-1 infection in Haitian women. JAMA 1992;267(15):2062–6.
60. Chao A, Bulterys M, Musanganire F, et al. Risk factors associated with prevalent HIV-1 infection among pregnant women in Rwanda. National University of Rwanda-Johns Hopkins University AIDS Research Team. Int J Epidemiol 1994; 23(2):371–80.
61. Penkower L, Dew MA, Kingsley L, et al. Behavioral, health and psychosocial factors and risk for HIV infection among sexually active homosexual men: the Multicenter AIDS Cohort Study. Am J Public Health 1991;81(2):194–6.
62. Wojna V, Robles L, Skolasky RL, et al. Associations of cigarette smoking with viral immune and cognitive function in human immunodeficiency virus seropositive women. J Neurovirol 2007;13(6):561–8.

63. Nieman RB, Fleming J, Coker RJ, et al. The effect of cigarette smoking on the development of AIDS in HIV-1-seropositive individuals. AIDS 1993;7(5):705–10.
64. Feldman JG, Minkoff H, Schneider MF, et al. Association of cigarette smoking with HIV prognosis among women in the HAART era: a report from the women's inter-agency HIV study. Am J Public Health 2006;96(6):1060–5.
65. Eskild A, Petersen G. Cigarette smoking and drinking of alcohol are not associated with rapid progression to acquired immunodeficiency syndrome among homosexual men in Norway. Scand J Soc Med 1994;22(3):209–12.
66. Galai N, Park LP, Wesch J, et al. Effect of smoking on the clinical progression of HIV-1 infection. J Acquir Immune Defic Syndr Hum Retrovirol 1997;14(5):451–8.
67. Craib KJ, Schechter MT, Montaner JS, et al. The effect of cigarette smoking on lymphocyte subsets and progression to AIDS in a cohort of homosexual men. Clin Invest Med 1992;15(4):301–8.
68. Webber MP, Schoenbaum EE, Gourevitch MN, et al. A prospective study of HIV disease progression in female and male drug users. AIDS 1999;13(2):257–62.
69. Kuhlman JE, Knowles MC, Fishman EK, et al. Premature bullous pulmonary damage in AIDS: CT diagnosis. Radiology 1989;173(1):23–6.
70. Diaz PT, King ER, Wewers MD, et al. HIV infection increases susceptibility to smoking-induced emphysema. Chest 2000;117(90051):285S.
71. Diaz PT, King MA, Pacht ER, et al. Increased susceptibility to pulmonary emphysema among HIV-seropositive smokers. Ann Intern Med 2000;132(5):369–72.
72. Crothers K, Butt AA, Gibert CL, et al. Increased COPD Among HIV-positive compared to HIV-negative veterans. Chest 2006;130(5):1326–33.
73. Petrache I, Diab K, Knox KS, et al. HIV associated pulmonary emphysema: a review of the literature and inquiry into its mechanism. Thorax 2008;63(5):463–9.
74. Rabe KF, Hurd S, Anzueto A, et al. Global strategy for the diagnosis, management, and prevention of chronic obstructive pulmonary disease: GOLD executive summary. Am J Respir Crit Care Med 2007;176(6):532–55.
75. Salvi SS, Barnes PJ. Chronic obstructive pulmonary disease in non-smokers. Lancet 2009;374(9691):733–43.
76. Shaheen SO, Barker DJ, Shiell AW, et al. The relationship between pneumonia in early childhood and impaired lung function in late adult life. Am J Respir Crit Care Med 1994;149(3 Pt 1):616–9.
77. Martin CJ, Hallett WY. The diffuse obstructive pulmonary syndrome in a tuberculosis sanatorium. II. Incidence and symptoms. Ann Intern Med 1961;54:1156–64.
78. Willcox PA, Ferguson AD. Chronic obstructive airways disease following treated pulmonary tuberculosis. Respir Med 1989;83(3):195–8.
79. Dheda K, Booth H, Huggett JF, et al. Lung remodeling in pulmonary tuberculosis. J Infect Dis 2005;192(7):1201–9.
80. Plit ML, Anderson R, Van Rensburg CE, et al. Influence of antimicrobial chemotherapy on spirometric parameters and pro-inflammatory indices in severe pulmonary tuberculosis. Eur Respir J 1998;12(2):351–6.

Extensively Drug-resistant Tuberculosis: Epidemiology and Management Challenges

Keertan Dheda, MBBcH, FCP(SA), FCCP, PhD(Lond), FRCP(Lond)[a,b,c,*],
Robin M. Warren, PhD[d],
Alimuddin Zumla, FRCP, PhD(Lond), FRCPath[c],
Martin P. Grobusch, MD, MSc, DTM&H, FRCP(Lond)[e,f]

KEYWORDS

• Extensively drug-resistant tuberculosis • Human
• Epidemiology • Survival • HIV

This work and KD were supported by a TBsusgent grant from the European Commission (EU-FP7), the European and Developing Countries Clinical Trials Partnership, a South African Medical Research Council Career Development Award, and a National Research Foundation/-South African Research Chairs Initiative award.

[a] Lung Infection and Immunity Unit, Division of Pulmonology and Clinical Immunology & UCT Lung Institute, Department of Medicine, University of Cape Town, Cape Town, South Africa
[b] Institute of Infectious Diseases and Molecular Medicine, University of Cape Town, Cape Town, South Africa
[c] Department of Infection, Centre for Infectious Diseases and International Health, Windeyer Institute of Medical Sciences, UCL Medical School, 46 Cleveland Street, London W1T 4JF, UK
[d] DST/NRF Centre of Excellence for Biomedical Tuberculosis Research/MRC Centre for Molecular and Cellular Biology, Division of Molecular Biology and Human Genetics, Faculty of Health Sciences, Stellenbosch University, Tygerberg, South Africa
[e] Infectious Diseases, Tropical Medicine and Aids, Amsterdam Medical Centre, University of Amsterdam, The Netherlands
[f] Medical Research Unit, Albert Schweitzer Hospital, B.P. 118, Lambaréné, Gabon
* Corresponding author. Department of Medicine, H floor (Old Main Building), Groote Schuur Hospital, Observatory, Cape Town 7925, South Africa.
E-mail address: keertan.dheda@uct.ac.za

Infect Dis Clin N Am 24 (2010) 705–725
doi:10.1016/j.idc.2010.05.001
0891-5520/10/$ – see front matter © 2010 Elsevier Inc. All rights reserved.

The phenomenon of multidrug-resistant tuberculosis (MDR-TB) emerged as a clinical entity in the early 1990s after a couple of decades of widespread use of rifampin. A World Health Organization (WHO)-associated global laboratory surveillance network detected an increase in the global caseload of MDR-TB from ~ 274,000 in 2000 to ~ 500, 000 cases in 2007 (5% of the global case burden of TB).[1–3] MDR-TB diverts resources from existing TB control programs and has poorer outcomes than drug-sensitive TB.[4] Eclipsing this alarming trend in MDR-TB is the recent widespread emergence of extensively drug-resistant TB (XDR-TB) (with bacillary resistance, at least, to rifampin and isoniazid, plus any fluoroquinolone and any of the injectable agents [amikacin, kanamycin, or capreomycin]). XDR-TB is more expensive to treat than MDR-TB and outcomes are poorer, particularly in patients who are positive for the human immunodeficiency virus (HIV).[5] Several aspects of XDR-TB have been described in recent reviews.[5–11] This review, however, focuses on the clinical and molecular epidemiology of XDR-TB and what insights they provide, outlines the clinical challenges to clinicians in diagnosing and managing cases of XDR-TB, and the ethical dilemmas health care workers (HCWs) have to face in high- and low-TB–burden settings. To facilitate interpretation of the relevant data by practicing clinicians the article provides some background to the molecular epidemiologic techniques and diagnostic technologies discussed. Other important aspects of DR-TB, including the use and monitoring of treatment-specific regimens, contact tracing, HCW screening, and infection control interventions, have recently been discussed elsewhere.[5]

INSIGHTS FROM CLINICAL EPIDEMIOLOGY

Results from the fourth round of the Global Project on Anti-Tuberculosis Drug Resistance Surveillance,[3] based on data from more than 90,000 patients from 83 countries, indicate that the median prevalence of resistance to any drug in newly identified TB cases is currently about 11%. The prevalence of MDR-TB is increasing most strongly in South Korea and certain areas of the former Soviet Union. Almost 40 countries (ie, approximately 50% of those countries contributing representative data globally) report the prevalence of XDR-TB.

In general, Wright and colleagues[3] reported low absolute numbers of XDR-TB from Central and Western Europe, the Americas, Asia, and most African countries surveyed. Case numbers are highest in areas of high MDR-TB prevalence, peaking in regions of the former Soviet Union. Data on drug resistance are missing for many countries, particularly from sub-Saharan Africa, where a lack of funding and facilities for second-line drug sensitivity testing prevails. With regard to the African situation, Amor and colleagues[12] hypothesize, from MDR-TB rates obtained for 39 of 46 countries, that *Mycobacterium tuberculosis* with higher degrees of resistance is likely to be more prevalent than previously reckoned. More recent data indicate high rates of MDR-TB in several prevalence surveys. Recent surveys from Ethiopia (retreatment cases),[13] Nigeria (tertiary hospital),[14] Zambia (prison),[15] and Rwanda (retreatment cases)[16] indicate MDR-TB prevalence rates of 26%, 54%, 9.5%, and 9.4%, respectively. Thus, additional well-conducted and comprehensive surveys from Africa are urgently needed. In South Africa, however, surveillance and diagnostic capacity has been dramatically increased in the wake of the so-called Tugela Ferry outbreak reported in 2006,[17] which identified Southern Africa as a hitherto un(der)recognized hotbed of XDR-TB on the global map. Thus, a mortality of almost 100% and evidence of extensive nosocomial spread in a cohort of patients coinfected with HIV and XDR-TB was brought to the attention of the global community.

A compartmental difference-equation mathematical model focusing on looking into how improved diagnosis could improve DR TB management in a setting of high HIV/TB coinfection rates was developed by Dowdy and colleagues.[18] Using South African data it was predicted that performing culture and drug-susceptibility testing (DST) in 37% of new cases and in 85% of previously treated cases could yield a 17% reduction in TB mortality, avert 14% of MDR, and prevent almost 50% of MDR-TB deaths. If used alone, expanded culture and DST are not helpful in curbing the XDR-TB spread, for which additional tools such as improved treatment on a broad scale are required. Further mathematical modeling of the transmission dynamics in rural KwaZulu-Natal/South Africa suggested that nosocomial clusters of transmission may lead to community-based epidemics under prevailing conditions (high levels of HIV coinfection, poor resources, and dense yet decentralized rural populations).[19] Using branching process mathematics, and in line with what common sense suggests, early community-based DST and effective XDR-TB therapy were identified as the most effective tools helping to curtail ongoing transmission. However, and as shown for MDR-TB,[11] effective treatment hinges on individualized treatment regimens accounting for significant comorbidity, strong patient support, and treatment follow-up systems, let alone access to drugs and appropriate treatment facilities.

Nosocomial transmission often seems to play a lead role in XDR-TB transmission in resource-poor settings.[17] Based on this observation, another approach in mathematical modeling has suggested that a synergistic combination of available (yet often not easily applicable) nosocomial infection control strategies could prevent nearly half of XDR-TB cases on its own.[20] However, the difficulty with all mathematical modeling lies with the accuracy of its underlying assumptions. For example, in the South African setting, early reports of XDR-TB mortality reached almost 100%,[17] whereas current pooled data from various centers across the country and worldwide suggest an overall mortality of around 20% to 50%,[21–23] even when taking into account HIV coinfection, thus rendering mathematical modeling susceptible to gross errors.

INSIGHTS FROM MOLECULAR EPIDEMIOLOGY

Classic epidemiology continues to provide valuable insights into the epidemiology of TB. However, these analytical methods have assumed that the phenotype of the causative agent (M tuberculosis) does not directly influence the epidemiology of disease. This notion has been challenged with the discovery of polymorphic genetic elements, which allow for the classification of M tuberculosis strains and their spatial and temporal analysis in different epidemiologic settings.

Numerous genotyping methods have been developed, each with their own level of discrimination and applicability to answer epidemiologic questions. Three of these methods are internationally standardized. The most widely used genotyping method is spoligotyping, which allows the genetic classification of strains according to the number of direct variable repeat sequences that are present in the direct repeat region of the M tuberculosis chromosome.[24] Strains are grouped into lineages according to the presence of defined spoligotype signatures.[25] Currently, 22 lineages have been described, of which the Beijing lineage has been most frequently reported followed by the Latin American-Mediterranean (LAM) lineage.[26] The internationally standardized IS6110 DNA fingerprinting is based on the quantification of the number of IS6110 elements located within the chromosome of a strain and their position relative to a specific endonuclease restriction site (PvuII), which determines the physical size of the fragment when electrophoretically fractionated in an agarose gel.[27] This method is widely accepted as the gold standard but has proved to be cumbersome, requiring growth of the bacilli, DNA extraction, Southern blotting, and hybridization, which implies that this method cannot be used in a real-time manner to investigate epidemiologic events. Despite this limitation, IS6110 DNA fingerprinting continues to be the most informative method for the classification of clinical isolates of M tuberculosis. In an attempt to overcome this limitation a polymerase chain reaction (PCR)-based method, which amplifies mycobacterial interspersed repetitive-unit-variable-number tandem-repeat (MIRU-VNTR) sequences has been developed.[28] This method has several different formats, with the 15 MIRU-VNTR combination being proposed as the new standard for molecular epidemiology.[29] In certain settings this method has proved more informative than IS6110 DNA fingerprinting in that a more precise correlation between genotype and epidemiologic contact was observed.[30] However, the suitability of this method to define the epidemiology of TB in high-incidence settings has recently been challenged by the observed discordance between the definition of a strain when using the MIRU-VNTR typing method compared with the IS6110 DNA fingerprinting method.[31]

Molecular epidemiologic calculations, using the methods mentioned earlier, are based on the assumption that the genomes of M tuberculosis strains are in constant flux and thus strains that show identical genotypes (within a defined geographic region) reflect a recent epidemiologic event (**Fig. 1**).[32] Conversely, strains that show different genotypes imply that sufficient time has elapsed, allowing the genotypes to

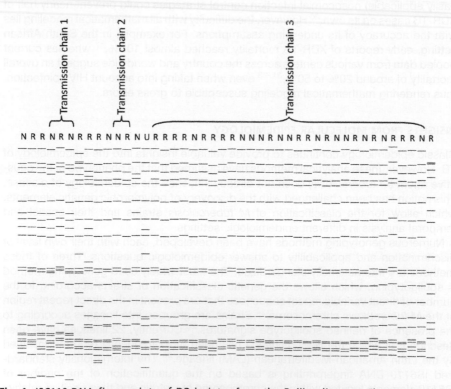

Fig. 1. IS6110 DNA fingerprints of DR isolates from the Beijing lineage. Clustered isolates reflecting recent transmission are bracketed. Clustered cases include patients who have a previous history of anti-TB treatment suggesting reinfection. N, new case; R, retreatment case; U, unknown history of previous treatment.

evolve, and thus these cases are believed to be epidemiologically unrelated.[32] These definitions allow TB cases to be grouped into 2 categories (see **Fig. 1**): clustered cases (identical genotypes representing recent transmission) and unique cases (nonidentical genotypes representing reactivation, infection outside the study site, or failure to identify the index case). Using these simple definitions it has been possible to challenge numerous classic epidemiologic dogmas. Some of the major advances that have been achieved include (1) identifying the population structure of M tuberculosis in different geographic settings[33,34]; (2) quantification of the contribution of casual contact to ongoing transmission[32,35]; (3) defining the mechanism leading to recurrent TB[36]; (4) identification of outbreaks[37]; (5) demonstrating that DR M tuberculosis strains can be transmitted[37]; (6) challenging the interpretation of drug surveillance studies[38]; (7) understanding human-animal and animal-human transmission of TB[39]; (8) understanding where transmission occurs (ie, household)[40]; (9) proving nosocomial transmission of M tuberculosis[41]; (10) proving multiple infection in patients in a high-incidence community[42]; (11) demonstrating laboratory cross-contamination[43]; and that smear-negative cases contribute to transmission.[44]

Perhaps the most significant finding is that recurrence can occur through reinfection.[36] This finding not only challenges the concept that previous infection confers protective immunity against a subsequent infection but also questions the interpretation of drug-resistance surveillance data, which initially failed to recognize the concept of reinfection. Before the development of genotyping methods, patients with DR TB were grouped according to their previous history of exposure to anti-TB drugs.[45] Patients without previous exposure were interpreted to have developed DR TB through transmission (primary resistance), whereas patients with a previous history of TB treatment were interpreted to have developed DR TB when poor regimens and/or adherence allowed for the selection of spontaneously occurring DR mutants (acquired resistance). The relative proportion of each category was then used as a measure of the efficacy of the TB control program. The strong association between retreatment and drug resistance has been interpreted to reflect poor adherence, placing the patient at fault. However, the observation that a significant proportion of DR TB cases are clustered, irrespective of their previous history of TB treatment, shows the importance of reinfection as a mechanism leading to the development of DR TB (see **Fig. 1**).[37,46,47] Reinfection may occur either following cure of a previous episode, during a current episode (while on treatment), or as a consequence of multiple infections before the development of disease followed by antibiotic selection.[48] Together, these finding emphasize the importance of transmission as a mechanism exacerbating the DR TB epidemic. This finding is supported by numerous studies, which used DNA fingerprinting to show the spread of DR TB.[37,49,50]

These molecular epidemiologic observations have also questioned the longstanding dogma that the evolution of drug resistance is associated with a fitness cost.[51] Accordingly, it was believed that the evolution of resistance to several anti-TB drugs would further attenuate pathogenicity and such strains would fail to propagate through transmission. However, compensatory mutations may accumulate during a disease episode, thereby ameliorating the fitness cost of the initial resistance, causing mutation(s) leading to the evolution of highly transmissible DR strains.[52] This finding may explain outbreaks of DR TB. An alternative explanation has been that the genetic background confers a high fitness phenotype.[52] The association between the Beijing genotype (genetic background) and drug resistance is well documented.[53] However, it is not known whether this genotype is able to acquire resistance more readily (mutator phenotype) or transmit resistance more efficiently. Alternatively, successful spread may be linked to an inefficient TB control program or the immune status of the human population.[17,54] Transmission of DR TB among HIV-infected individuals has been well documented and explained the rapid spread of MDR-TB in New York in the early 1990s.[49] Concern over the spread of MDR-TB had continued for the previous 15 years, with research focusing on the identification of mutations conferring resistance, with the view to developing molecular-based diagnostics.[55]

More recently, concern was raised about the emergence of resistance to second-line anti-TB drugs.[56] This concern was heightened by the report from Tugela Ferry, KwaZulu-Natal (KZN), South Africa, which showed high mortality associated with bacillary resistance to at least isoniazid, rifampicin, fluoroquinolones, and either aminoglycosides or capreomycin and HIV coinfection,[17] thus leading to the revised definition of XDR-TB.[46] Genotyping, using a combination of IS6110 DNA fingerprinting and spoligotyping, grouped 85% of the strains into the F15/LAM4/KZN lineage.[57] Accordingly, the investigators suggested that the grouping of these strains implied ongoing transmission. This suggestion was supported by the observation that 55% of the XDR-TB cases had no previous history of TB and that a further 15% had been reinfected after being cured from a previous disease episode. Spoligotyping of M tuberculosis cultures taken from different episodes confirmed the importance of reinfection as a mechanism leading to the emergence of MDR-TB and XDR-TB in previously treated TB cases.[47] Subsequently the investigators showed that the F15/LAM4/KZN was the most prevalent MDR-TB strain in the province and that the first documented case of XDR-TB occurred in 2001.[57] However, the resistance profile of this XDR-TB strain differed from the Tugela Ferry XDR-TB outbreak strain. Together this suggests that XDR-TB may have evolved on separate occasions in strains belonging to the F15/LAM4/KZN lineage as well as in non-F15/LAM4/KZN lineage strains and thereafter had been transmitted either nosocomially or in community settings.[57] The relative proportion of acquired versus transmitted XDR-TB in the KZN Province remains to be determined.

Following the disclosure of the Tugela Ferry outbreak 11 published studies have investigated the relationship between strain genotype and XDR resistance to determine the mechanisms underlying this new epidemic.[22,58–68]

South Africa

Spoligotyping of XDR-TB isolates collected retrospectively, by Mlambo and colleagues,[58] from cases resident in 4 of 9 provinces of South Africa identified 17 strains belonging to 7 lineages during the period June 2005 to December 2006. The observed combination of genetic diversity and the broad geographic distribution of these strains suggested that between 63% and 75% of the cases had developed XDR-TB through acquisition. This notion was confirmed in a recent clinical study[22] and is linked to the high default rate among patients receiving MDR-TB treatment. The study by Mlambo and coworkers[58] showed that XDR-TB was largely associated with the Beijing lineage (34%) and only 3 cases outside KZN had the F15/LAM4/KZN strain.

Estonia

A combination of IS6110 DNA fingerprinting and spoligotyping was used to describe the population structure of XDR-TB strains in Estonia during the period January 2003 to December 2005.[59] In this setting, MDR-TB and XDR-TB were strongly associated with the Beijing genotype but this did not influence treatment outcome.

China

The genetic background of 13 XDR-TB isolates cultured from patients resident in Beijing during the period January 2002 to December 2005 was determined by a combination of spoligotyping and MIRU-VNTR typing.[60] As expected 77% were from the Beijing lineage, whereas the remaining isolates were from the T1 lineage. Only 2 isolates (15%) were clustered, showing that XDR-TB was emerging independently, possibly as a result of nonadherence. However, in a second study VNTR typing showed that 73% of XDR-TB isolates were clustered indicating ongoing transmission in Shanghai during the period March 2004 to November 2007.[61] This finding was supported by the observation that 55% of the patients were new cases, and a previous study that had shown that 84% of previously treated cases were reinfected with circulating MDR-TB strains.[46]

Japan

During the period 2001 to 2004, isolates from 29 cases with XDR-TB were genotyped by IS*6110* DNA fingerprinting and MIRU-VNTR typing.[62] Of these, 20 (69%) were clustered, suggesting ongoing transmission when transmission was strongly associated with the *kat*GS315T mutation, which confers high-level isoniazid resistance. In a second study Iwamoto and colleagues[63] investigated the relationship between XDR-TB and Beijing sublineages in isolates collected between January 2001 and December 2006. This analysis showed an association between sublineages ST3 and ST26, and XDR-TB, whereas clustering by MIRU-VNTR typing suggested transmission rates of 65% and 71%, respectively. The investigators conclude that strains from the different sublineages may have evolved unique properties, which enable them to overcome fitness cost associated with the evolution of resistance, and therefore it is important to prevent the spread of these strains.

Uzbekistan

IS*6110* DNA fingerprint analysis allowed investigators to determine the mechanisms leading to the evolution of ofloxacin resistance in 18 patients receiving treatment of MDR-TB.[9] Resistance to ofloxacin and other second-line anti-TB drugs was acquired in 13 patients, whereas 3 patients were reinfected with an existing XDR-TB strain. This study shows the complexity of scaling up the treatment of MDR-TB and the need to prevent the emergence and spread of XDR-TB during treatment.

Iran

Second-line DST identified 12 XDR-TB cases between January 2003 and January 2005, which could be grouped into 2 clusters according to IS*6110* DNA fingerprinting.[65] Both clusters reflected family and community transmission. In a subsequent study between October 2006 and October 2008 a further 23 cases were analyzed, of which 8 had XDR-TB and 15 had totally DR TB (MDR-TB in association with resistance to all second-line drugs).[66] Spoligotyping in combination with VNTR typing failed to identify transmission chains, suggesting acquisition. This finding, in association with the observation that 95% of these patients had been previously treated, suggests inadequate diagnosis and inappropriate treatment.

Poland

Only one case of XDR-TB has been documented in Poland, which was shown by spoligotyping to be a member of the T11558 cluster.[67]

Portugal

MIRU-VNTR typing in combination with DNA sequencing of genes conferring resistance showed a high level of mutational diversity in MIRU-VNTR defined clusters, suggesting amplification of resistance in existing MDR-TB strains in 2003.[68] Analysis of mutations conferring second-line resistance revealed that 56% of MDR-TB cases were XDR-TB cases. However, this study did not calculate the relative proportion of transmitted versus acquired XDR resistance, and only speculated about the evolution of XDR-TB strains from persistently circulating MDR-TB strains.

Our knowledge regarding the molecular epidemiology of XDR-TB remains sparse; different settings report different levels of transmission. One clear theme that seems to be emerging from these cumulative studies is that highly prevalent MDR-TB strains seem to evolve to become XDR-TB strains, which then spread. This subsequent spread of XDR-TB strains needs to be interrogated using a combination of DNA fingerprinting and mutational analysis because it is not always possible to rely on drug-susceptibility patterns; many different mutations may confer the same resistance phenotype.

DIAGNOSIS OF MDR AND XDR-TB

A definitive diagnosis of MDR-TB and XDR-TB depends on identification of the presence of M tuberculosis and the DST thereof. Thus, the accuracy of the laboratory-based DST is crucial for diagnosis of MDR-TB or XDR-TB, with profound implications for the individual patient. This diagnosis can be achieved only if laboratory quality-assurance programs are implemented. The gold standard for DST is the indirect proportion method on agar medium.[69,70] This method requires obtaining a pure culture of M tuberculosis followed by inoculation onto solid agar medium containing the critical concentration of a specific anti-TB drug (the drug concentration that differentiates bacillary resistance from susceptibility) (Table 1). Bacillary resistance is generally defined by using the proportion method, the absolute concentration method, or the resistance ratio method.[71] However, the indirect proportional may take 4 to 8 weeks following standard culture, which has significant implications for the patient (higher morbidity and mortality) and TB control (transmission of DR TB). Liquid-based culture methods (BACTEC460 and BACTEC960; BD BioSciences, Spacks, MD, USA) can reduce the turnaround time of DST to 2 to 4 weeks when using the indirect method[72] and are particularly reliable for the first-line drugs isoniazid and rifampin.[69,70] The reliability of ethambutol DST has been questioned and pyrazinamide DST is rarely performed.[73,74] The diagnostic delay period can be further reduced using the direct method (inoculation directly into liquid medium); however, the indirect method is preferred because the potential for bacterial contamination and the presence of nontuberculous mycobacteria is significantly reduced.

Second-line DST is not standardized and surveys of current practices have revealed important differences including the methodology, the critical drug concentrations, and the critical proportions of resistance.[75–77] Laboratory techniques, including medium, pH, incubation temperature, filter sterilization, and incomplete dissolution, may influence DST results.[78] A further complicating factor is that the critical drug concentration may be close to the minimum inhibitory concentration, leading to possible misclassification and poor reproducibility of DST results. DST for aminoglycosides, polypeptides, and fluoroquinolones show good reliability and reproducibility (see Table 1). However, data on the remaining second-line anti-TB drugs are sparse or have not been established (see Table 1).[79]

DNA sequencing has shown that drug resistance evolves as a consequence of mutations in specific genes,[80] when different mutations may lead to different levels of resistance.[81] Thus the detection of specific mutations conferring resistance may define whether an anti-TB drug should be included in the treatment regimen or used at a higher dose.[82,83] However, the correlation between in vitro resistance (specific

Table 1
Methodology and critical drug concentrations for second-line DST

Drug	DST Method	Critical Drug Concentrations (µg/ml)					
		Lowenstein-Jensen[a]	Middlebrook 7H10[a]	Middlebrook 7H11[a]	BACTEC460	BACTEC960	BACTEC960
Isoniazid	Solid/liquid	0.2	0.2	0.2	0.1	0.1	1.0
Rifampicin	Solid/liquid	40.0	1.0	1.0	2.0	1.0	1.0
Ethambutol	Solid/liquid	2.0	5.0	7.5	2.5	5.0	5.0
Pyrazinamide	Liquid	–	–	–	100.0	100.0	–
Streptomycin	Solid/liquid	4.0	2.0	2.0	2.0	1.0	1.0
Kanamycin	Solid/liquid	30.0	5.0	6.0	4.0	–	–
Amikacin	Liquid	–	–	–	1.0	1.0	1.0
Capreomycin	Solid/liquid	40.0	10.0	10.0	1.25	2.5	5.0
Viomycin	None	–	–	–	–	–	–
Ciprofloxacin	Solid/liquid	2.0	2.0	2.0	2.0	1.0	–
Ofloxacin	Solid/liquid	2.0	2.0	2.0	2.0	2.0	2.0
Levofloxacin	Solid/liquid	–	2.0	–	–	2.0	–
Moxifloxacin	Liquid	–	–	–	0.5	0.25	–
Gatifloxacin	Solid	–	1.0	–	–	–	–
Ethionamide	Solid/liquid	40.0	5.0	5.0	2.5	5.0	2.5
Prothionamide	Solid/liquid	40.0	–	–	1.25	2.5	–
Cycloserine	Solid	40.0	–	–	–	–	–
Terizidone	None	–	–	–	–	–	–
PAS	Solid/liquid	1.0	2.0	8.0	2.0	–	–
Thioacetazone	None	–	–	–	–	–	–
Clofazimine	Liquid	–	–	–	4.0	–	–
Amoxicillin/clavulanate	None	–	–	–	–	–	–
Clarithromycin	None	–	–	–	–	–	–
Linezolid	Liquid	–	–	–	1.0	1.0	1.0

[a] Indirect proportion method.
Data from WHO. Guidelines for surveillance of drug resistance in tuberculosis, 4th edition. France, WHO. 2009. Available at: http://whqlibdoc.who.int/publications/2009/9789241598675_eng.pdf. Accessed May 4, 2010; Springer B, Lucke K, Calligaris-Maibach R, et al. Quantitative drug susceptibility testing of *Mycobacterium tuberculosis* by use of MGIT 960 and epicenter instrumentation. J Clin Microbiol 2009;47(6):1773–80.

mutations) and clinical response has not been well established for second-line anti-TB drugs and therefore the predictive value of these laboratory-based tests for prognosis remains unclear.[79] One such test is the line-probe assay, which is not well validated in smear-negative TB, although the results are encouraging.[84–86] These assays amplify a resistance-containing gene segment (eg, the rpoB gene hotspot) and the PCR products are hybridized to oligonucleotide probes on a nitrocellulose strip (line probe; this is an open system).[85] A variation, the Hain MDRplus sl version, can rapidly detect resistance to several drugs (**Fig. 2**). An ideal test would be one that can accurately and rapidly detect drug resistance regardless of smear status. The Gene Xpert (Cepheid, Sunnyvale, CA, USA) is a user-friendly closed (the PCR products remain within the cassette or tube) nested real-time PCR platform that can rapidly diagnose TB and detect bacillary resistance to rifampin (**Fig. 3**). It is likely that this platform will be rapidly expanded to include testing for isoniazid, aminoglycosides, fluoroquinolones, and other drugs. Particularly encouraging are the preliminary performance outcomes in smear-negative TB[87] and the potential for use of this technology as point-of-care test in microscopy centers and district hospitals.

Microscopic observation DST (MODS) relies on identifying the characteristic cording of *M tuberculosis* in liquid medium using an inverted light microscope (**Fig. 4**).[88] It is cheap, accurate, and DST results are available with 7 to 10 days.[88] The main drawback is that it is labor intensive. Thin-layer agar (TLA) microscopically detects early growth of *M tuberculosis* on a thin layer of agar; the platform can be simplified and standardized to colorimetrically detect resistance.[87] The nitrate reductase assays (NRA) rely on an *M tuberculosis*-produced nitrite-induced color change (Griess reaction) to detect growth in selective media.[89] NRA and TLA are cheap and accurate alternatives to the molecular biologic assays, which are prone to problems of

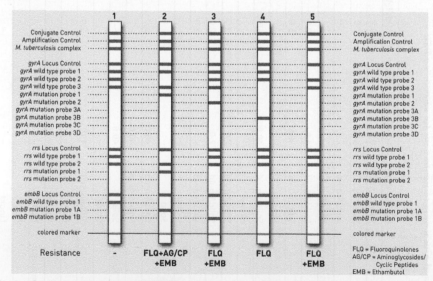

Fig. 2. The Hain GenoType MTBDRs*l* assay, in addition to rifampicin and isoniazid resistance confirmed by the GenoType MTBDR*plus* version of the assay, identifies additional resistance to fluoroquinolones, aminoglycosides, capreomycin, and ethambutol. The turnaround time of both tests from sample collection to result acquisition is about 2 to 3 days. Thus, XDR-TB may be rapidly diagnosed in patients with suspected DR TB. (*Courtesy of* Hain Lifescience GmbH, Nehren, Germany; with permission.)

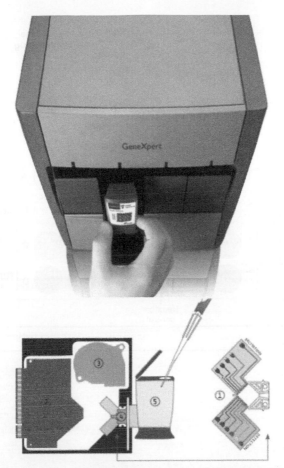

Fig. 3. The TB GeneXpert System (Cepheid) is a closed, self-contained, fully integrated, and automated nested real-time PCR platform for rapid diagnosis of TB and simultaneous confirmation of rifampicin resistance. The system is designed to purify, concentrate, detect, and identify targeted *Mtb*-specific nucleic acid sequences, thereby delivering answers directly from unprocessed samples. The sample is placed into a cartridge (5) and the targeted sequence is amplified by PCR (4); the optical PCR block detects and quantifies 6 different nucleic acid targets (1), and the circuitry (2) passes the information to a computer for display. The technology is suitable for use as a potential point-of-care test for use in microscopy centers and district hospitals. The key advantage, in contrast to the Hain assay, is a lower risk of contamination. (*From* Cepheid: www.cepheid.com; with permission.)

contamination, particularly when open systems are used. Novel approaches include the high resolution melt (HRM) assay, which is able to identify clinical isolates harboring mutations conferring rifampin resistance by comparing DNA melt profiles of their rifampin resistance determining region to the DNA melt profiles of a wild type standard (**Fig. 5**).[90,91]

Patients may harbor multiple bacillary strains[48] and transient clinical improvement may be seen in patients with MDR-TB when on standard short-course therapy for drug-sensitive TB. The same phenomena may explain discordant DST results at different times from the same patient, and this must be distinguished from the high

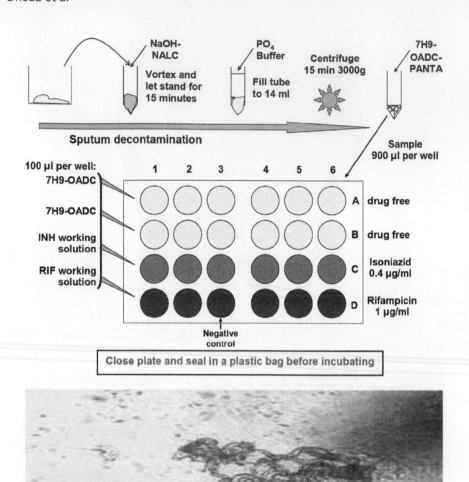

Fig. 4. The MODS assay relies on recognition of the characteristic cording pattern of *M tuberculosis* (*bottom panel*) using an inverted microscope; simultaneous susceptibility testing is performed through incubation in selective media (*top panel*) and the results are available within a median time of 7 days. The plate is sealed in a plastic bag and thus the postinoculation infection risk is minimal. The technology is cheap but labor intensive. (*From* Brady MF, Coronel J, Gilman RH, Moore DA. The MODS method for diagnosis of tuberculosis and multidrug resistant tuberculosis. J Vis Exp 2008;11:845; with permission.)

interlaboratory variability and stochastic results seen with second-line DST. Furthermore, because a sizeable proportion of patients with MDR-TB have no previous risk factors such as previous TB treatment or contact with known DR TB cases, it is rational to screen all smear-positive cases with culture or rapid molecular biologic tests such as the line-probe assays.[84] This approach is also likely to be cost-effective in many settings.[18]

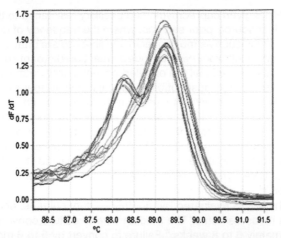

Fig. 5. Derivative of the intensity of fluorescence of the DNA duplexes at different temperatures using the HRM assay. Isolates were scored as drug-susceptible to rifampicin according to the presence of a single derivative peak within a defined temperature range (89–89.5°C). Isolates were scored as DR to rifampicin according to the presence of 2 derivative peaks in defined temperature ranges (88–88.5°C and 89–89.5°C). Thus, the amplicons with and without the relevant rifampicin-defining mutations have differing DNA melting temperatures.

MANAGEMENT CHALLENGES

The first step is to make the correct diagnosis. In settings of appreciable drug resistance, a laboratory result may reflect sample contamination or administrative error. As outlined earlier, because of several reasons, second-line DST information from different laboratories may yield different results. It is also possible that one may be sampling a subpopulation of pulmonary bacilli that are of a different strain and have a different DST profile. In a patient failing a first-line drug regimen care should be taken to re-evaluate the diagnosis and exclude, where appropriate and where no culture results are available, other possibilities such as interstitial lung disease, pneumoconioses, and cavitating malignancy.

Once the diagnosis is confirmed by the DST and there is contextual fidelity, the next step is to choose an effective and suitable regimen. A detailed outline of the specific putative drug regimens, their doses, and associated adverse event profiles has recently been given elsewhere[5] and is not covered here. For MDR-TB and XDR-TB, the clinician is guided by the DST results and previous drug usage. In general, MDR treatment regimens comprise a backbone of a fluoroquinolone and aminoglycoside with 2, or preferably 3, additional drugs to which the organism is susceptible and preferably which the patient has not previously used. A single drug should not be added to a failing regimen. The XDR-TB treatment regimen similarly depends on DST results but often contains a backbone of para-aminosalicylic acid (PAS) and capreomycin to which other drugs are added. XDR-TB regimens are difficult to construct for several reasons. First, bacillary resistance testing for PAS and capreomycin is unreliable and second, often if there has been previous MDR-TB treatment, there are few drugs with which to construct an effective regimen. Often remaining drugs such as amoxicillin/clavulanate, clarithromycin, clofazimine, and dapsone have weak antimycobacterial activity.[92,93] A recent study in South Africa found that approximately 60% of patients with XDR-TB given capreomycin had bacillary resistance to the drug at treatment initiation.[22] In resource-poor settings, where the frequency of drug resistance is often the highest, drugs such as moxifloxacin and linezolid are unavailable. Our recent data suggested that moxifloxacin was an independent predictor of survival in XDR-TB, despite ofloxacin resistance in all the enrolled patients, and we therefore suggest, in the absence of specific drug-susceptibility data and until further data become available, that consideration be given to using moxifloxacin in an XDR-TB treatment regimen in specific settings.[22] Further studies are urgently needed to clarify the prevailing cross-resistance between the different fluoroquinolone and the role of the second-generation quinolones in XDR-TB. There is evidence of incomplete cross-resistance within the quinolone class, possibly explained by differential drug-specific binding to DNA gyrase.[82] High-dose isoniazid is another cheap and effective therapeutic option.[94]

Response to therapy is evaluated by monthly sputum cultures, chest radiography, and body weight measurements. The median time to culture conversion in MDR-TB cases is approximately 6 to 8 weeks.[4] Failure to convert by 5 to 6 months of therapy suggests that the regimen is failing. Similar parameters can be used to monitor patients with XDR-TB. We recently showed that patients with XDR-TB who weighed less than 50 kg had poorer outcomes than those who weighed more than 50 kg.[22] Almost 90% of all patients who culture converted did so by month 9 of XDR therapy.[22]

In patients who are compliant with their treatment, the outcomes for MDR-TB are reasonable and therefore medical therapy should be tried in the first instance.[4] In treatment failures compliance should be carefully reassessed, copathologies should be excluded, and the patient should be evaluated for surgical resection if possible. An alternative regimen needs to be constructed once these issues have been addressed. By contrast XDR-TB has poorer treatment-related outcomes. In a cohort of 227 patients with XDR-TB who had inpatient intensive therapy with a capreomycin and PAS-based regimen, the overall outcomes were poor (19% overall conversion and an overall mortality of approximately 36%).[22] Thus, we recommend that patients who have adequate cardiopulmonary status and are failing an MDR-TB treatment regimen, or all patients with XDR-TB, should be evaluated for surgical lung resection when possible. However, the capacity to perform cardiothoracic surgery is severely limited in settings with a high TB burden.

The frequency of adverse drug reactions is high.[22] Specific adverse drug reactions and how therapy should be monitored have been outlined elsewhere.[5] Use of the aminoglycosides should be accompanied by monitoring of renal function and audiometry. The same applies to capreomycin, which may cause hypokalemia and hypomagnesemia, and result in renal failure at any stage of therapy. Patients with pre-XDR-TB (resistance to rifampin, isoniazid, and a fluoroquinolone or aminoglycoside [not both]) should be managed in the same way as patients with XDR-TB.

ETHICAL DILEMMAS

In high-burden settings, given the extent of the TB pandemic and poor treatment outcomes, increasing numbers of patients with MDR and particularly XDR-TB fail medical therapy. These patients may have limited or extensive bilateral disease, are not suitable candidates for surgery, have high-grade bacillary resistance with no option for additional agents, have had other copathologies ruled out, and have failed to culture convert after 12 months of intensive inpatient therapy, after which the chance of culture conversion is minimal.[22] Can treatment be suspended in these patients if cure is deemed highly unlikely? In the Western Cape Province of South Africa the decision to suspend treatment is taken by a multidisciplinary review committee after all other options have been exhausted. In some cases the patients are not critically ill. However, bed space in DR TB hospitals is overwhelmed and urgently needed for new cases, and there are no dedicated hospice or isolation facilities in which patients may be nursed. Can these patients be justifiably discharged back to their homes, where often families live in single rooms or informal housing? In the Western Cape Province of South Africa a home assessment is first conducted and the family counseled about infection control and the nature of the illness before patients are discharged to their homes. Resource limitations leave open no alternative options. Should these patients, who fail treatment and remain infectious, be permanently isolated from society, where should they be isolated, and can we prioritize the right of the community over the right of the individual?[95,96]

Equally difficult is the decision to withdraw therapy in chronic defaulters, often with substance abuse problems, who already have high-grade bacillary resistance. Is it justifiable to incarcerate these patients who are a threat to the wider community?[96] Currently no such facilities exist in high-burden settings and the legal framework lacks clarity to deal with this scenario. In the Western Cape, the review committee has withdrawn therapy in cases of persistent ongoing default when there is high risk of further increasing drug resistance, alternative copathologies have been ruled out. and there are no further therapeutic or management options. The rationale here is to limit further development of drug resistance in the face of little hope of successful treatment. Equally difficult is the management of pregnant patients with XDR-TB or single parents with infants when there are no available alternative caregivers and overwhelmed social services.

With the increasing burden of disease these eventualities will become more common in resource-poor settings, and urgent attention will have to be focused on providing funding and other appropriate resources for dedicated hospices, community treatment facilities, and isolation centers for patients with XDR-TB who have little chance of cure.

SUMMARY

The prevalence of MDR-TB has increased globally in the past decade and likely will continue to increase in many areas within resource-poor settings like India, China, territories within the former Soviet Union, and Africa. This increase has the capacity to destabilize TB control, and additional prevalence data on MDR-TB and XDR-TB are urgently needed from these regions. Molecular epidemiologic studies suggest MDR-TB and XDR-TB are predominantly acquired with subsequent horizontal spread within communities. A 2-pronged strategy is required to tackle this global epidemic. First, existing cases need to be actively found, rapidly diagnosed, and aggressively treated to minimize transmission of disease. This strategy requires funding to access the appropriate second-line drugs, rapid diagnostic tools, infection control interventions, and increased laboratory capacity. However, in parallel aggressive preventative strategies need to be undertaken, which include programmatic strengthening, roll-out of rapid diagnostics, expanding laboratory testing capacity, improved case finding and access to appropriate drug therapy, and strategies to deal with incurable cases. However, perhaps most important is the alleviation of poverty, the main driver of TB and associated drug resistance, and the prevention and treatment of HIV infection. This goal is attainable only through appropriate funding, political will, and downscaling of war and political conflicts in resource-poor settings.

REFERENCES

1. WHO. Anti-tuberculosis drug resistance in the world: the WHO/IUATLD Global Project on Anti-Tuberculosis Drug Resistance Surveillance. Geneva (Switzerland): WHO; 2008.
2. WHO. Global tuberculosis control 2009: epidemiology, strategy, financing. Geneva (Switzerland): WHO; 2009.
3. Wright A, Zignol M, Van Deun A, et al. Epidemiology of antituberculosis drug resistance 2002–07: an updated analysis of the global project on anti-tuberculosis drug resistance surveillance. Lancet 2009;373(9678):1861–73.
4. Yew W, Leung C. Management of multidrug-resistant tuberculosis: update 2007. Respirology 2008;13(1):21–46.
5. Schaaf HS, Moll AP Dheda K. Multidrug- and extensively drug-resistant tuberculosis in Africa and South America: epidemiology, diagnosis and management in adults and children. Clin Chest Med 2009;30(4):667–83.
6. LoBue P. Extensively drug-resistant tuberculosis. Curr Opin Infect Dis 2009;22(2): 167–73.
7. Madariaga MG, Lalloo UG, Swindells S. Extensively drug-resistant tuberculosis. Am J Med 2008;121(10):835–44.
8. Jassal M, Bishai WR. Extensively drug-resistant tuberculosis. Lancet Infect Dis 2009;9(1):19–30.
9. Scano F, Vitoria M, Burman W, et al. Management of HIV-infected patients with MDR- and XDR-TB in resource-limited settings. Int J Tuberc Lung Dis 2008; 12(12):1370–5.
10. Sotgiu G, Ferrara G, Matteelli A, et al. Epidemiology and clinical management of XDR-TB: a systematic review by TBNET. Eur Respir J 2009;33(4):871–81.
11. Orenstein E, Basu S, Shah N, et al. Treatment outcomes among patients with multidrug-resistant tuberculosis: systematic review and meta-analysis. Lancet Infect Dis 2009;9(3):153–61.
12. Ben Amor Y, Nemser B, Singh A, et al. Underreported threat of multidrug-resistant tuberculosis in Africa. Emerg Infect Dis 2008;14(9):1345–52.
13. Meskel DW, Abate G, Lakew M, et al. Anti-tuberculosis drug resistance among retreatment patients seen at St Peter Tuberculosis Specialized Hospital. Ethiop Med J 2008;46(3):219–25.
14. Kehinde AO, Obaseki FA, Ishola OC, et al. Multidrug resistance to Mycobacterium tuberculosis in a tertiary hospital. J Natl Med Assoc 2007;99(10): 1185–9.
15. Habeenzu C, Mitarai S, Lubasi D, et al. Tuberculosis and multidrug resistance in Zambian prisons, 2000–2001. Int J Tuberc Lung Dis 2007;11(11):1216–20.
16. Umubyeyi AN, Vandebriel G, Gasana M, et al. Results of a national survey on drug resistance among pulmonary tuberculosis patients in Rwanda. Int J Tuberc Lung Dis 2007;11(2):189–94.
17. Gandhi NR, Moll A, Sturm AW, et al. Extensively drug-resistant tuberculosis as a cause of death in patients co-infected with tuberculosis and HIV in a rural area of South Africa. Lancet 2006;368(9547):1575–80.
18. Dowdy DW, Chaisson RE, Maartens G, et al. Impact of enhanced tuberculosis diagnosis in South Africa: a mathematical model of expanded culture and drug susceptibility testing. Proc Natl Acad Sci U S A 2008;105(32): 11293–8.
19. Basu S, Friedland G, Medlock J, et al. Averting epidemics of extensively drug-resistant tuberculosis. Proc Natl Acad Sci U S A 2009;106(18):7672–7.

20. Basu S, Andrews J, Poolman E, et al. Prevention of nosocomial transmission of extensively drug-resistant tuberculosis in rural South African district hospitals: an epidemiological modelling study. Lancet 2007;370(9597):1500–7.

21. Bonilla CA, Crossa A, Jave HO, et al. Management of extensively drug-resistant tuberculosis in Peru: cure is possible. PLoS One 2008;3(8):e2957.

22. Dheda K, Shean K, Zumla A, et al. Early treatment outcomes and HIV status of patients with extensively drug-resistant tuberculosis in South Africa: a retrospective cohort study. Lancet 2010;375(9728):1798–807.

23. Mitnick CD, Shin SS, Seung KJ, et al. Comprehensive treatment of extensively drug-resistant tuberculosis. N Engl J Med 2008;359(6):563–74.

24. Kamerbeek J, Schouls L, Kolk A, et al. Simultaneous detection and strain differentiation of *Mycobacterium tuberculosis* for diagnosis and epidemiology. J Clin Microbiol 1997;35(4):907–14.

25. Streicher EM, Victor TC, van der Spuy G, et al. Spoligotype signatures in the *Mycobacterium tuberculosis* complex. J Clin Microbiol 2007;45(1):237–40.

26. Brudey K, Driscoll JR, Rigouts L, et al. *Mycobacterium tuberculosis* complex genetic diversity: mining the fourth international spoligotyping database (SpolDB4) for classification, population genetics and epidemiology. BMC Microbiol 2006;6:23.

27. van Embden JD, Cave MD, Crawford JT, et al. Strain identification of *Mycobacterium tuberculosis* by DNA fingerprinting: recommendations for a standardized methodology. J Clin Microbiol 1993;31(2):406–9.

28. Supply P, Allix C, Lesjean S, et al. Proposal for standardization of optimized mycobacterial interspersed repetitive unit-variable-number tandem repeat typing of *Mycobacterium tuberculosis*. J Clin Microbiol 2006;44(12):4498–510.

29. Oelemann MC, Diel R, Vatin V, et al. Assessment of an optimized mycobacterial interspersed repetitive- unit-variable-number tandem-repeat typing system combined with spoligotyping for population-based molecular epidemiology studies of tuberculosis. J Clin Microbiol 2007;45(3):691–7.

30. Allix-Beguec C, Fauville-Dufaux M, Supply P. Three-year population-based evaluation of standardized mycobacterial interspersed repetitive-unit-variable-number tandem-repeat typing of *Mycobacterium tuberculosis*. J Clin Microbiol 2008;46(4):1398–406.

31. Hanekom M, van der Spuy GD, Gey van Pittius NC, et al. Discordance between mycobacterial interspersed repetitive-unit-variable-number tandem-repeat typing and IS6110 restriction fragment length polymorphism genotyping for analysis of *Mycobacterium tuberculosis* Beijing strains in a setting of high incidence of tuberculosis. J Clin Microbiol 2008;46(10):3338–45.

32. Small PM, Hopewell PC, Singh SP, et al. The epidemiology of tuberculosis in San Francisco. A population-based study using conventional and molecular methods. N Engl J Med 1994;330(24):1703–9.

33. Hermans PW, Messadi F, Guebrexabher H, et al. Analysis of the population structure of *Mycobacterium tuberculosis* in Ethiopia, Tunisia, and the Netherlands: usefulness of DNA typing for global tuberculosis epidemiology. J Infect Dis 1995;171(6):1504–13.

34. Warren R, Hauman J, Beyers N, et al. Unexpectedly high strain diversity of *Mycobacterium tuberculosis* in a high-incidence community. S Afr Med J 1996;86(1):45–9.

35. Alland D, Kalkut GE, Moss AR, et al. Transmission of tuberculosis in New York City. An analysis by DNA fingerprinting and conventional epidemiologic methods. N Engl J Med 1994;330(24):1710–6.

36. van Rie A, Warren R, Richardson M, et al. Exogenous reinfection as a cause of recurrent tuberculosis after curative treatment. N Engl J Med 1999;341(16):1174–9.

37. van Rie A, Warren RM, Beyers N, et al. Transmission of a multidrug-resistant *Mycobacterium tuberculosis* strain resembling "strain W" among noninstitutionalized, human immunodeficiency virus-seronegative patients. J Infect Dis 1999; 180(5):1608–15.

38. Van Rie A, Warren R, Richardson M, et al. Classification of drug-resistant tuberculosis in an epidemic area. Lancet 2000;356(9223):22–5.

39. Michalak K, Austin C, Diesel S, et al. *Mycobacterium tuberculosis* infection as a zoonotic disease: transmission between humans and elephants. Emerg Infect Dis 1998;4(2):283–7.

40. Verver S, Warren RM, Munch Z, et al. Proportion of tuberculosis transmission that takes place in households in a high-incidence area. Lancet 2004;363(9404):212–4.

41. Heyns L, Gie RP, Goussard P, et al. Nosocomial transmission of *Mycobacterium tuberculosis* in kangaroo mother care units: a risk in tuberculosis-endemic areas. Acta Paediatr 2006;95(5):535–9.

42. Richardson M, Carroll NM, Engelke E, et al. Multiple *Mycobacterium tuberculosis* strains in early cultures from patients in a high-incidence community setting. J Clin Microbiol 2002;40(8):2750–4.

43. Small PM, McClenny NB, Singh SP, et al. Molecular strain typing of *Mycobacterium tuberculosis* to confirm cross-contamination in the mycobacteriology laboratory and modification of procedures to minimize occurrence of false-positive cultures. J Clin Microbiol 1993;31(7):1677–82.

44. Behr MA, Warren SA, Salamon H, et al. Transmission of *Mycobacterium tuberculosis* from patients smear-negative for acid-fast bacilli. Lancet 1999;353(9151):444–9.

45. Weyer K. Survey of tuberculosis drug resistance; Western Cape. Available at: http://www.sahealthinfo.org/tb/tbdrugresistance.htm. Accessed September 2009.

46. Li X, Zhang Y, Shen X, et al. Transmission of drug-resistant tuberculosis among treated patients in Shanghai, China. J Infect Dis 2007;195(6):864–9.

47. Andrews JR, Gandhi NR, Moodley P, et al. Exogenous reinfection as a cause of multidrug-resistant and extensively drug-resistant tuberculosis in rural South Africa. J Infect Dis 2008;198(11):1582–9.

48. van Rie A, Victor TC, Richardson M, et al. Reinfection and mixed infection cause changing *Mycobacterium tuberculosis* drug-resistance patterns. Am J Respir Crit Care Med 2005;172(5):636–42.

49. Bifani PJ, Mathema B, Liu Z, et al. Identification of a W variant outbreak of *Mycobacterium tuberculosis* via population-based molecular epidemiology. JAMA 1999;282(24):2321–7.

50. Victor TC, Streicher EM, Kewley C, et al. Spread of an emerging *Mycobacterium tuberculosis* drug-resistant strain in the Western Cape of South Africa. Int J Tuberc Lung Dis 2007;11(2):195–201.

51. Andersson DI. The biological cost of mutational antibiotic resistance: any practical conclusions? Curr Opin Microbiol 2006;9(5):461–5.

52. Gagneux S, Long CD, Small PM, et al. The competitive cost of antibiotic resistance in *Mycobacterium tuberculosis*. Science 2006;312(5782):1944–6.

53. European Concerted Action on New Generation Genetic Markers and Techniques for the Epidemiology and Control of Tuberculosis. Beijing/W genotype *Mycobacterium tuberculosis* and drug resistance. Emerg Infect Dis 2006;12(5):736–43.

54. Strauss OJ, Warren RM, Jordaan A, et al. Spread of a low-fitness drug-resistant *Mycobacterium tuberculosis* strain in a setting of high human immunodeficiency virus prevalence. J Clin Microbiol 2008;46(4):1514–6.

55. Johnson R, Streicher EM, Louw GE, et al. Drug resistance in *Mycobacterium tuberculosis*. Curr Issues Mol Biol 2006;8(2):97–111.
56. Centers for Disease Control and Prevention (CDC). Emergence of *Mycobacterium tuberculosis* with extensive resistance to second-line drugs–worldwide, 2000–2004. MMWR Morb Mortal Wkly Rep 2006;55(11):301–5.
57. Pillay M, Sturm AW. Evolution of the extensively drug-resistant F15/LAM4/KZN strain of *Mycobacterium tuberculosis* in KwaZulu-Natal, South Africa. Clin Infect Dis 2007;45(11):1409–14.
58. Mlambo CK, Warren RM, Poswa X, et al. Genotypic diversity of extensively drug-resistant tuberculosis (XDR-TB) in South Africa. Int J Tuberc Lung Dis 2008;12(1): 99–104.
59. Kliiman K, Altraja A. Predictors of poor treatment outcome in multi- and extensively drug-resistant pulmonary TB. Eur Respir J 2009;33(5):1085–94.
60. Sun Z, Chao Y, Zhang X, et al. Characterization of extensively drug-resistant *Mycobacterium tuberculosis* clinical isolates in China. J Clin Microbiol 2008; 46(12):4075–7.
61. Zhao M, Li X, Xu P, et al. Transmission of MDR and XDR tuberculosis in Shanghai, China. PLoS One 2009;4(2):e4370.
62. Ano H, Matsumoto T, Suetake T, et al. Relationship between the isoniazid-resistant mutation KATGS315 T and the prevalence of MDR-/XDR-TB in Osaka, Japan. Int J Tuberc Lung Dis 2008;12(11):1300–5.
63. Iwamoto T, Yoshida S, Suzuki K, et al. Population structure analysis of the *Mycobacterium tuberculosis* Beijing family indicates an association between certain sublineages and multidrug resistance. Antimicrobial Agents Chemother 2008; 52(10):3805–9.
64. Cox HS, Sibilia K, Feuerriegel S, et al. Emergence of extensive drug resistance during treatment for multidrug-resistant tuberculosis. N Engl J Med 2008; 359(22):2398–400.
65. Masjedi MR, Farnia P, Sorooch S, et al. Extensively drug-resistant tuberculosis: 2 years of surveillance in Iran. Clin Infect Dis 2006;43(7):841–7.
66. Velayati AA, Masjedi MR, Farnia P, et al. Emergence of new forms of totally drug-resistant tuberculosis bacilli: super extensively drug-resistant tuberculosis or totally drug-resistant strains in Iran. Chest 2009;136(2):420–5.
67. Augustynowicz-Kopec E, Zwolska Z. [Tuberculosis caused by XDR resistant *Mycobacterium tuberculosis* in Poland. Microbiological and molecular analysis]. Pneumonol Alergol Pol 2007;75(1):32–9 [in Polish].
68. Perdigao J, Macedo R, Joao I, et al. Multidrug-resistant tuberculosis in Lisbon, Portugal: a molecular epidemiological perspective. Microb Drug Resist 2008; 14(2):133–43.
69. Drobniewski F, Rusch-Gerdes S, Hoffner S. Antimicrobial susceptibility testing of *Mycobacterium tuberculosis* (EUCAST document E.Def 8.1)–report of the Subcommittee on Antimicrobial Susceptibility Testing of *Mycobacterium tuberculosis* of the European Committee for Antimicrobial Susceptibility Testing (EUCAST) of the European Society of Clinical Microbiology and Infectious Diseases (ESCMID). Clin Microbiol Infect 2007; 13(12):1144–56.
70. Kim SJ. Drug-susceptibility testing in tuberculosis: methods and reliability of results. Eur Respir J 2005;25(3):564–9.
71. Sirgel FA, Wiid I, van Helden PD. Measuring inhibitory concentrations in mycobacteria. In: Parish T, Brown AC, editors. Methods in molecular biology: mycobacterium protocols. New York: The Human Press Inc; 2008. p. 173–86.

72. Perkins MD, Cunningham J. Facing the crisis: improving the diagnosis of tuberculosis in the HIV era. J Infect Dis 2007;196(Suppl 1):S15–27.
73. Johnson R, Jordaan AM, Pretorius L, et al. Ethambutol resistance testing by mutation detection. Int J Tuberc Lung Dis 2006;10(1):68–73.
74. Gandhi NR, Nunn P, Dheda K, et al. Multidrug-resistant and extensively drug-resistant tuberculosis: a threat to global control of tuberculosis. Lancet 2010; 375(9728):1830–43.
75. Kruuner A, Yates MD, Drobniewski FA. Evaluation of MGIT 960-based antimicrobial testing and determination of critical concentrations of first- and second-line antimicrobial drugs with drug-resistant clinical strains of *Mycobacterium tuberculosis*. J Clin Microbiol 2006;44(3):811–8.
76. Pfyffer GE, Bonato DA, Ebrahimzadeh A, et al. Multicenter laboratory validation of susceptibility testing of *Mycobacterium tuberculosis* against classical second-line and newer antimicrobial drugs by using the radiometric BACTEC 460 technique and the proportion method with solid media. J Clin Microbiol 1999; 37(10):3179–86.
77. Rusch-Gerdes S, Pfyffer GE, Casal M, et al. Multicenter laboratory validation of the BACTEC MGIT 960 technique for testing susceptibilities of *Mycobacterium tuberculosis* to classical second-line drugs and newer antimicrobials. J Clin Microbiol 2006;44(3):688–92.
78. Hawkins JE. Drug susceptibility testing. In: Kubica GP, Wayne LG, editors. The mycobacteria. A sourcebook. Part a. New York: Marcel Dekker; 1984. p. 177–93.
79. WHO. Guidelines for surveillance of drug resistance in tuberculosis. 4th edition. France: WHO; 2009. Available at: http://whqlibdoc.who.int/publications/2009/9789241598675_eng.pdf. Accessed May 4, 2010.
80. Sandgren A, Strong M, Muthukrishnan P, et al. Tuberculosis drug resistance mutation database. PLoS Med 2009;6(2):e2.
81. Springer B, Lucke K, Calligaris-Maibach R, et al. Quantitative drug susceptibility testing of *Mycobacterium tuberculosis* by use of MGIT 960 and epicenter instrumentation. J Clin Microbiol 2009;47(6):1773–80.
82. Kam KM, Yip CW, Cheung TL, et al. Stepwise decrease in moxifloxacin susceptibility amongst clinical isolates of multidrug-resistant *Mycobacterium tuberculosis*: correlation with ofloxacin susceptibility. Microb Drug Resist 2006;12(1):7–11.
83. Warren RM, Streicher EM, van Pittius NC, et al. The clinical relevance of mycobacterial pharmacogenetics. Tuberculosis (Edinb) 2009;89(3):199–202.
84. Ling DI, Zwerling AA, Pai M. Genotype MTBDR assays for the diagnosis of multidrug-resistant tuberculosis: a meta-analysis. Eur Respir J 2008;32(5): 1165–74.
85. Pai M, Kalantri S, Dheda K. New tools and emerging technologies for the diagnosis of tuberculosis: part II. Active tuberculosis and drug resistance. Expert Rev Mol Diagn 2006;6(3):423–32.
86. Barnard M, Albert H, Coetzee G, et al. Rapid molecular screening for multidrug-resistant tuberculosis in a high-volume public health laboratory in South Africa. Am J Respir Crit Care Med 2008;177(7):787–92.
87. O'Brien R. New diagnostic methods for tuberculosis. APHL 5th National Conference on Laboratory Aspects of Tuberculosis San Diego 11–13 2008. Available at: http://www.aphl.org/profdev/conferences/proceedings/Documents/2008TBconference/009-OBrien.pdf. Accessed May 5, 2010.
88. Moore DA, Evans CA, Gilman RH, et al. Microscopic-observation drug-susceptibility assay for the diagnosis of TB. N Engl J Med 2006;355(15):1539–50.

89. Martin A, Panaiotov S, Portaels F, et al. The nitrate reductase assay for the rapid detection of isoniazid and rifampicin resistance in *Mycobacterium tuberculosis*: a systematic review and meta-analysis. J Antimicrob Chemother 2008;62(1):56–64.

90. Hoek KG, Gey van Pittius NC, Moolman-Smook H, et al. Fluorometric assay for testing rifampin susceptibility of *Mycobacterium tuberculosis* complex. J Clin Microbiol 2008;46(4):1369–73.

91. Pietzka AT, Indra A, Stoger A, et al. Rapid identification of multidrug-resistant *Mycobacterium tuberculosis* isolates by RPOB gene scanning using high-resolution melting curve PCR analysis. J Antimicrob Chemother 2009;63(6): 1121–7.

92. Moll AP, Friedland G, Gandhi N, et al. Extensively drug-resistant tuberculosis (XDR-TB). In: Schaaf SH, Zumla AI, editors. Tuberculosis. A comprehensive clinical reference. 1st edition. St Louis (MO): Elsevier; 2009. p. 551–7.

93. WHO. Guidelines for the programmatic management of drug-resistant tuberculosis: emergency update 2008. Geneva (Switzerland): WHO; 2008.

94. Katiyar S, Bihari S, Prakash S, et al. A randomised controlled trial of high-dose isoniazid adjuvant therapy for multidrug-resistant tuberculosis. Int J Tuberc Lung Dis 2008;12(2):139–45.

95. Bateman C. XDR TB–humane confinement 'a priority'. S Afr Med J 2007;97(11): 1026 28, 30.

96. Singh JA, Upshur R, Padayatchi N. XDR-TB in South Africa: no time for denial or complacency. PLoS Med 2007;4(1):e50.

Childhood Tuberculosis: An Emerging and Previously Neglected Problem

Ben J. Marais, MRCP (Paed UK), FCP (Paed SA), MMed (Paed), PhD*,
H. Simon Schaaf, MMed (Paed), MD (Paed)

KEYWORDS

- Childhood • Pediatric • Tuberculosis

Of the estimated 8.3 million new cases of active tuberculosis (TB) diagnosed in 2000, 884,019 (11%) were in children less than 15 years of age.[1] However, this figure is outdated and almost certainly represents an underestimate of the current situation, because an estimated 10.4 million episodes of TB (first and subsequent) occurred during 2007.[2] Poor case ascertainment, absence of active case finding in most TB-endemic areas, and limited surveillance data hamper efforts to accurately quantify the global pediatric TB disease burden.[3] In a community based survey performed in Cape Town, South Africa, children less than 13 years of age contributed 13.7% of the total disease burden, with a calculated TB incidence of 408/100,000/y; nearly 50% of the total adult TB incidence (840/100,000/y) reported during the same period.[4] It is estimated that with accurate diagnosis and good reporting systems children less than 15 years old are likely to contribute 15% to 20% of the disease burden in areas where the TB epidemic is poorly controlled. In developed countries the burden of childhood TB is greatly reduced (<5%) as a result of minimal TB transmission and differences in the population age structure with fewer children compared with adults.[5]

A common misperception was that children are not severely affected by the global TB epidemic and that they rarely develop life-threatening disease. This impression resulted from observations in developed countries, where diligent contact tracing and active case finding ensures that children either receive adequate preventive therapy or are diagnosed early in their disease course. However, this is not the case

Conflicts of interest: None to declare.
Department of Paediatrics and Child Health, Faculty of Health Sciences, Tygerberg Children's Hospital, Stellenbosch University, PO Box 19063, Tygerberg 7505, South Africa
* Corresponding author.
E-mail address: bjmarais@sun.ac.za

Infect Dis Clin N Am 24 (2010) 727–749
doi:10.1016/j.idc.2010.04.004
0891-5520/10/$ – see front matter © 2010 Elsevier Inc. All rights reserved.

id.theclinics.com

in TB-endemic areas, where children often present with advanced disease and TB is a major contributor to morbidity and mortality of children under 5 years of age. An autopsy study conducted in Zambia showed that TB rivals bacterial pneumonia as a major cause of death from respiratory disease, in human immunodeficiency virus (HIV)-infected and -uninfected children.[6] Although the generalizability of these autopsy results has been questioned, observations from a more recent South African study confirmed the contribution of TB to respiratory disease among children in TB-endemic areas. The study documented identifiable causes of respiratory disease in children with community-acquired pneumonia not responding to first-line antibiotics; *Mycobacterium tuberculosis* was commonly identified irrespective of the child's HIV status.[7] The spectrum of disease observed in children who present with TB to health care facilities in endemic areas shows advanced disease in most cases,[8] which is in contrast to the experience in developed countries.

EVIDENCE OF EMERGENCE

Diagnosing a young child with TB represents a sentinel event that reflects recent transmission within a limited circle of social contact. Because most disease manifestations in children occur within 1 year of primary infection, the incidence of pediatric TB provides an accurate measure of ongoing transmission within communities.[9] Therefore, accurate quantification of the pediatric TB disease burden provides a key parameter of epidemic control. Conversely, the pediatric disease burden can also be estimated from accurate adult data because the number of children affected is proportional to the number of infectious adult cases; taking the population age distribution, diagnostic delay, and the provision of preventive therapy into account. In general, the total adult TB incidence (new and retreatment TB) provides a close approximation of the expected pediatric disease burden (estimated at roughly 50% of total adult TB incidence) in TB-endemic settings with poor access to preventive therapy.

Great strides have been made in the last 15 years to scale up diagnostic and treatment services, but the effect on the epidemic remains limited in endemic areas, particularly in areas worst affected by the HIV epidemic and/or resistance to first-line TB drugs.[10] Because the pediatric TB disease burden follows adult prevalence trajectories, childhood TB is most common in those parts of the world where epidemic control remains poor and incidence rates high. Although incidence rates per capita are starting to decrease in all of the World Health Organization (WHO) subregions, the absolute number of cases continues to increase because of increases in population size.[2] Incidence rates in HIV-endemic countries are also showing a slow decline from peak rates achieved in 2004, but remain at high levels.[2] A striking observation is the dichotomy that exists between developed countries, where incidence rates are less than 10/100,000 population, and low-income TB-endemic countries, where incidence rates still exceed 100/100,000 population, up to levels exceeding 1000/100,000 population in some high-burden areas.[2]

Within developed countries transmission is limited and most cases of active TB occur among immigrant populations, socially destitute or elderly people. Although most of the disease burden is confined to immigrant populations, the available evidence suggests little spill-over into resident communities,[11] although a few institutional outbreaks involving young children have been described.[12] Children rarely contribute to disease transmission unless they develop cavitary and/or sputum smear-positive disease, which occurs most frequently in older adolescent children (>8–10 years of age) and forms only a small fraction of all pediatric cases.[9] However, high rates of transmission are sustained in TB-endemic areas by many adult and adolescent cases that remain undiagnosed,[2] prolonged diagnostic and treatment delay among those who do ultimately receive treatment, as well as ineffective treatment of cases with undiagnosed drug-resistant disease. Annual risk of TB infection (ARTI) studies provide an estimate of the infection pressure that exists within communities. A major limitation of ARTI surveys is the selection bias introduced by age restriction; participation is usually limited to children aged 6 to 10 years. Highly selective ARTI surveys performed among primary-school children probably underestimate the infection pressure that exists among adolescents and adults within the same community, especially among those with high-risk social behavior. Because most adults in TB-endemic areas are already infected with M tuberculosis and none of the current tests is able to register a reinfection event in a nondiseased individual, it is impossible to quantify the true infection pressure that exists among high-risk groups. Molecular epidemiology studies demonstrated that exogenous reinfection is the most common cause of recurrent TB in highly endemic areas.[13,14] ARTI studies conducted at the same site also demonstrated high and increasing levels of infection among children,[15] confirming the high infection pressure that exists in these communities and reflecting worsening epidemic control.

Effect of HIV

The HIV epidemic has had a major negative effect on TB control efforts. The absolute number of adult patients with TB continues to show an alarming increase in HIV-affected areas, predominantly among those with sputum smear-negative disease.[16,17] In addition to increased absolute numbers of TB patients, HIV induced a marked age and gender shift among adult TB cases, with more young people and women of child-bearing age developing TB, which probably reflects that HIV infection in TB-endemic areas is more prevalent among younger adults and females.[16] The implication for children is that more parents with young families at home are developing active TB, drastically increasing the exposure of young and vulnerable children in these communities. Exceptionally high levels of TB exposure have been documented in infants born to HIV-infected mothers. Documented TB exposure was an exclusion criteria for enrolment into a randomized placebo-controlled isoniazid (INH) prevention trial conducted in South Africa. During enrolment screening 74/769 (9.4%) of 3- to 4-month-old infants living in HIV-affected households reported TB exposure and had to be excluded from the study.[18]

Effect of Drug Resistance

Because of the paucibacillary nature of pediatric TB (in those without cavitary disease or extensive lung infiltration), children are less likely to acquire drug resistance and/or transmit drug-resistant organisms than adults. However, although children contribute little to the creation of the drug-resistant epidemic they are greatly affected by it. The fact that incident cases of childhood TB reflect recent transmission implies that drug resistance patterns observed among child TB cases reflect primary (transmitted) drug resistance within the community.[19] Globally the emergence of the drug-resistant TB epidemic has been identified as a major threat to TB control.[20] The unavailability of effective second-line drugs and long delays before drug-resistant TB is identified imply that many patients are initially treated with ineffective regimens, which leads to acquisition of additional drug resistance and continued transmission of drug-resistant organisms within their communities.

The impression that drug-resistant organisms are likely to be less fit and therefore less transmissible and/or pathogenic (able to cause disease) than drug-susceptible strains is contradicted by recent observations. The fitness cost associated with the acquisition of drug resistance seems variable and strain dependent.[21,22] In addition, compensatory evolution may account for significantly higher fitness in clinical strains compared with their progenitors or laboratory strains.[21] Successful transmission is suggested by the geographic clustering of drug-resistant cases, evidence of clonal expansion, and drug-resistant disease in children.[22–24] The number of multidrug-resistant (MDR)-TB cases is on the increase and was estimated at 511,000 cases in 2007. Of these 289,000 were among new (no previous treatment or treatment of <1 month) cases (3.1% of all new cases) and 221,000 among previously treated cases (19% of all previously treated cases).[2] Drug-resistant TB among children usually mirrors trends observed in adults.[25] A prospective surveillance study from South Africa documented a marked increase in drug-resistant, especially MDR, TB among children from 1994 to 2007, most likely reflecting increased MDR-TB among adults in the area.[26] Unless effective measures are urgently implemented to limit transmission, the emergence of drug-resistant TB is likely to accelerate and affect greater numbers of children in the near future.

INCREASED AWARENESS

Awareness regarding the massive TB disease burden suffered by children in TB-endemic areas is increasing, but as yet this has not been translated into improved service delivery. Recognition that patients with sputum smear-negative TB may suffer severe disease and justify treatment, despite the fact that they are less infectious and therefore pose less of a public health risk than sputum smear-positive patients, benefitted children indirectly. Because sputum smear-negative TB is a common cause of death among HIV-infected patients, efforts to improve access to accurate diagnosis and effective treatment have been greatly expanded. Increased public awareness regarding the relevance of sputum smear-negative TB also benefitted children, because they were effectively sidelined by an exclusive emphasis on sputum smear-positive disease. The Stop TB Strategy formulated an inclusive goal: to treat "all TB patients, infectious or non-infectious, adults and children, with/without HIV infection, with/without drug-resistant disease." This served as a catalyst for WHO to compile its first comprehensive guidance on the management of childhood TB in 2006; it also requested countries to include pediatric TB data, specifically for the age bands 0 to 4 and 5 to 14 years, in all future reports.[27]

Drug-susceptible TB responds remarkably well to standard first-line treatment, but until recently few resource-limited countries had access to child-friendly drug formulations. The Global Drug Facility (GDF) has made great strides to improve the provision of quality-assured fixed-dose combination tablets to adults in poor countries. Since its establishment in 2001 the GDF has distributed treatment to approximately 20% of patients with TB treated worldwide, including in 15 of the 22 high-burden countries. Until 2008 no child-friendly formulations had been distributed; however, with funding support from UNITAID the GDF has approved grant applications from 55 countries for the provision of child-friendly TB formulations and distributed approximately 115,000 treatments free of charge to children in poor countries during 2008.[28] Indications are that the GDF initiative will be sustained and expanded in future. Although these efforts improved the availability of child-friendly drug formulations, reliable access to quality-assured drugs remains a concern in many countries and huge programmatic barriers still limit the availability of these drugs. In addition it has become apparent that existing treatment guidelines and fixed-dose combination preparations for children may be suboptimal when age-dependent pharmacokinetic profiles are taken into account.[29-31] Guidance on optimal drug dosages for first-line drugs has been finalized, but drug companies require time to develop and test new child-friendly combination products. Most children respond well to current treatment regimens, although there is concern about the response of severely immune-compromised HIV-infected children in the absence of highly active antiretroviral therapy (HAART).[32]

PROGRAMMATIC BARRIERS
Lack of Political Commitment and Adequate Monitoring

Although global political commitment to reduce the prevalence and severity of pediatric TB in endemic areas is increasing, a lot remains to be done. Many health care workers and policy makers remain poorly informed regarding childhood TB. A practical first step to enhance awareness and service delivery may be a requirement that all national and/or international TB guidelines should include a child TB section as part of the main body of the document. This strategy should assist in increasing awareness among health care workers and policy makers, although more creative and sustained efforts are required to ensure implementation.

Improved service delivery does not follow changes in policy recommendations unless clear evaluation systems are developed in parallel to monitor and reward actual implementation. A good example is the provision of INH-preventive therapy to young and vulnerable children in close contact with an infectious adult source. Most national TB guidelines state that child TB contacts should be actively traced and screened to exclude disease, before providing preventive therapy to those at high risk of progression to disease. With rare exceptions, implementation of these guidelines is nearly nonexistent in TB-endemic areas. Current standardized reporting systems do not include any measure that reflects service delivery to children, which is essential to change behavior at the local level. Pragmatic operations research is required to identify key performance indicators that can be easily monitored, without compromising the quality of routine data collected.

Overburdened Health Care Services

In many resource-limited settings, especially in those coping with dual TB and HIV epidemics, existing TB services are overburdened by the provision of directly observed therapy (DOT) to huge numbers of adult patients with sputum smear-positive disease. In these settings, there is reluctance to take on new responsibilities unless additional resources are made available. Although early and effective treatment of the most infectious (sputum smear-positive) patients should remain the priority from a public health perspective, there is an urgent need to align service delivery models with the inclusive goals defined by the Stop TB Strategy. This requires the allocation of substantially more resources to TB control efforts, from national governments and international agencies.

TB has always been a disease of poor and marginalized people. TB services are traditionally linked to public health and epidemic control efforts, with little regard for the need to develop a patient-centered approach. In contrast, HIV services developed a strong patient-centered approach and used vocal activism to help mobilize resources for service delivery and essential technological advances. The constructive role that patient activism can play in improving service delivery and addressing socioeconomic inequalities that underlie the TB epidemic has not been fully harnessed, but progress has been made in recent years. The need to dedicate more resources to address the problem and achieve much-needed technological breakthroughs is now well recognized, although governments in endemic areas have been slow to respond and significant advances remain elusive.

DIAGNOSTIC DILEMMA
Inability to Screen for TB Disease

Addressing the dichotomy that exists between written guidelines and practice requires creative solutions to provide the best possible care to children under suboptimal circumstances. Current WHO guidelines advise that all children less than 5 years of age and all HIV-infected children in close contact with a sputum smear-positive index case should be actively traced, screened for TB, and provided with preventive chemotherapy once TB disease has been ruled out.[27] The International Standards for TB Care made the same recommendation.[33] Most national TB guidelines still regard the tuberculin skin test (TST) and chest radiograph (CXR) as prerequisite screening tests to exclude disease in child TB contacts. This strategy serves as a barrier to access preventive therapy in resource-limited settings in which these tests are not readily available. The contribution made by the TST in routine contact screening is limited, and the decision to initiate preventive therapy following recent TB exposure should not be influenced by the TST result. Symptom-based screening as suggested by WHO (**Fig. 1**) seems safe and feasible.[34] However, in settings in which health systems are severely overburdened it may be more feasible to restrict preventive therapy to those who are at greatest risk of disease following documented TB exposure and/or infection (<3 years of age and/or HIV-infected), as suggested in **Fig. 2**.[35]

It is important to understand differences in the underlying rationale that motivates discrepant approaches in developed countries with adequate resources where TB eradication is an achievable goal and TB-endemic areas with limited resources where the primary aim is to reduce TB-associated morbidity and mortality and to achieve epidemic control (limit transmission).[36] In developed countries the provision of preventive chemotherapy to everyone with documented TB infection is promoted to assist TB eradication. Resource constraints are minimal and eradicating the pool of latent TB infection (LTBI) is important to prevent future reactivation disease, which is the most common cause of adult TB in these settings. In TB-endemic areas, the converse is true. Limited resources require careful priority setting. Poor epidemic control implies ongoing transmission and frequent reinfection, which makes it impossible to eradicate

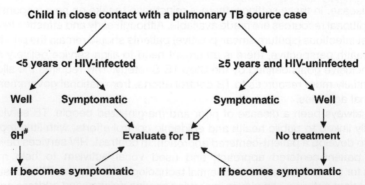

Fig. 1. Suggested approach to contact management when CXR and tuberculin skin testing are not readily available. #INH 10/mg/kg daily for 6 months. (*Adapted from* WHO Guidance for National Tuberculosis Programs on the Management of Tuberculosis in Children. Geneva, Switzerland: WHO guidance. p. 17; with permission.)

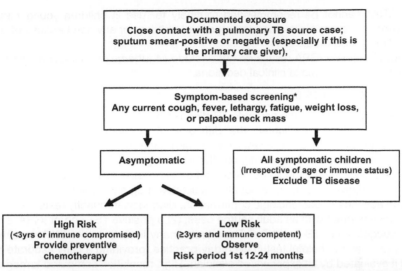

Fig. 2. Proposed algorithm to screen children with documented exposure to a pulmonary TB source case in resource-limited settings. (*Adapted from* Marais BJ, Pai M. New approaches and emerging technologies in the diagnosis of childhood tuberculosis. Paediatr Respir Rev 2007;8:131; with permission.)

the pool of latent infection. Reinfection rather than reactivation is the major cause of adult TB and therefore the primary aim is to limit ongoing transmission, which sustains the epidemic. Prevention is restricted to the most vulnerable subgroups to try to limit TB-associated morbidity and mortality.

Interferon-γ Release Assays

Interferon-γ release assays (IGRAs) are T-cell assays that measure interferon-γ released after stimulation by *M tuberculosis*-specific antigens. Two assays are currently available as commercial kits: the T-SPOT.*TB* (Oxford Immunotec, Oxford, UK) and the QuantiFERON-TB Gold in-tube assay (Cellestis Limited, Victoria, Australia). In general these tests are regarded as more specific and potentially more sensitive than the traditional TST, although pediatric studies remain limited and results inconsistent. Following documented TB exposure the first priority remains the provision of preventive therapy to high-risk contacts irrespective of the IGRA result. The 2009 American Academy of Pediatrics (AAP) Red Book (http://aapredbook. aappublications.org/) recommendations for use of IGRAs in children are as follows:

- For immune-competent children 5 years of age and older, IGRAs can be used in place of a TST to confirm cases of TB or cases of LTBI and likely will yield fewer false-positive test results.
- Children with a positive result from an IGRA should be considered infected with *M tuberculosis* complex. A negative IGRA result cannot universally be interpreted as absence of infection.
- Because of their higher specificity and lack of cross-reaction with bacille Calmette-Guérin (BCG), IGRAs may be useful in children who have received BCG vaccine. IGRAs may be useful to determine whether a BCG-immunized child with a reactive TST more likely has LTBI or has a false-positive TST reaction caused by the BCG.

- IGRAs cannot be recommended routinely for use in children younger than 5 years of age or for immunocompromised children of any age because of a lack of published data.
- Indeterminate IGRA results do not exclude *M tuberculosis* infection and should not be used to make clinical decisions.

Inability to Confirm TB Disease

Increased awareness of the pediatric TB disease burden and improved availability of child-friendly drugs highlighted the difficulty of accurate disease diagnosis in resource-limited settings. Bacteriologic confirmation is often considered to be of limited use because of poor yields, but the yield is greatly increased in children with advanced disease and should be pursued if at all possible because a positive culture not only confirms the diagnosis but also facilitates drug susceptibility testing.[35]

In the absence of bacteriologic confirmation, diagnosis frequently rests on the triad of (1) close contact with an adult source case, (2) a positive TST and/or IGRA, and (3) signs suggestive of TB on CXR.[36] Despite its many limitations the CXR remains the most practical and helpful test in everyday practice, providing a fairly accurate diagnosis if evaluated by an experienced clinician. High-resolution computed tomography is more sensitive to detect early signs of disease, but particular caution is required when interpreting the relevance of these findings in children with absent or minimal symptoms, because transient adenopathy is common following recent primary infection.[36] It is important to take the presence of additional signs and symptoms suggestive of TB into account and not to base a TB diagnosis solely on the radiographic findings.

However, in many TB-endemic areas even a CXR may not be readily available and a variety of clinical scoring systems have been developed to diagnose TB in children. A critical review of these scoring systems concluded that their value is severely limited by the absence of standard symptom definitions and inadequate validation.[37] Accurate symptom definition is essential to differentiate TB from other common conditions. The most helpful symptoms include: (1) persistent, nonremittent cough or wheeze of more than 2 weeks' duration, (2) documented failure to thrive or weight loss despite food supplementation (if food security is a concern), and (3) fatigue or reduced playfulness; clinical follow-up is safe and adds specificity in older children who are at low risk of rapid disease progression.[38] Adolescent children (>8–10 years of age) frequently develop cavitary disease and can be diagnosed using traditional methods.[36] The most common extrathoracic manifestation of TB in children is cervical adenitis. A simple clinical algorithm that identified children with a persistent (>4 weeks) cervical mass of 2 × 2 cm or greater, without a visible local cause or response to first-line antibiotics, showed excellent diagnostic accuracy in a TB-endemic area.[39] It may be less accurate in nonendemic areas, where cervical adenitis is mainly caused by nontuberculous mycobacteria (NTM). Establishing a definitive tissue and/or culture diagnosis remains preferable and this can be achieved by fine needle aspiration biopsy (FNAB).[40]

New Advances

Immune-based diagnosis is complicated by the wide spectrum of disease and other factors that influence the host immune response such as BCG vaccination, exposure to NTM, and HIV coinfection.[35] A recent systematic review showed that current serologic tests have highly variable sensitivity and specificity and have not been validated for clinical use,[41] despite being marketed in TB-endemic countries with poor regulatory control. Current T-cell assays (IGRAs) also fail to differentiate *M tuberculosis* infection from disease. Identifying novel ways to differentiate latent infection from incipient and active disease and finding the correct application for these novel tools in TB-endemic areas remain top research priorities.

A positive culture is regarded as the gold standard test to establish a definitive diagnosis of TB in a symptomatic child. The fact that organisms may be isolated from non-diseased (asymptomatic) children shortly after primary infection may pose a major case definition dilemma in prospective studies, but this is rarely a concern in clinical practice when children present with symptoms suspicious of TB.[36] A recent pediatric study reported reduced time to detection and possible increased bacteriologic yield with the addition of a nutrient broth to standard liquid media.[42] Novel culture-based approaches include simple colorimetric systems, but their accuracy and robustness in field conditions have not been confirmed. The microscopic observation drug susceptibility (MODS) assay uses an inverted light microscope to detect microcolony formation in liquid growth media. It is an inexpensive method that has performed well under field conditions (in adults and children).[43,44] The test is not widely available, remains highly operator dependent, and is labor intensive. Further research is required to identify optimal growth conditions for paucibacillary TB, which can be linked to a variety of detection systems.

Other innovative organism-based approaches include the detection of TB-specific antigens such as lipoarabinomannan in sputum and/or urine. Initial field trials were not promising mainly because of poor sensitivity; improved sensitivity was achieved in HIV-infected adults and those with disseminated disease.[45] No results from pediatric studies have been reported. The phage amplification assay uses bacteriophages to infect live M tuberculosis and is commercially available as FASTPlaque-TB; a variant (FASTPlaque-TB Response) was designed for the rapid detection of rifampin (RMP) resistance. Phage-based assays are cumbersome to perform and cross-contamination has been a major problem in field trials, it has now been superseded by nucleic acid amplification tests (NAATs). **Table 1** summarizes traditional and novel diagnostic approaches, their potential application and the perceived problems, and/or benefits of each. The latest developments on novel diagnostic tests are available at http://www.tbevidence.org/.

NAATs amplify regions specific to M tuberculosis complex and have high specificity, but modest and variable sensitivity, especially in sputum smear-negative TB. Line-probe assays present a major breakthrough in rapid detection of drug resistance. Two commercially available assays are currently approved: INNOLiPA (Innogenetics, Ghent, Belgium) labeled for use on M tuberculosis isolates from solid culture, as well as Genotype MTBDR and DRplus (Hain Lifescience, Nehren, Germany) labeled for use on isolates from solid and liquid culture and directly on sputum smear-positive specimens. These assays show high specificity, help to confirm a TB diagnosis, and detect mutations associated with RMP resistance, but generally require preculture and/or sputum smear-positive disease.[46,47] Genotype MTBDRplus also has the ability to identify mutations associated with INH resistance, but sensitivity remains suboptimal given the variety of possible mutations; additional susceptibility testing for second-line drugs is currently being evaluated.[48] More recent developments include the loop-mediated isothermal amplification (Eiken Chemical Co Ltd, Tokyo, Japan) assay, a simplified manual NAAT designed for peripheral laboratory facilities, and the Xpert MTB/RIF assay (Cepheid, Sunnyvale, CA, USA), a fully automated NAAT platform that can detect M tuberculosis complex as well as RMP resistance. These tests show great promise, and published reports as well as studies in children are eagerly awaited. Transrenal excretion of DNA fragments offer an exciting alternative avenue to diagnose extrapulmonary TB and simplify specimen collection.[49]

Table 1
Various diagnostic approaches: potential application and perceived problems/benefits

	Application	Problems/Benefits	Validation
Traditional approaches			
TB culture using solid or liquid broth media	Bacteriologic confirmation of active disease	Slow turnaround time, expensive poor sensitivity in children	Accepted gold standard
Chest radiography	Diagnosis of probable active TB	Difficult to interpret if asymptomatic; Rarely available in endemic areas with limited resources; accurate disease classification important	Marked inter- and intraobserver variability; reliable in expert hands and in presence of suspicious symptoms
Symptom-based approaches	Diagnosis of probable active TB	Poor symptom definition	Poorly validated
TST	Diagnosis of M tuberculosis infection	Not available in many areas; does not differentiate LTBI from active disease; insensitive in immune-compromised children; No laboratory infrastructure required	Different cutoffs advised in different settings
Novel approaches			
Organism-based			
Colorimetric culture systems	Bacteriologic confirmation of active TB	Simple and feasible, limited resources required; potential for contamination in field conditions	Not validated in children
Phage-based tests	Diagnosis of probable active TB; detection of RMP resistance	Requires laboratory infrastructure; performs poorly when used on clinical specimens	Not well validated in children; evidence from adults suggests suboptimal performance
MODS assay	Diagnosis of probable active TB; detection of drug resistance	Simple and feasible, limited resources required	Evidence from adults look promising

NAATs	Diagnosis of probable active TB; detection of RMP resistance	Rarely available; sensitivity poor in paucibacillary TB, specificity usually good; strict quality control essential	Extensively evaluated, but evidence not in favor of widespread use
Antigen-based assays	Diagnosis of probable active TB	Simple, point-of-care testing; limited clinical data on accuracy	Evidence from adults shows inconsistent performance
Immune-based			
Antibody-based assays MPB64 skin test	Diagnosis of probable active TB Diagnosis of active TB	Simple, point-of-care testing, variable accuracy Simple, point-of-care testing	Evidence from adults not in favor of routine use Not sufficiently validated
T-cell assays	Diagnosis of LTBI	Limited data in children, inability to differentiate LTBI from TB; require 3–5 mL blood; expensive; may have relevance in high-risk children	Evidence inconsistent; no strong evidence of being superior to TST in endemic countries
Symptom-based			
Symptom-based screening	Screening child contacts of adult TB cases	Should improve access to preventive chemotherapy for asymptomatic high-risk contacts in endemic areas	Additional validation preferable
Refined symptom-based diagnosis	Diagnosis of probable active TB	Should improve access to chemotherapy in resource-limited settings; poor performance in HIV-infected children	Additional validation preferable

Adapted from Marais BJ, Pai M. New approaches and emerging technologies in the diagnosis of childhood tuberculosis. Paediatr Respir Rev 2007;8:128; with permission.

Specimen Collection

Specimen collection presents a significant challenge in young children who are unable to expectorate. Routine specimens collected include gastric aspirates and induced sputum, which can be performed in children of any age. Collection of fasting gastric aspirates is cumbersome and usually requires hospitalization, whereas hypertonic-saline–induced sputum requires a shorter period of fasting and can be performed as an outpatient procedure.[35] Collecting a gastric aspirate and an induced sputum specimen on the same day seems to provide the most feasible option.[50] The string test is an innovative method that proved superior to induced sputum in HIV-infected adults with sputum smear-negative TB.[51] A major limitation is the inability of young children to swallow the string-containing capsule; studies are under way to find creative ways of string introduction and retrieval. FNAB is a robust and simple technique that provides a rapid and definitive diagnosis. In a comparative study FNAB specimens provided superior yields compared with standard respiratory specimens in child TB suspects with a palpable lymph node mass.[52] The use of a small 23-gauge needle is well tolerated and associated with minimal side effects and the technique can be performed as an outpatient procedure. **Table 2** provides a summary of specimen collection methods and the perceived problems and/or benefits of each.

TB AND HIV COINFECTION

HIV-related immune compromise is one of the main risk factors for TB development following infection. Among HIV-infected children TB is a major cause of morbidity and mortality.[53] However, because few children are infected with HIV in settings with well-functioning prevention of mother-to-child transmission programs and very young children are highly vulnerable irrespective of their HIV status, most child TB cases remain uninfected with HIV.[54] International guidelines recognize that HIV-infected children remain at high risk of developing TB and recommend provision of preventive therapy, following documented TB exposure and exclusion of active disease, to all HIV-infected children, irrespective of their age (see **Fig. 1**). Preventive therapy should be provided repeatedly in case of repeated TB exposure, but current evidence does not support the provision of continuous INH prophylaxis. It is uncertain if children with adequate immune reconstitution following HAART initiation could be treated similar to HIV-uninfected children. The frequency with which children in settings in which TB/HIV coinfection is common are exposed to adults with sputum smear-negative pulmonary TB and the transmission risk that this may pose is cause for concern. It seems prudent to consider contact with a primary caregiver who has sputum smear-negative pulmonary TB (diagnosed on culture or CXR) as a significant exposure risk and to provide preventive therapy because of the likelihood of prolonged and intimate contact.

The diagnostic challenge is particularly pronounced in HIV-infected children because[54]:

HIV-infected adult patients are more likely to have sputum smear-negative TB and may not be identified as a potential source case

The TST and IGRAs have reduced sensitivity in HIV-infected children, with the TST positive in the minority of HIV-infected children with bacteriologically confirmed TB despite using an induration size cutoff of 5 mm or greater

Chronic pulmonary symptoms from other HIV-related conditions are common and failure to thrive is a typical feature of TB and HIV, which greatly reduces the specificity of symptom-based diagnostic approaches

Table 2
Specimen collection methods: perceived problems/benefits and potential clinical application

Specimen Collection Method	Problems/Benefits	Potential Clinical Application
Sputum	Not feasible in very young children; assistance and supervision may improve the quality of the specimen	Routine sample to be collected in children more than 7 y of age (all children who can produce a good-quality specimen)
Induced sputum	Increased yield compared with gastric aspirate; no age restriction; specialized technique, requires nebulization and suction facilities; potential transmission risk	To be considered in the hospital setting on an in- or outpatient basis
Gastric aspirate	Difficult and invasive procedure; not easily performed on an outpatient basis; requires prolonged fasting; sample collection advised on 3 consecutive days	Routine sample to be collected in hospitalized patients who cannot produce a good-quality sputum specimen
Nasopharyngeal aspiration	Less invasive than gastric aspirate; no fasting required; comparable yield to gastric aspirate	To be considered in primary health care clinics or on an outpatient basis
String test	Less invasive than gastric aspirate; tolerated well in older children (>4–5 y); bacteriologic yield and feasibility requires further investigation	Potential to become the routine sample collected in children who can swallow the capsule, but cannot produce a good-quality sputum specimen Innovative ways of string delivery required in young children
Bronchoalveolar lavage	Extremely invasive	Only for use in patients who are intubated or who require diagnostic bronchoscopy
Urine/stool	Not invasive; excretion of *M tuberculosis* well documented	To be considered with novel sensitive bacteriologic or antigen-based tests
Blood/bone marrow	Bone marrow seems best source to consider in children with uncertain disseminated TB	To be considered for the confirmation of probable disseminated TB in hospitalized patients
CSF	Fairly invasive; important diagnostic procedure although bacteriologic yield low; contraindicated if signs of raised intracranial pressure	To be considered in any child with signs suggestive of meningitis
FNAB	Minimally invasive using a fine 23-G need e; excellent bacteriologic yield, minimal side effects	Procedure of choice in children with superficial lymphadenopathy

Adapted from Marais BJ, Pai M. Specimen collection methods in the diagnosis of childhood tuberculosis. Indian J Med Microbiol 2006;24:250; with permission.

Rapid disease progression may also occur, thereby reducing the sensitivity of diagnostic approaches that focus on persistent, nonremitting symptoms

CXR interpretation is complicated by comorbid conditions such as bacterial pneumonia, lymphocytic interstitial pneumonitis, and bronchiectasis, as well as the atypical presentation of TB in immune-compromised children.

Immune reconstitution inflammatory syndrome (IRIS) has emerged as an important complication to consider after the introduction of HAART in HIV-infected, immunocompromised patients. The temporary exacerbation of TB-associated symptoms and/or signs can be ascribed to improved immune function and does not indicate treatment failure, although drug-resistant TB or other causes of exacerbation should be actively excluded. Administration of the BCG vaccine is contraindicated in children known to be infected with HIV, mainly because of the high risk of disseminated BCG disease.[55] However, BCG IRIS is also common and usually presents with right axillary adenitis following recent HAART initiation in HIV-infected infants who received routine BCG vaccination at birth (as is the practice in most developing countries). Treatment is rarely required, although severe cases may require aspiration of the cold abscess for pain relief.

As in adults it is imperative to combine HIV and TB management in children who are dually infected. Both are chronic diseases needing long-term management and regular health care visits. Often the parents or caregivers are themselves affected, and a comprehensive, family-oriented combined HIV and TB service decreases the number of visits and improves the quality of care these patients receive. However, effective infection control measures are crucial, and highly infectious (sputum smear-positive) patients should not share a waiting room or consulting space with vulnerable HIV-infected patients and children. Child TB cases are rarely sputum smear-positive. For those with sputum smear-positive disease care can be transferred to an integrated family clinic as soon as sputum smear conversion has been confirmed.

TREATING CHILDREN WITH TB

TB treatment aims to cure the individual patient with minimal adverse effects. From a public health perspective it is important to rapidly terminate transmission and prevent the emergence of drug resistance. Bactericidal drugs kill most bacilli that are actively metabolizing, which improves clinical symptoms, terminates transmission, and prevents the emergence of drug resistance. Sterilizing drugs prevents disease relapse by eradicating organisms with intermittent spurts of metabolism and those that reside in an acid pH environment. The need to ensure eradication of these hypometabolic bacilli determines the total duration of therapy. INH has the most potent bactericidal activity and kills most rapidly metabolizing bacilli within the first few days of treatment.[56] RMP has good bactericidal activity but is particularly effective in eradicating slower-growing bacilli. Pyrazinamide (PZA) contributes by killing bacilli that persist within the acidic centers of caseating granulomas. In the presence of a high bacterial load any drug given in isolation is vulnerable to spontaneously occurring drug-resistant mutants, but the use of multiple drugs in combination reduces this risk. Drugs with the most potent bactericidal activity provide the greatest protection to companion drugs.[56]

Practical operational issues, such as access to early and accurate diagnosis, the uninterrupted provision of quality-assured drugs that are stored and dispensed appropriately, and the establishment of systems to ensure treatment adherence are important. Quality-assured fixed-dose combination tablets should be used whenever possible to reduce the risk of drug resistance and to improve simplicity and adherence. The DOT, short-course (DOTS) strategy addresses most of the important operational issues, although the emphasis on sputum smear-positive disease excludes most children with TB, and comprehensive support should be provided to try to ensure adherence.

Preventive Therapy

INH monotherapy for 6 to 9 months is the best-studied preventive therapy regimen, to reduce the TB risk following documented exposure.[57] Efficacy is variable in different studies, but believed to be as high as 90% with good adherence and in the absence of drug resistance.[58] However, poor adherence is a major concern. The effectiveness of preventive therapy in everyday clinical practice reflects efficacy under trial conditions, real-life adherence and the prevalence of drug resistance. The use of a 3-month INH plus RMP regimen is well established and showed equivalent efficacy and improved adherence compared with 6 to 9 months of INH monotherapy.[59,60] Disadvantages include increased drug cost and drug interactions in HIV-infected children on HAART. Evaluating efficacy, adherence, and adverse event profiles of novel short-course preventive therapy regimens remains an important area for future research.

Vaccination with BCG is the most widely used preventive strategy, although studies have shown highly variable protection.[61] Factors such as variations in strain-specific immunogenicity, timing and technique of vaccine administration, host genetic factors, the presence or absence of NTM, and multiple reinfection events may contribute to this variability. BCG vaccination seems to offer significant protection against disseminated (miliary) disease and tuberculous meningitis (TBM) in very young children, but no protection against adult-type TB.[62] A controversial area is the risk versus benefit that BCG provides in HIV-infected children, in whom benefit has not been established and the risk of disseminated BCG disease is substantial.[53] The development of novel vaccines with improved efficacy and safety remains a major research challenge.

Curative Treatment

With drug-susceptible TB the main variables that influence treatment success include the bacterial load, anatomic distribution of bacilli, and competence of host immunity. Sputum smear-negative disease is usually paucibacillary, the risk of acquired drug resistance is low, and drug penetration into the anatomic sites involved is good. The success of 3 drugs (INH, RMP, PZA) during the 2-month intensive phase and 2 drugs (INH, RMP) during the 4-month continuation phase is well established.[56] In the presence of extensive radiographic disease or severe immune compromise, the addition of ethambutol (EMB) during the intensive phase is advised to improve outcome and reduce the risk of acquiring drug resistance.[27] The optimal duration of therapy in immune-compromised patients and the efficacy of shorter treatment durations in immune-competent children with minimal disease require further evaluation.

Sputum smear-positive disease implies a high organism load. Selecting MDR mutants is a particular concern when INH monoresistance is prevalent. The use of 4 drugs (INH, RMP, PZA, EMB) during the 2-month intensive phase should reduce this risk. Once the organism load is sufficiently reduced, daily or intermittent (2–3 times/wk) therapy with INH and RMP during the 4-month continuation phase seems sufficient to ensure organism eradication.[56] However, intermittent therapy is not advised by WHO and should not be used if adherence cannot be ensured, especially in those with cavitary disease, because missing a single dose leads to prolonged periods of suboptimal drug levels. Caution should be exercised when initial treatment response has been suboptimal and in HIV-infected children. It is essential to consider the cerebrospinal fluid (CSF) penetration of drugs used in the treatment of TBM or disseminated (miliary) disease. INH and PZA penetrate the CSF well. RMP and streptomycin penetrate the CSF poorly, but may achieve therapeutic levels in the presence of meningeal inflammation, whereas EMB hardly penetrates the CSF at all.[63] Ethionamide shows good CSF penetration and has been used successfully as the fourth drug in short-course TBM treatment regimens.[64]

Drug Dosing

Previous WHO drug dosing guidelines recommended a uniform INH dose of 4 to 6 mg/kg for adults and children. However, children achieve lower serum INH levels with a similar dose/kg body weight, which may lead to significant underdosing, particularly in settings in which most of the population are rapid acetylators of INH.[29] Studies also showed reduced serum concentrations in children compared with adults receiving identical mg/kg body weight dosages for other first-line drugs including RMP, PZA, and EMB.[30,31,65] Revised dosage recommendations have been formulated to take these findings into account. Recommended single daily doses are: INH 10 to 15 mg/kg (max 300 mg), RMP 10 to 20 mg/kg (max 600 mg), PZA 30 to 40 mg/kg (max 2000 mg), and EMB 15 to 25 mg/kg (max 2000 mg). AAP dosage recommendations for INH have always been higher, at 10 to 15 mg/kg. For intermittent (2–3 times/wk) dosing the recommended doses are: INH 20 to 35 mg/kg (max 900 mg), RMP 10 to 20 mg/kg (max 600 mg), PZA 50 mg/kg (max 2000 mg), and EMB 30 to 50 mg/kg (max 2500 mg).

Retreatment

The most likely cause of treatment failure in the absence of drug-resistant disease is poor adherence. Following treatment interruption most children may be restarted on the original treatment regimen provided adequate supervision is available, because the risk of developing acquired drug resistance is small. If an immune-competent child presents with a new episode of TB, then it most likely represents reinfection disease and standard first-line treatment is appropriate. There is no indication to use escalated retreatment regimens. With genuine treatment failure (absence of clinical response to supervised treatment or relapse soon after treatment completion) drug susceptibility testing and comprehensive history taking to exclude exposure to a drug-resistant source case is of paramount importance.

DRUG RESISTANCE

The clinical and radiologic presentation of drug-resistant and drug-susceptible TB cases is similar and the principles guiding the management of drug-resistant disease remain unchanged. High-risk children in contact with MDR-TB cases should be protected with appropriate preventive therapy, whereas accurate disease classification and drug susceptibility test results of the child's isolate, or in absence thereof, the source case's isolate, should guide therapy in those with TB disease.[66]

The term MDR-TB implies resistance to INH and RMP, with or without resistance to other TB drugs.

Second-line drugs are generally more toxic, but with correct dosing few serious adverse effects are seen in children. Treatment should best be discussed with an expert in the field. A rational guide for preventive therapy in high-risk MDR contacts is to use at least 2 drugs to which the organism is susceptible, for at least 6 months.[67] Basic treatment principles include:[68]

Box 1
Summary of research priorities for childhood tuberculosis

Exposure and infection

1. Role of IGRAs and skin tests with inclusion of novel antigens to differentiate between latent infection, incipient, and active disease, as well as the ability to register a reinfection event

2. Finding pragmatic ways to identify children in need of preventive therapy

3. Randomized control trials for short-course combination preventive therapy

4. Evaluate interventions to improve adherence to preventive therapy

5. Identify optimal preventive therapy for contacts of MDR- and XDR-TB cases

6. Feasibility of implementing a contact register to encourage/monitor provision of preventive therapy

7. Identify barriers to provision of preventive therapy

8. Prospective evaluation of risk/benefit of BCG in HIV-exposed children (HIV-infected on HAART)

9. Develop and evaluate new TB vaccines

10. Preventing TB in highly vulnerable populations (eg, HIV-infected pregnant women)

Diagnosis

1. Improved methods for specimen collection

2. Role of more sophisticated imaging modalities to assist diagnosis and improve understanding of disease pathology

3. Role of bronchoscopy and other invasive methods in complicated TB cases

4. Value of rapid *M tuberculosis* identification and drug resistance testing in children

5. Improving the diagnosis in the absence of sophisticated tests

6. Early detection of TB meningitis, before irreversible damage is done

Treatment

1. Pharmacokinetics and -dynamics of all TB drugs in children, including all relevant age bands

2. Safety and adverse effects of second-line and new TB drugs

3. Optimal duration and drug combinations/doses for different disease manifestations (eg, TB meningitis and spinal TB)

4. Optimal duration of MDR- and XDR-TB treatment in children with early or advanced disease

5. Optimal duration of treatment in HIV-infected children on/off HAART, with early or advanced disease

6. Interventions to improve adherence

7. Optimal/safe treatment of pregnant women with MDR-TB

8. Document frequency/presentation of IRIS caused by TB, BCG, or NTM; effect of early HAART; optimal management

9. Drug interactions between antiretroviral and TB drugs (first- and second-line)

10. Value of post-TB treatment INH prophylaxis in HIV-infected children; influence of HAART

Other interventions

1. What is the role of surgery in: nodal compression of the airways/children with MDR-/XDR-TB/spinal TB
2. Role of steroids in lymph node compression of airways/IRIS
3. Value of cotrimoxazole prophylaxis in HIV-infected children with TB on HAART; influence of CD4 count
4. Value of and feasible strategies for nutritional support

Recording/reporting

1. Collecting and reporting accurate data on smear-positive and -negative TB in children in 2 age groups (<5 years and 5 to 14 years) as requested by WHO
2. Documenting and reporting HIV test results in all children treated for TB (should be performed in all TB suspects)
3. Identify barriers to HIV testing and making the result available for optimal patient management

Infection control

1. Infection control measures applied in pediatric inpatient ward; consider parents/caretakers with possible TB, children with cavitary disease
2. Monitoring of staff working in neonatal/pediatric wards for possible TB
3. Infection control in primary care and TB treatment clinics; exposure of vulnerable children

Other issues

1. Understanding disease pathology. What causes the change from primary TB in children to adult-type TB in adolescents, and the reverse in adults with advanced HIV infection?
2. Documenting emergence of transmitted drug resistance and dominant strains using children with TB as a marker of recent transmission/epidemic control
3. Identify best practices to care for adolescent children with TB

BCG, bacille Calmette-Guérin; HAART, highly active antiretroviral therapy; HIV, human immunodeficiency virus; IGRA, interferon gamma release assay; IRIS, immune reconstitution inflammatory syndrome; MDR, multidrug-resistant; NTM, nontuberculous mycobacteria; TB, tuberculosis; XDR, extremely drug resistant.

(1) Collect multiple specimens for culture and drug susceptibility testing, preferably before treatment initiation
(2) Provisionally treat the child according to the drug susceptibility pattern of the likely source case's isolate
(3) Give 3 or more drugs to which the isolate is susceptible and/or naive (preferably more if the child has extensive or cavitary disease); never add one drug to a failing regimen
(4) Use daily DOT only
(5) Schedule regular follow-up visits to monitor response to therapy and adverse events
(6) Treatment should continue for an extended period after the first negative culture (at least 12 months in early primary disease and at least 18 months in cavitary, extensive pulmonary, or disseminated disease).

Extensive drug-resistant (XDR)-TB can be defined as MDR-TB with additional resistance to fluoroquinolones and one or more of the second-line injectable agents kanamycin, amikacin, or capreomycin. Currently preventive therapy for high-risk XDR contacts is not advised, but in the light of possible low- or intermediate-level INH resistance, high-dose INH (15–20 mg/kg) may provide some protection.[69,70] High-risk contacts should receive diligent follow-up for a minimum of 2 years. Once a patient has been diagnosed with MDR-TB it is essential to perform second-line drug susceptibility testing to optimize treatment and prevent the development of additional resistance. Fluoroquinolone resistance often applies to the whole class of drugs, but susceptibility to moxifloxacin may still be present. Newer drugs, such as linezolid, have been used with success in children with XDR-TB, but are expensive and adverse events are common with prolonged therapy.[71]

RESEARCH PRIORITIES

Children are frequently excluded from drug trials because there is a perception of additional risk and limited financial return. Many drugs remain unlicensed for use in children or become available for pediatric use only long after initial registration. Children were almost completely excluded from the initial clinical trials on TB treatment. As a result, nearly 40 years after the development of short-course regimens for adults, fundamental uncertainties about optimal dosing and treatment duration persist.[72] It is essential that children should be included in the evaluation of novel TB drugs, as soon as initial safety and efficacy studies have been concluded. There are difficulties that complicate their inclusion in efficacy trials and it seems reasonable to extrapolate efficacy data from adult studies. However, because of the existence of unique age-related pharmacokinetic and toxicity profiles it is essential to include children in safety and dose ranging studies and to develop child-friendly formulations before product registration. A summary of research priorities is provided in **Box 1**.

SUMMARY

Optimizing access to preventive and curative treatment is essential to reduce the morbidity and mortality associated with pediatric TB. Children develop TB where adults continue to spread the infection, and TB disease burdens predominantly reflect global socioeconomic disparities. Strong political commitment to comprehensive health initiatives such as the Millennium Developmental Goals (MDGs), together with local community involvement and ongoing advocacy, are required to meet the daunting challenge posed by the global TB epidemic.

REFERENCES

1. Nelson LJ, Wells CD. Global epidemiology of childhood tuberculosis. Int J Tuberc Lung Dis 2004;8:636–47.
2. World Health Organization. Global tuberculosis control: epidemiology, strategy, financing: WHO Report 2009. Geneva (Switzerland): World Health Organization; 2009.
3. Newton SM, Brent AJ, Anderson S, et al. Paediatric tuberculosis. Lancet Infect Dis 2008;8:499–510.
4. Marais BJ, Hesseling AC, Gie RP, et al. The burden of childhood tuberculosis and the accuracy of routine surveillance data in a high-burden setting. Int J Tuberc Lung Dis 2006;10:259–63.
5. Donald PR. Childhood tuberculosis: out of control? Curr Opin Pulm Med 2002;8: 178–82.

6. Chintu C, Mudenda V. Lucas S et.al. Lung diseases at necropsy in African children dying from respiratory illnesses: a descriptive necropsy study. Lancet 2002;360:985–90.

7. McNally LM, Jeena PM, Gajee K, et al. Effect of age, polymicrobial disease, and maternal HIV status on treatment response and cause of severe pneumonia in South African children: a prospective descriptive study. Lancet 2007;369:1440–51.

8. Marais BJ, Gie RP, Schaaf HS, et al. The spectrum of childhood tuberculosis in a highly endemic area. Int J Tuberc Lung Dis 2006;10:732–8.

9. Marais BJ, Gie RP, Schaaf HS, et al. The natural history of childhood intra-thoracic tuberculosis – a critical review of the pre-chemotherapy literature. Int J Tuberc Lung Dis 2004;8:392–402.

10. Nunn P, Reid A, De Cock KM. Tuberculosis and HIV infection: the global setting. J Infect Dis 2007;196(Suppl 1):S5–14.

11. Dahle UR, Eldholm V, Winje BA, et al. Impact of immigration on the molecular epidemiology of Mycobacterium tuberculosis in a low-incidence country. Am J Respir Crit Care Med 2007;176:930–5.

12. Gillman A, Berggren I, Bergström SE, et al. Primary tuberculosis infection in 35 children at a Swedish day care center. Pediatr Infect Dis J 2008;27:1078–82.

13. Van Rie A, Warren R, Richardson M, et al. Exogenous reinfection as a cause of recurrent tuberculosis after curative treatment. N Engl J Med 1999;341:1174–9.

14. Verver S, Warren RM, Beyers N, et al. Rate of reinfection tuberculosis after successful treatment is higher than rate of new tuberculosis. Am J Respir Crit Care Med 2005;171:1430–5.

15. Kritzinger FE, den Boon S, Verver S, et al. No decrease in annual risk of tuberculosis infection in endemic area in Cape Town, South Africa. Trop Med Int Health 2009;14:136–42.

16. Lawn SD, Bekker LG, Middelkoop K, et al. Impact of HIV infection on the epidemiology of tuberculosis in a peri-urban community in South Africa: the need for age-specific interventions. Clin Infect Dis 2006;42:1040–7.

17. Churchyard GJ, Scano F, Grant AD, et al. Tuberculosis preventive therapy in the era of HIV infection: overview and research priorities. J Infect Dis 2007;196:S52–62.

18. Cotton MF, Schaaf HS, Lottering G, et al. Tuberculosis exposure in HIV-exposed infants in a high-prevalence setting. Int J Tuberc Lung Dis 2008;12:225–7.

19. Schaaf HS, Marais BJ, Hesseling AC, et al. Childhood drug-resistant tuberculosis in the Western Cape Province of South Africa. Acta Paediatr 2006;95:523–8.

20. Wright A, Zignol M, Van Deun A, et al. Epidemiology of antituberculosis drug resistance 2002-07: an updated analysis of the Global Project on Anti-Tuberculosis Drug Resistance Surveillance. Lancet 2009;373:1861–73.

21. Gagneux G, Long CD, Small PM, et al. The competitive cost of antibiotic resistance in Mycobacterium tuberculosis. Science 2006;312:1944–6.

22. Moss AR, Alland D, Telzak E, et al. A city-wide outbreak of a multiple-drug-resistant strain of Mycobacterium tuberculosis in New York. Int J Tuberc Lung Dis 1997;1:115–21.

23. Drobniewski F, Balabanova Y, Nikolayevsky V, et al. Drug-resistant tuberculosis, clinical virulence and the dominance of the Beijing strain family in Russia. JAMA 2005;293:2726–31.

24. Marais BJ, Victor TC, Hesseling AC, et al. Beijing and Haarlem genotypes are over-represented among children with drug resistant tuberculosis in the Western Cape Province of South Africa. J Clin Microbiol 2006;44:3539–43.

25. Steiner P, Rao M. Drug-resistant tuberculosis in children. Semin Pediatr Infect Dis 1993;4:275–82.

26. Schaaf HS, Marais BJ, Hesseling AC, et al. Surveillance of antituberculosis drug resistance among children from the Western Cape Province of South Africa - an upward trend. Am J Public Health 2009;99:1486–90.

27. World Health Organization. Guidance for national tuberculosis programmes on the management of tuberculosis in children. Geneva (Switzerland): World Health Organization; 2006. WHO/HTM/TB/2006.371.

28. Gie RP, Matiru RH. Supplying quality-assured child-friendly anti-tuberculosis drugs to children. Int J Tuberc Lung Dis 2009;13:277–8.

29. McIlleron H, Willemse M, Werely CJ, et al. Isoniazid plasma concentrations in a cohort of South African children with tuberculosis: implications for international pediatric dosing guidelines. Clin Infect Dis 2009;48:1547–53.

30. Schaaf HS, Willemse M, Cilliers K, et al. Rifampin pharmacokinetics in children, with and without human immunodeficiency virus infection, hospitalized for the management of severe forms of tuberculosis. BMC Med 2009;7(1):19.

31. Graham SM, Bell DJ, Nyirongo S, et al. Low levels of pyrazinamide and ethambutol in children with tuberculosis and impact of age, nutritional status and human immunodeficiency virus infection. Antimicrob Agents Chemother 2006;50:407–13.

32. Schaaf HS, Krook S, Hollemans DW, et al. Recurrent culture-confirmed tuberculosis in human immunodeficiency virus-infected children. Pediatr Infect Dis J 2005;24:685–91.

33. Hopewell PC, Pai M, Maher D, et al. International standards for tuberculosis care. Lancet Infect Dis 2006;6:710–25.

34. Kruk A, Gie RP, Schaaf HS, et al. Symptom-based screening of child tuberculosis contacts: improved feasibility in resource-limited settings. Pediatrics 2008;121: e1646–52.

35. Marais BJ, Pai M. New approaches and emerging technologies in the diagnosis of childhood tuberculosis. Paediatr Respir Rev 2007;8:124–33.

36. Marais BJ, Gie RP, Schaaf HS, et al. Childhood pulmonary tuberculosis – old wisdom and new challenges. Am J Respir Crit Care Med 2006;173:1078–90.

37. Hesseling AC, Schaaf HS, Gie RP, et al. A critical review of diagnostic approaches used in the diagnosis of childhood tuberculosis. Int J Tuberc Lung Dis 2002;6:1038–45.

38. Marais BJ, Gie RP, Schaaf HS, et al. A refined symptom-based approach to diagnose pulmonary tuberculosis in children. Pediatrics 2006;118:e1350–9.

39. Marais BJ, Wright C, Gie RP, et al. Etiology of persistent cervical adenopathy in children: a prospective community-based study in an area with a high incidence of tuberculosis. Pediatr Infect Dis J 2006;25:142–6.

40. Wright CA, Warren RW, Marais BJ. Fine needle aspiration biopsy: an undervalued diagnostic modality in pediatric mycobacterial disease. Int J Tuberc Lung Dis 2009;13:1467–75.

41. Steingart KR, Henry M, Laal S, et al. A systematic review of commercial serological antibody detection tests for the diagnosis of extrapulmonary tuberculosis. Thorax 2007;83:705–12.

42. Brittle EW, Marais BJ, Hesseling AC, et al. Improved mycobacterial yield and reduced time-to-detection in pediatric samples using a nutrient broth growth supplement. J Clin Microbiol 2009;47:1287–9.

43. Moore DAJ, Evans CAW, Gilman RH, et al. Microscopic-observation drug-susceptibility assay for the diagnosis of TB. N Engl J Med 2006;355:1539–50.

44. Oberhelman RA, Soto-Castellares G, Caviedes L, et al. Improved recovery of Mycobacterium tuberculosis from children using the microscopic observation and drug susceptibility method. Pediatrics 2006;118:e100–6.

45. Shah M, Variava E, Holmes CB, et al. Diagnostic accuracy of a urine lipoarabino-mannan test for tuberculosis in hospitalized patients in a high HIV prevalence setting. J Acquir Immune Defic Syndr 2009;52(2):145–51.
46. World Health Organization. Molecular line probe assays for rapid screening of patients at risk of multidrug-resistant tuberculosis (MDR-TB). WHO Policy Statement 27 June 2008. Geneva (Switzerland): World Health Organization; 2008.
47. Barnard M, Albert H, Coetzee G, et al. Rapid molecular screening for multidrug-resistant tuberculosis in a high-volume public health laboratory in South Africa. Am J Respir Crit Care Med 2008;177:787–92.
48. Hillemann D, Rusch-Gerdes S, Richter E. Feasibility of the genotype MTBDRsl assay for fluoroquinolone, amikacin-capreomycin, and ethambutol resistance testing of Mycobacterium tuberculosis strains and clinical specimens. J Clin Microbiol 2009;47:1767–72.
49. Green C, Huggett JF, Talbot E, et al. Rapid diagnosis of tuberculosis through the detection of mycobacterial DNA in urine by nucleic acid amplification methods. Lancet Infect Dis 2009;9:505–11.
50. Hatherill M, Hawkridge T, Zar HJ, et al. Induced sputum or gastric lavage for community-based diagnosis of childhood pulmonary tuberculosis? Arch Dis Child 2009;94:195–201.
51. Vargas D, Garcia L, Gilman RH, et al. Diagnosis of sputum-scarce HIV-associated pulmonary tuberculosis in Lima, Peru. Lancet 2005;365:150–2.
52. Wright CA, Hesseling AC, Warren RW, et al. Fine needle aspiration biopsy – a first line diagnostic procedure in pediatric tuberculosis suspects with peripheral lymphadenopathy. Int J Tuberc Lung Dis 2009;13:1373–9.
53. Hesseling AC, Cotton MF, Jennings T, et al. High incidence of tuberculosis among HIV-infected infants: evidence from a South African population-based study highlights the need for improved tuberculosis control strategies. Clin Infect Dis 2009; 48:108–14.
54. Marais BJ, Cotton M, Graham S, et al. Diagnosis and management challenges of childhood TB in the era of HIV. J Infect Dis 2007;196(Suppl 1):S76–85.
55. Hesseling AC, Johnson LF, Jaspan H, et al. Disseminated bacille Calmette–Guérin disease in HIV-infected South African infants. Bull World Health Organ 2009;87:505–11.
56. Marais BJ, Schaaf HS, Donald PR. Pediatric tuberculosis: issues related to current and future treatment options. Future Microbiol 2009;4:661–75.
57. Smieja MJ, Marchetti CA, Cook DJ, et al. Isoniazid for preventing tuberculosis in non-HIV infected persons. Cochrane Database Syst Rev 2000;2:CD001363.
58. Marais BJ, Ayles H, Graham SM, et al. Screening and preventive therapy for tuberculosis. Chest Clin N Am 2009;30:827–46.
59. Ena J, Valls V. Short course therapy with rifampicin plus isoniazid, compared with standard therapy with isoniazid, for latent tuberculosis: a meta-analysis. Clin Infect Dis 2005;40:670–6.
60. Spyridis NP, Spyridis PG, Gelesme A, et al. The effectiveness of a 9-month regimen of isoniazid alone versus 3- and 4-month regimens of isoniazid plus rifampin for treatment of latent tuberculosis infection in children: results of an 11-year randomized study. Clin Infect Dis 2007;45:715–22.
61. Fine PE, Carneiro IAM, Milstien JB, et al. Issues relating to the use of BCG in immunization programmes. A discussion document. Geneva (Switzerland): Department of Vaccines and Biologicals. World Health Organization; 1999: 1–33.

62. Trunz BB, Fine P, Dye C. Effect of BCG vaccination on childhood tuberculous meningitis and miliary tuberculosis worldwide: a meta-analysis and assessment of cost-effectiveness. Lancet 2006;367:1122–4.

63. Ellard GA, Humphries MJ, Allen BW. Cerebrospinal fluid drug concentrations and the treatment of tuberculous meningitis. Am Rev Respir Dis 1993;148:650–5.

64. Donald PR, Schoeman JF, van Zyl LE, et al. Intensive short course chemotherapy in the management of tuberculous meningitis. Int J Tuberc Lung Dis 1998;2: 704–11.

65. Donald PR, Maher D, Maritz JS, et al. Ethambutol dosage for the treatment of children: literature review and recommendations. Int J Tuberc Lung Dis 2006;10: 1318–30.

66. Mukherjee J, Schaaf HS. Multidrug-resistant tuberculosis in children. In: Schaaf HS, Zumla A, editors. Tuberculosis: a comprehensive clinical reference. 1st edition. St Louis (MO): Saunders Elsevier; 2009. p. 532–8.

67. Schaaf HS, Gie RP, Kennedy M, et al. Evaluation of young children in contact with adult multidrug-resistant pulmonary tuberculosis: a 30-month follow-up. Pediatrics 2002;109:765–71.

68. Schaaf HS. Drug-resistant tuberculosis in children. S Afr Med J 2007;97(Part 2): 995–7.

69. Schaaf HS, Victor TC, Engelke E, et al. Minimal inhibitory concentration of isoniazid in isoniazid-resistant *Mycobacterium tuberculosis* isolates from children. Eur J Clin Microbiol Infect Dis 2007;26:203–5.

70. Moulding TS. Should isoniazid be used in retreatment of tuberculosis despite acquired isoniazid resistance? Am Rev Respir Dis 1981;123:262–4.

71. Schaaf HS, Willemse M, Donald PR. Long-term linezolid treatment in a young child with extensively drug-resistant tuberculosis. Pediatr Infect Dis J 2009;28: 748–50.

72. Burman WJ, Cotton MF, Gibb DM, et al. Ensuring the involvement of children in the evaluation of new tuberculosis treatment regimens. PLoS Med 2008;5(8):e176.

Tuberculosis in the Global Aging Population

Toru Mori, MD, PhD[a],*, Chi Chiu Leung, MBBS, FCCP[b]

KEYWORDS

• Tuberculosis • Aging • Epidemiology • Prevention

EPIDEMIOLOGIC TRANSITION OF TUBERCULOSIS
Aging of the Tuberculosis Patient Population

Tuberculosis (TB) can attack people of any sex, age, or socioeconomic class. In reality, TB is likely to claim its greatest toll from certain strata of the population, and it is important to identify these for the purpose of planning and implementing TB control. **Fig. 1** presents the age-specific incidence rate of TB and the age distribution of TB patients in the United States[1] and Africa[2] (countries belonging to the African Region of the World Health Organization), representing countries with a low and high prevalence of TB, respectively. Here, "TB" refers to smear-positive TB for Africa, and TB of all forms for the United States. Also, for the United States it is limited to TB in whites, as 58% of the TB patients in the United States are foreign-born and have clearly distinct epidemiologic characteristics.

The epidemiologic situations with respect to TB in Africa and the United States are tremendously different, with incidence rates of smear-positive TB for the entire population of 124 and 1.1, respectively. A similar difference appears with regard to age-specific statistics. The incidence rate curve in Africa has a peak at 25 to 44 years of age that goes downward thereafter, whereas in the United States it goes up monotonically with age. As for the age composition of the patients, in Africa the age group of 15 to 44 years comprises 74% of the population, whereas in the United States it is only 24%, and instead the age group of 65 years and older occupies 35% (vs only 4% in Africa). It is apparent that in high-prevalence settings TB is badly affecting the most productive age groups. On the other hand, TB is now becoming a serious health issue of elderly persons in low-prevalence countries.

[a] Research Institute of Tuberculosis, Japan Anti-Tuberculosis Association, 3-1-24, Matsuyama, Kiyose, Tokyo 204-8533, Japan
[b] TB and Chest Service, Department of Health, Wanchai Chest Clinic, Wanchai, Hong Kong, China
* Corresponding author.
E-mail address: tmori-rit@jata.or.jp

Infect Dis Clin N Am 24 (2010) 751–768
doi:10.1016/j.idc.2010.04.011
0891-5520/10/$ – see front matter © 2010 Elsevier Inc. All rights reserved.

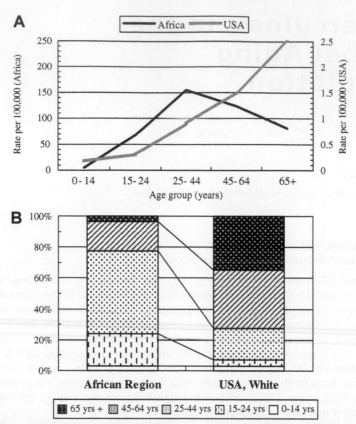

Fig. 1. (*A*) Age-specific notification rate (Africa: smear-positive TB; United States, white: all forms, 2007). (*B*) Newly notified cases according to age groups (Africa: smear-positive TB; United States, white: all forms, 2007). (*Data from* CDC. Reported tuberculosis in the United States, 2007. Atlanta (GA): US Department of Health and Human Services, CDC; 2008; and World Health Organization. Global tuberculosis control: epidemiology, strategy, financing. Geneva: WHO report; 2009. WHO/HTM/TB/2009.411.)

A similar comparison can be observed in the historical changes of TB within the same population. In Japan, TB mortality has changed dramatically in its level and age pattern from 1940 through 1990 (**Fig. 2**). **Fig. 3** presents the TB notification rates as well as the age composition of newly notified patients for the years 1962 and 2005 in Japan.[3] The notification rate for all ages was 303 (per 100,000 population) in 1962 and had fallen greatly to 22 by 2005. At the same time, the age strata of the population affected by the disease have changed drastically. The age-specific notification rate increased continuously with age during both years, but the gap between the young and the aged groups has recently become wider. Also, in 1962 a majority (65%) of the patients were aged 20 to 59 years, whereas in 2005 this group was replaced by those aged 60 years or older (60%), a group that accounted for only 16% in 1962.

When TB was prevalent globally, covering Europe and the United States during the nineteenth and early twentieth centuries, it was a problem of youth or middle age and was supposed to be rare in old age.[4,5] Such is characteristic of the current situation in Africa and that of the Japan in the past. When the level of epidemics is reduced, the problem of old age emerges to a varying extent.

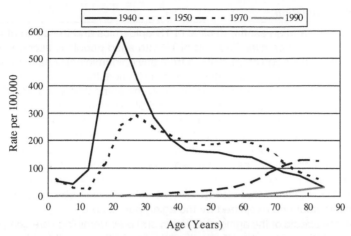

Fig. 2. Age-specific tuberculosis mortality rate of selected years, Japan. (*Data from* Ministry of Health, Labor & Welfare of Japan. Tuberculosis surveillance annual report 2006.)

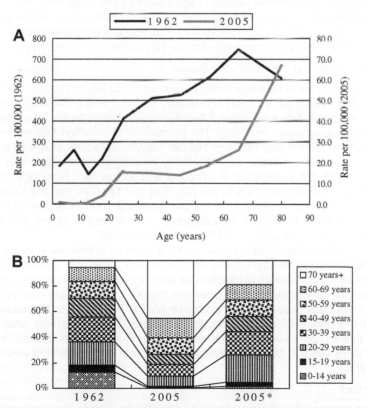

Fig. 3. (*A*) Case notification rates for 1962 and 2005, Japan, TB of all forms. (*B*) Distribution of notified cases according to age group, Japan, 1962 and 2005, TB of all forms. (*Data from* Ministry of Health, Labor & Welfare of Japan. Tuberculosis surveillance annual report 2006. Tokyo: Japan Anti-Tuberculosis Association; 2006.)

Aging of the Population

In many countries and areas, the decline of TB epidemics and the aging of the population are occurring in parallel. The drift of TB into aged people is ascribed greatly to the aging of the entire population, distinct from any epidemiologic changes. Taking the aforementioned example of the United States and Africa, the proportion of population older than 65 years is 13% and 6%, respectively, meaning that a considerable part of the predominance of the aged seen in the United States could be attributed to its aged population. Similarly, in Japan the proportion of those older than 60 years has increased from 9% in 1962 to 28% in 2005. The impact of this change is illustrated in **Fig.** 3B, in which the age composition of new cases in 2005 was adjusted by applying the age-specific rates of that year to the population structure of 1962. If it were not for the population aging, the proportion of those 60 years and older would have been 31%, meaning that about half (but not all) of the observed proportion of elderly patients could be explained by the aging population.

However, the effects of the aging population on TB epidemiology are complicated. If the aged population grows together with a decline in the overall incidence rate, the latter may slow down due to the higher level and slower decline of incidence in the elderly, as observed in Japan after the 1980s. As a result, the decline of infection sources within the population may be hampered. Infection can be transmitted to all age groups, thereby retarding the decline in age-specific case rates. Also, in the growing elderly population segment, there are more subjects with various health problems, such as underlying illnesses or risk factors that would predispose them to TB, and these may in turn have repercussions on the TB problem for the entire population.

Burden of Infection in the Older Age Group

The most basic index of TB epidemiology is annual risk of infection (ARI). The accumulated effect of ARI on each cohort is indicated by the age-specific prevalence of TB infection, as seen in **Fig.** 4 for Japan.[6] This estimate is based on the tuberculin survey results and mathematical modeling. The prevalence of infection thus estimated for 1950, when the TB mortality rate was 146 per 100,000, was 50% at age 20 and older, and 90% at age 60. In those days, mortality was highest in the 20s and 30s age groups. In 2005, the prevalence of infection was as low as 1% at age 20, but as high as 56% in the 60s and 70% in the 70s. This trend implies that the current aging of TB disease rates is a reflection of the overwhelming concentration of the infected into the older age segments of the population. In 2005, out of all infected subjects, 74% were 60 years or older, and 91% were older than 50.

At the same time, the risk of progression from infection to disease is not excessively high in the older subjects as compared with those of younger age. By dividing the incidence rate by the prevalence of infection for each age group, one can derive the risk of progression to clinical disease. As shown in **Fig.** 4B, an age-dependent profile with a young adult peak is seen, rather similar to what is observed for TB incidence rate in high-prevalence settings (see **Fig.** 2). The gradually declining risk after the 30s may be due to the passing of time after the primary infection. Indeed, for those aged 70 to 74 years in 2005, it is estimated that 80% of the infection was acquired before 1950.

Cohort Effect

Apart from the changing pattern of the age-specific prevalence of infection in the face of declining epidemics, the generation or cohort effect is another important epidemiologic mechanism that drives the change in age pattern of TB with time. This theory assumes that a generation of people born during a certain time period, that is, a cohort,

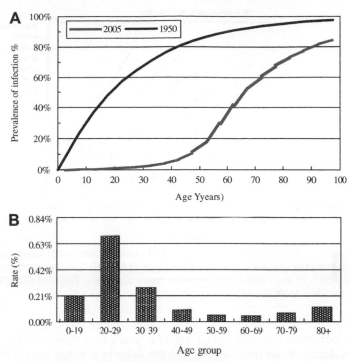

Fig. 4. (A) Estimated age-specific prevalence of infection, Japan, 1950 and 2005. (B) Estimated rate of development of TB from the infected, Japan, 2005. (*Data from* Mori T. Some recent aspects of tuberculosis infection in Japan (2). Kekkaku 1988;63:39–48 [In Japanese].)

shares the same age-dependent risk of disease development as cohorts born at other time. However, if the exposure level decreases with time, a higher burden of infection remains in the older cohorts, which is manifest by increasing disease risk with age at cross-sectional analysis. Thus, high levels of disease risk in old age indicate the residual effects of higher risks of infection earlier in life.[7] As Powell has said,[8] the fact that the pool of infected persons from which cases of disease arise is becoming older signifies the continuing success of the battle against TB.

Not Just Cohort Effect

However, there are some cases that indicate a deviation from the cohort model when analyzed closely. Tocque and colleagues[9] performed cohort analyses of the TB notification rates in Hong Kong and in England and Wales. In Hong Kong, each birth cohort exhibited a similar age pattern of notification rates, peaking in the 25 to 39 age group and gradually declining thereafter. After 1978, all cohorts exhibited an increase in rates with increasing age (**Fig. 5**). For England and Wales, the decline of the rates with age ceased in 1984. A similar discontinuation of the decline in the incidence rate in later life was observed in Japan after 1990. As shown in **Fig. 4**B, there is also an increase in the risk of developing disease after 60 years of age, even after controlling for difference in the prevalence of infection. Regarding the reasons for this recent irregular trend, Tocque and colleagues argued for the possibility of immunologic incompetence due to the pattern of aging leading to exogenous reinfection and reactivation. In England

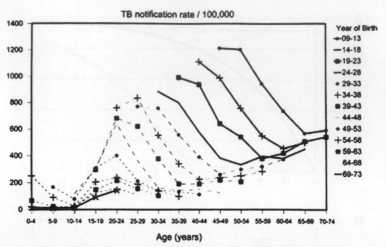

Fig. 5. Age-specific pattern of TB in 13 cohorts born between 1909 to 1913 and 1969 to 1973 in Hong Kong males. (*From* Tocque K, Bellis MA, Tam CM, et al. Long-term trends in tuberculosis. Comparison of age-cohort data between Hong Kong and England and Wales. Am J Respir Crit Care Med 1998;158:485; with permission.)

and Wales, increased infection during the War years is suspected as a possible cause.[10] For Japan, it has been argued that the cohorts infected around the end of the War under conditions of serious malnutrition may run a higher risk of disease that has lasted to the present day. A more plausible reason that could explain such a phenomenon across different localities might have been the attenuation of the natural selective forces for survival with the continuing socioeconomic development and improvement in health care. Whereas only few of the fittest could have survived beyond 70 years in the early part of the last century, most children born nowadays are expected to live beyond that age in developed countries. With the increasing prevalence of chronic degenerative diseases among the elderly nowadays, it is perhaps not surprising to see a rising incidence of TB at this extreme of age nowadays. The effect of tobacco smoking on TB has been established,[11] and differences in prevalence of this habit among cohorts could also have contributed.

RISK FACTORS FOR TB
Demographic Factors

Aging itself is generally not an important risk factor of TB disease. As remote infection is much more likely in elderly subjects, they often run a lower risk of developing disease, primarily due to the longer time lapse since the primary infection and their status as selected survivors. However, at the same time they are likely to have various risk factors commonly associated with aging that may enhance the risk of disease development, or modify/complicate the clinical picture of TB.

As cited by Perez-Guzman and colleagues[12] in their meta-analysis of comparative studies between elderly and nonelderly TB patients, most of the available studies reported a male predominance among elderly TB patients. For Japan in 2005, notification rates of males and females per 100,000 population considered separately were 10.2 versus 8.7 for 0 to 39 years, 24.5 versus 9.0 for 40 to 59 years, and 70.5 versus 30.2 for 60 years and older,[3] indicating a remarkable sex difference beyond the age of 40 years. For the United States in 2007, the rates were 4.0 versus 3.1 for age group of 0 to 44 years, 7.4 versus 3.3 for 45 to 64 years, and 9.4 versus 4.9 for 65 years and older,[1] also demonstrating a wider gap after the age of 45 years. The similar male predominance was reported from Hong Kong.[13] The reason for this male predominance in the TB rate may be at least partly ascribed to the more extensive social activity of males, exposing them to infection and in turn leading to TB disease.[12]

Smoking and Comorbidities

In a prospective study of older subjects on the risk of TB development, Leung and colleagues[14] found that TB incidence was clearly higher in current smokers (2.6 times that of nonsmokers). These investigators also calculated that 33% of male TB cases and 9% of female TB cases is attributable to smoking, which may partly explain these sex differences. Moreover, the recent deviations in the cohort pattern of notification rates can be related to recent changes in smoking habits within the cohorts.

Other factors analyzed by Perez-Guzman and colleagues[12] that were found to be significantly more common in elderly patients included cardiovascular diseases, chronic obstructive pulmonary disease, diabetes mellitus, a history of gastrectomy, and malignancy. These diseases or conditions are more common in the elderly than in the general population, and the contribution of diabetes, gastrectomy, and malignancy to TB has been well documented.

As for diabetes, Ponce-de-Leon and colleagues[15] found in a survey in Mexico that subjects with diabetes had a prevalence rate of TB 6.8 times higher than the general population. In a prospective study conducted in Korea from 1988 to 1990, people with diabetes were found to have an incidence rate of TB 3.47 times higher (5.15 times for bacteriologically confirmed TB) than those without diabetes.[15,16] In Japan's surveillance report, the proportion of reported diabetes cases among newly notified TB patients was 7.0% for those younger than 60 years but 15.2% for those aged 60 years and older.[17] The contribution of diabetes to TB appears not only in its higher disease development but also in causing rapid progress of the illness, a poor treatment response,[18] and a greater risk of relapse.

In Hong Kong, TB patients older than 60 years were known to have more underlying diseases, including diabetes (in 16.6%, compared with 6.2% for those younger than 60 years), silicosis (2.3% vs 1.0%), liver disease (2.1% vs 1.4%), lung cancer (1.6% vs 0.3%), and other malignancies (1.2% vs 0.2%).[19] Korzeniewska-Kosela and colleagues[20] also reported that elderly patients had cancers other than lung cancer 3.94 times more frequently than younger patients.

Interacting Effects/Environment

The changes in immunity associated with advanced age is well known from many observations of waning tuberculin reactions, or even anergy, among both TB patients and healthy subjects at the upper extreme of age.[21,22] All of the illnesses or conditions cited above are supposed to promote these immunity changes, thus creating a predisposition for the development of clinically manifest disease.

Finally, there is the issue of elderly subjects living in nursing homes or other congregate facilities. In such facilities in the United States, tuberculin positivity has been reported at higher levels and outbreaks of TB have not been rare.[23,24] Staff members at these facilities are also known to have a higher risk of TB. Similar observations were made in Hong Kong as well.[25] However, no such problem was found in similar facilities in Canada.[26] Further studies are warranted to address this issue properly.

PREVENTIVE TREATMENT
Goal of Intervention

Infection is the prerequisite for development of disease. Preventive treatment for TB generally refers to the screening and treatment of latent TB infection (LTBI). Like that for other infectious diseases, it serves 2 main functions: personal protection and public health control.

TB is a chronic infection. Although the risk of disease is highest in the first 2 years after infection, considerable magnitude of risk persists for their lifetime.[27] As discussed earlier, there is generally excess risk of LTBI among the elderly segment of the indigenous population in developed countries,[28,29] likely reflecting the much higher burden of TB in the past decades. With the waning immunity associated with advance age and increasing prevalence of multiple comorbidities, there is often an excess risk for the development of clinical disease. Indeed in Hong Kong, there is up to a 100-fold risk differential between elderly men aged 75 or older and those aged 14 or younger (**Fig. 6**).[30] Smoking,[13] low body mass index,[31] and poorly controlled diabetes mellitus[32] have been associated with an increased risk of TB among an elderly cohort in the same locality. Furthermore, TB often presents atypically among the elderly.[12,13] Delay in diagnosis and treatment, coupled with poorer drug tolerance, accounts for the much higher mortality among this group.[13] Screening and treatment of LTBI can, at least in theory, help to avert morbidity and mortality in this age group.

TB is an airborne infectious disease and a major killer in the history of mankind. There is, perhaps, a more important public health dimension in the screening and treatment of LTBI. It is estimated that 2 billion people worldwide have LTBI.[33] There is little doubt that treatment of active disease by DOTS (Directly Observed Treatment Short-course) remains the key strategy to bring the transmission risk under rapid control in most high-incidence countries. However, such a strategy alone cannot

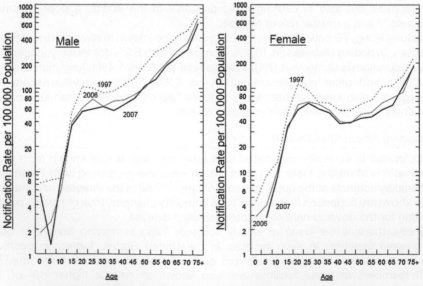

Fig. 6. Sex- and age-specific tuberculosis notification rate in Hong Kong, 1997, 2006 and 2007. (*Data from* Tuberculosis and Chest Service. Annual Report of Tuberculosis and Chest Service 2007. Hong Kong (China): Department of Health; 2009.)

tackle the continuing development of disease by endogenous reactivation among those latently infected. In many intermediate burden areas, where the transmission risk has been brought under control either by natural decline or the introduction of effective chemotherapy, endogenous reactivation of LTBI among the elderly segment of the population accounts for the increasing proportion of TB cases.[30,34] In contrast to the treatment of active disease by DOTS, screening and treatment of LTBI, if implemented on a population scale, has the potential to tackle the large pool of infected individuals across successive birth cohorts, and thereby to bring the disease under more rapid control. However, the limitations of existing diagnostic and treatment tools must be overcome before such an ambitious goal can be realized.

Screening Tools for LTBI

With a very low bacillary load and in the absence of clinical manifestations, the diagnosis of LTBI involves measurement of the specific host immune responses to the pathogen. Serologic tests have contributed remarkably in the diagnosis of many viral infections, even when the there is difficulty in isolating the causative organism. For TB, the situation is much more complex. The human body appears to rely mainly on cellular immune response to defend against the tubercle bacillus. Humoral responses are variable and inconsistent. No serologic test has been conclusively found to be useful for the diagnosis of either TB infection or disease.[27,35,36] The diagnosis of LTBI therefore relies on the measurement of cellular responses to TB antigens, either in vivo with the tuberculin skin test or in vitro with the interferon-γ release assays (IGRAs). **Table 1** summarizes the characteristics of the currently available diagnostic tools for TB infection. The tuberculin skin test (TST), which measures the in vivo cellular immune response to intradermally injected purified protein derivatives (PPD) of the human tubercle bacillus, has been the gold standard test for diagnosis of LTBI for many years. As TST is cross-reactive to bacillus Calmette-Guérin (BCG) and nontuberculous mycobacteria, a relatively high specificity is attainable often at the expense of sensitivity, especially among BCG-vaccinated populations. However, cross-reactivity to BCG is usually not a major issue among the elderly, as few of them would have the opportunity of being vaccinated with BCG during their childhood. On the other hand, the immunologic response to the injected antigens does vary with age and host immunologic status. Multiple cut-offs are therefore recommended to give the best predictive values under different clinical[27] and epidemiologic situations.[27,30,37] The tuberculin response is often found to be diminished among the elderly,[22,38] but substantial disease risk is still found among those with a negative tuberculin response, especially among those with a body mass index (weight in kilograms divided by height in meters squared) below 18.5.[29] The need for a separate test-reading visit and potential boosting of response on serial testing also affect its field application, especially in marginalized population segments or institutional settings.[27] Although repeat testing within 2 weeks is sometimes recommended to pick up infected negatives among the elderly, this has been found to decrease the specificity of TST in identifying active TB on follow-up in a recent Hong Kong study.[29]

With advances in immunology and genomics, several relatively specific antigens have been discovered in the pathogenic *Mycobacterium tuberculosis* complex. These antigens include the early secretory antigen target 6 (ESAT-6) and culture filtrate protein 10 (CFP-10), which are encoded by genes located in the Region of Difference (RD-1) of the bacillary genome, and are absent in all BCG strains and most environmental mycobacteria (with the exception of *Mycobacterium szulgai*, *Mycobacterium marinum*, *Mycobacterium flavescens*, and *Mycobacterium kansasii*). The newly introduced IGRAs, QuantiFERON TB Gold (QFT-G), QuantiFERON TB Gold in-Tube

Table 1
Comparison of available tests for TB infection

	Tuberculin Skin Test	QuantiFERON TB-Gold/IT	T-Spot.TB
Antigens	Complex: purified protein derivative Cross reaction: BCG, other mycobacteria	Specific:ESAT6, CFP10, TB7.7 Absent in BCG and most NTM	Specific: ESAT6, CFP10 Absent in BCG and most NTM
Test method	Skin test: intradermal/multiple puncture; 2 visits	Whole blood interferon assay; single visit	Blood monocyte spot test; single visit
Laboratory support	No; clinic/bedside procedure	High; fresh blood delivery	Highest; fresh blood delivery
Cell separation	No	No	Yes
Cost	Relatively low	High	Highest
Interference by BCG	Yes	No	No
Booster effect	Yes (2 tests >1 wk to exclude booster)	No (good for serial testing)	No (good for serial testing)
Choice of cut-off	5, 10, 15 mm in different clinical scenarios Trade-off: sensitivity and specificity Higher disease risk with larger induration	Single Not fully clarified yet Not fully clarified yet	Single Not fully clarified yet Not fully clarified yet
Conversion	Criterion established for recent conversion	Not fully clarified yet	Not fully clarified yet
Infection or disease	Do not distinguish	Do not distinguish	Do not distinguish
Recent versus remote	Do not distinguish	Do not distinguish adequately	Do not distinguish adequately
Exposure correlation	Some	Higher	Higher/highest
Immune compromise	Affected significantly	Less affected	Least affected
Advance age	Significantly affected	Less affected	Less affected
Proxy sensitivity[a]	71%-82%	QFT-Gold: 73%-82%; QFT-Gold IT: 63%-78%	86%-93%
Proxy specificity[b]	No BCG: 95%-99%; BCG: low and heterogeneous	No BCG: 98%-100%; BCG: 94%-98%	86%-100%
Longitudinal data	Abundant	Scant	Scant

Abbreviations: BCG, bacillus Calmette-Guérin; NTM, nontuberculous mycobacteria.
[a] Positive rate among patients with culture confirmed tuberculosis.
[b] Negative rate among low risk individuals.

(QFT-G-IT) (Cellestis Ltd, Carnegie, Victoria, Australia), and the T-SPOT.TB test (Oxford Immunotec, Oxford, UK) measure the release of interferon-γ by blood monocytes on stimulation by these specific antigens. In the absence of a gold standard for LTBI, surrogate measures like positive rate among culture-confirmed TB (for sensitivity) and negative rate among subjects with low risk for TB infection (for specificity) were used in most of the available studies evaluating the performance of TST and IGRAs.[39] The performance of IGRA has also been evaluated by correlating test results with TB exposure factors[40] and BCG status.[39] In general, studies have demonstrated similar levels of specificity for IGRAs and independence from BCG status.[39] The sensitivity of IGRAs has been shown to be at least equivalent to that of TST and superior with T-SPOT.TB among human immunodeficiency virus (HIV)-infected children, the severely malnourished, and children younger than 3 years. The IGRAs also appear to be less affected by advance age in comparison with the TST.[41–44] It should be noted, however, that the IGRAs still measure the host's immunologic reaction to the tubercle bacillus. As such, they might be affected by the host immune status, though possibly by a lesser degree than TST. Although they have several operational advantages, such as completion of test in one visit, results available in 24 hours, absence of inter- and intraobserver divergence, detection of potential immunodepression, and avoidance of the booster phenomenon, the need for delivery of fresh blood, lengthy laboratory processes, and high costs may limit their large-scale application in most TB-endemic areas.

In the clinical application of both TST and IGRAs, it is of importance that clinically manifest disease only develops in a minority of infected subjects after a highly variable latent period. Using development of active disease as the end point, the predictive values of all available LTBI tests are necessarily low. None of these tests are able to distinguish satisfactorily between recent and remote infection, latent infection and active disease, or untreated and treated infection/disease. Remote infection generally carries a much lower risk of disease development than recent infection.[27] The prevalence of background infection tends to increase with advance age and varies greatly between different places and settings, depending on past disease incidence and exposure pattern. These factors must be taken into careful consideration in the implementation of LTBI screening, either with traditional TST or the more specific IGRAs, among the elderly, especially in high TB burden settings. Better cost-effectiveness can often be achieved by a more targeted approach, focusing on defined risk groups such as those with a higher chance of recent infection (eg, recent household or institutional contacts) or a higher risk of reactivation (eg, HIV-infected subjects, silicosis, and immunosuppressive therapy, and so forth).

While isolation of Mycobacterium tuberculosis complex is often regarded as the gold standard in the diagnosis of active TB disease, conventional cultures take a very long time and bacteriologic confirmation is never established in at least 15% to 20% of cases. As TB disease must be preceded by infection, attempts have been made to evaluate the potential roles of the new IGRAs in the diagnosis of active TB disease, especially among children[43] and the elderly.[22] Unfortunately, conflicting results are obtained depending on the prevalence of the target conditions in the study population and the background prevalence of LTBI.[45,46] Untreated active TB disease carries very substantial morbidity and mortality, especially among the elderly. The sensitivity and specificity of both TST and IGRAs are not adequate to rule in or rule out active disease,[27,39] even though a positive or negative result might affect the likelihood of the presence or absence of disease. Account must therefore be taken of the overall clinical and epidemiologic situation in reaching a sensible diagnosis.[47]

Treatment of LTBI

Isoniazid monotherapy, either daily or twice weekly, for 9 months is currently the recommended regimen for treatment of LTBI in United States,[27] while a 6-month regimen is adopted in Hong Kong.[30,48] In the International Union Against Tuberculosis (IUAT) Trial, a daily 52-week regimen of isoniazid was slightly more effective in reducing the risk of TB than a 24-week regimen (75% vs 65%) in persons with fibrotic lung disease.[49] The risk of hepatotoxicity with isoniazid was reported to be in the range of 0.5% to 1% in that trial and the United States Public Health Service (PHS) multicenter study.[50] The 24-week regimen prevented more cases of TB per case of drug-induced hepatitis in the IUAT trial,[51] and the cost per case of TB prevented by 6-month isoniazid was also shown to be half of that under the 12-month regimen.[52]

The risk of hepatotoxicity increases with age. In the PHS study, isoniazid-associated hepatitis occurred in 0% of those aged under 20, 0.3% from 20 to 34, 1.2% from 35 to 49, and 2.3% from 50 to 64 years.[50] In these early studies, the hospitalization rates were up to 5.0 per 1000 treatment initiations[49] and a mortality rate of 0.6 per 1000 persons was reported in the PHS study, even though liver cirrhosis might have been a confounding factor.[50] More recently, the rate of symptomatic hepatitis has been estimated to be 1 to 3 per 1000, and much lower hospitalization rates (0.1–0.2 per 1000) and mortality rates (0.0–0.3 per 1000) have been reported.[52,53]

Treatment with rifampicin at a dose of 10 mg/kg daily (maximum 600 mg) for 4 months is currently an acceptable alternative for treatment of LTBI.[27] Unlike isoniazid, there are only scant clinical data on its clinical efficacy, but hepatotoxicity risk appears to be low in the limited number of clinical studies.[48,54] The combination of rifapentine, 900 mg and isoniazid, 900 mg once weekly for 12 weeks was found to be well tolerated in a recent human trial.[55] Further clinical studies to address the tolerance and efficacy of this combination are ongoing. Despite initial favorable reports on the use of 2 months of rifampicin plus pyrazinamide in the treatment of LTBI among the HIV-infected persons,[56,57] such a regimen was associated with an unacceptably high incidence of hepatotoxicity in subsequent field surveillance[52] and clinical trials.[58,59] This result could not be entirely accounted for by risk factors like alcohol use or chronic viral hepatitis, but older age and concomitant use of other medications could have contributed.[59,60]

To minimize the risk of hepatotoxicity during the treatment of LTBI among the elderly, careful pretreatment assessment is needed to balance the benefit against the potential risk.[61] Close clinical monitoring is necessary during treatment. Patients should be thoroughly educated about the symptoms of hepatitis, and advised to report them promptly for early evaluation. Baseline and monthly (or biweekly) laboratory testing of liver enzymes is generally recommended for high-risk patients, especially for chronic alcohol users, HIV-infected persons, and those with chronic liver disease, or those taking concomitant hepatotoxic medications.[27,52] Isoniazid or rifampicin should be withheld as recommended if serum transaminase level is higher than 3 times the upper limit of normal in a symptomatic patient or 5 times the upper limit of normal in the absence of symptoms.[27,62]

OTHER PREVENTION STRATEGIES
Modification of Host Factors

As smoking[13] and poorly controlled diabetes mellitus[32] are proven risk factors for TB among the elderly, careful control of these risk factors by healthy lifestyle and careful management of comorbidities could make substantial contributions in reducing the TB morbidity and mortality among the elderly. Evidence is also accumulating in both human and animal studies that undernutrition is associated with increased risk and severity of TB.[31,63,64] Maintaining a balanced diet with adequate protein, calories, and micronutrient intake is therefore important not only for general health but also for protection against the human tubercle bacillus, at no additional cost or potential risk. Both macronutrient and micronutrient deficiencies should be aggressively treated. Vitamin D deficiency has been implicated as a risk factor for TB,[65] but the role of vitamin supplementation in the absence of clinical deficiency has yet to be clarified.[66]

Tuberculosis Control in Elderly Institutions

In elderly institutions, the concentration of both potential infectious sources and susceptible contacts is conducive to the spread of TB. Although TB is an airborne disease, its infectivity decreases rapidly with effective treatment unless there is significant drug resistance. Early identification, separation, and treatment of symptomatic infectious cases therefore play a key role in infection control. Maintaining good ventilation and avoiding overcrowding are also important in reducing the risk of transmission. For nursing homes and other health care facilities, the established hierarchy of administrative, environmental, and personal protective measures should be followed to contain the infectious sources, reduce the environmental pathogen level, and protect those at risk of exposure.[67] Although indiscriminate chest radiography screening is unlikely to be cost-effective, preadmission examination of both staff and clients may serve a dual purpose: to avoid inadvertent introduction of infectious cases into the high-risk environment and to provide baseline results for later comparison. As intradermal injection of antigens is not involved in the new IGRAs, they have an advantage over TST in the serial surveillance of LTBI among staff and/or clients in some of these high-risk settings. However, previous sensitization by the antigens used for TST might still affect their own interpretation. Further studies are required to clarify their exact role, especially in high-burden settings.

CLINICAL DISEASE AMONG THE ELDERLY
Clinical Presentation and Diagnosis

Most TB in elderly persons occurs as a result of endogenous reactivation of remote infections. However, in low-prevalence situations, it includes many more cases of clinical disease in immunologically compromised subjects as compared with the younger age strata. This scenario often affects the clinical presentation of TB in elderly persons. Among a total of 25,311 newly notified patients in Japan in 2007, 17% had TB in sites other than the lung in those aged 14 to 59 years, while it was 24% in those older than 60 years. Miliary TB accounted for 3.3% of all TB for those aged 60 years or older, which was significantly high compared with 0.9% for younger subjects. Schluger[68] also mentioned that elderly patients are more likely to have extrapulmonary TB including miliary disease, although this was not supported in recent United States statistics[69] or in Hong Kong.[19] In Japan, 74% of pulmonary TB patients were bacteriologically confirmed cases for the age group 15 to 59 years, compared with 86% for those aged 60 years or older. A similar tendency was also seen in Hong Kong[13,19] and in the meta-analysis by Perez-Guzman and colleagues.[12]

Regarding the clinical presentation of TB, the meta-analysis of Perez-Guzman and colleagues[12] suggested that fever, sweating, and hemoptysis were less frequent in older patients, but dyspnea was more frequent, while there was no significant difference for coughing, sputum, loss of body weight, and fatigue or malaise. Leung and colleagues[13] also reported the same findings in their systematic comparison of old and young patients in Hong Kong. Laboratory findings indicated that the tuberculin-positive rate, serum total protein level, and white blood cell counts were lower in elderly patients.[12,13] There was no difference between the two age groups in hemoglobin concentration or in liver transaminase activity.

Radiographic findings such as cavity formation and lesions in the upper lung area are supposed to be characteristic of the adult type (reactivation) TB. The meta-analysis by Perez-Guzman and colleagues[12] revealed that cavity formation is rare in elderly patients and that the upper zone predominance was similar for both age groups, whereas Leung and colleagues[13] found that the elderly patients have more extensive disease and lower zone involvement on chest radiograph. Chan-Yeung and colleagues[19] reported that cavitary lesions were seen in 16% of the aged patients, slightly lower than the 19% of younger patients. Morris[70] pointed out that the most common radiographic findings in the elderly or immunocompromised TB patients are opacity in the lower zone accompanied by basal effusion or thickening, and that the apical as well as lower lung cavity are rare. He also noted that disseminated lesions are rare but can occur in the absence of significant host reaction, resulting in an apparently normal radiograph.

The atypical clinical presentation of TB in the elderly can often make diagnosis difficult, and can be further complicated due to the coexistence of underlying illnesses. Diagnosis is sometimes made at a very late stage of the disease.[71] Perez-Guzman and colleagues[12] found a longer evolution time in elderly patients in their meta-analysis. The longer delay in presentation and start of treatment was seen in elderly patients in Hong Kong.[13] Thus, Iseman[72] stresses the importance of considering TB and careful history taking of exposure, followed by 3 sputum examinations. He also recommends sputum induction or gastric juice aspiration if voluntary production of sputum is difficult.

Treatment of Active Disease

In general, TB in elderly patients should be treated with the same treatment used for younger patients. However, special attention must be paid to preventing, detecting, and managing the adverse reactions of anti-TB drugs. Higher risk of hepatotoxicity is seen for isoniazid in those aged 50 years or older and in those with a previous history of liver disease. Similar caution should be taken when using rifampicin and pyrazinamide. Ethambutol can cause problems with the optic nerve, including disturbances of visual acuity and color sensation, which might be difficult to detect in presence of cataract or other preexisting causes of visual impairment often more common at this age. Although these visual disturbances are often assumed to be reversible, some reports indicate that there are irreversible changes that warrant special attention in the case of long-term use of the drug.[2]

The outcomes of treatment are not always favorable in elderly patients. The 12-month treatment success rate in the study of Chan-Yeung and colleagues[19] in Hong Kong was 83% for those younger than 60 years compared with 77% for the elderly, and the death rate was 1% (59 years and younger) and 9% (60 years and older). The treatment success rate in Hong Kong was only 72.5% and mortality 16% for those aged 65 or older.[13]

In Japan, the 9-month treatment success rate was 87% for young patient cohorts and 71% for elderly patient cohorts; the death rates were 21% (elderly) and 3% (young).[17] On the other hand, the death risk relative to that of the general population was 12.5 times higher for the 30 to 49 age group, 11.7 times for the 50 to 59 age group, 8.8 times for the 60 to 74 age group, and 4.5 times for the 75 and older age group. The lower relative risks at the upper age ranges reflect the high background mortality, rather than decreased lethality of TB, at these ages.

FUTURE PERSPECTIVE

Despite the decline in the overall incidence of TB in many developed countries, TB remains an important problem among the older population. The epidemiologic transition will take several decades in most of the intermediate-burden areas, as very high disease rates were observed in these areas in the middle of the last century. The control of TB in the elderly will remain a major challenge in the coming years because of the limitations of the existing tools for the diagnosis and treatment of both LTBI and clinically active disease. Diagnostic tests with better predictive values for the development of clinical disease will be required for tackling the large infection pool at this age. Shorter, more effective, and less toxic treatment regimens will also be required if any large-scale treatment of LTBI is to be contemplated among the elderly. Better diagnostic tools and new TB drugs are also required to manage patients with clinically active disease, especially in the face of the global emergence of drug resistance. Until these become available, a high index of suspicion will continue to be required to detect the often atypically presenting disease. A careful, holistic approach is also needed in the management of elderly TB patients because of the often late presentation, poorer drug tolerance, and sometimes less satisfactory outcome.

REFERENCES

1. CDC. Reported tuberculosis in the United States, 2007. Atlanta (GA): U.S. Department of Health and Human Services, CDC; 2008.
2. World Health Organization. Global tuberculosis control: epidemiology, strategy, financing. Geneva: WHO report; 2009. WHO/HTM/TB/2009.411.
3. Ministry of Health, Labour & Welfare of Japan. Tuberculosis surveillance annual report 2006. Tokyo: Japan Anti-Tuberculosis Association; 2006.
4. Meyers JA. Tuberculosis in the aged. Postgrad Med 1967;41:214–22.
5. Mori T. Role of tuberculosis control technologies in health transition of the productive population. In: Furukawa T, editor. High-technology, population wealth and health. Perspectives of advanced technology science 2. Tokyo: Maruzen Planet; 1995. p. 73–92.
6. Mori T. [Some recent aspects of tuberculosis infection in Japan (2)]. Kekkaku 1988;63:39–48 [in Japanese].
7. Frost WH. The age selection of mortality from tuberculosis in successive decades. Am J Hyg 1939;30:91–6.
8. Powell K. The rising age of the tuberculosis patients. The sign of success or failure. J Infect Dis 1980;142(6):946–8.
9. Tocque K, Bellis MA, Tam SM, et al. Long-term trends in tuberculosis. Comparison of age-cohort data between Hong Kong and England and Wales. Am J Respir Crit Care Med 1998;158:484–8.
10. Davies PDO. The slowing of the decline in tuberculosis notifications and HIV infections. Respir Med 1989;83:321–2.
11. A WHO/Union Monograph on TB and Tobacco Control. Joining efforts to control two related global epidemics. Geneva: WHO report; 2009. WHO/HTM/TB/2007,390.
12. Perez-Guzman C, Vargas MH, Torres-Cruz A, et al. Does aging modify pulmonary tuberculosis? A meta-analytical review. Chest 1999;116(4):961–7.
13. Leung CC, Yew WW, Chan CK, et al. Tuberculosis in older people: a retrospective and comparative study from Hong Kong. J Am Geriatr Soc 2002;50(7):1219–26.
14. Leung CC, Li T, Lam TH, et al. Smoking and tuberculosis among the elderly in Hong Kong. Am J Respir Crit Care Med 2004;170:1027–33.

15. Ponce-de-Leon A, Garcia-Garcia L, Garcia-Sancho MC, et al. Tuberculosis and diabetes in southern Mexico. Diabetes Care 2004;27(7):1584–90.
16. Kim SJ, Hong YP, Lew WJ, et al. Incidence of pulmonary tuberculosis among diabetics. Tuber Lung Dis 1995;76(6):529–33.
17. Ministry of Health, Labour & Welfare of Japan. Tuberculosis surveillance annual report 2007. Tokyo: Japan Anti-Tuberculosis Association; 2007.
18. Alisjahbana B, Sahiratmadja E, Nelwan EJ, et al. The effect of type 2 diabetes mellitus on the presentation and treatment response of pulmonary tuberculosis. Clin Infect Dis 2007;45:428–35.
19. Chan-Yeung M, Noertjojo K, Tan J, et al. Tuberculosis in the elderly in Hong Kong. Int J Tuberc Lung Dis 2002;6(9):771–9.
20. Korzeniewska-Kosela M, Krysl J, Muller N, et al. Tuberculosis in young adults and the elderly. A prospective comparison study. Chest 1994;106(1):28–32.
21. Grzybowski S, Allen EA. The challenge of tuberculosis in decline. A study based on the epidemiology of tuberculosis in Ontario, Canada. Am Rev Respir Dis 1964; 90:707–20.
22. Nisar M, Williams CSD, Ashby D, et al. Tuberculin testing in residential homes for the elderly. Thorax 1993;48:1257–60.
23. Stead WW, Lofgren JP, Warren E, et al. Tuberculosis as an endemic and nosocomial infection among the elderly in nursing homes. N Engl J Med 1985;312: 1483–7.
24. Prevention and control of tuberculosis in facilities providing long-term care to the elderly. Recommendations of the Advisory Committee for Elimination of Tuberculosis. MMWR Recomm Rep 1990;39(RR-10):7–13.
25. Woo J, Chan HS, Hazlett CB, et al. Tuberculosis among elderly Chinese in residential homes: tuberculin reactivity and estimated prevalence. Gerontology 1996;42(3):155–62.
26. MacArthur C, Enarson DA, Fanning A, et al. Tuberculosis among institutionalized elderly in Alberta, Canada. Int J Epidemiol 1992;21:1175–9.
27. CDC. Targeted tuberculin testing and treatment of latent tuberculosis infection. MMWR Recomm Rep 2000;49(No. RR-6):1–51.
28. Bennett DE, Courval JM, Onorato I, et al. Prevalence of tuberculosis infection in the United States population: the national health and nutrition examination survey, 1999-2000. Am J Respir Crit Care Med 2008;177:348–55.
29. Chan-Yeung M, Dai DL, Cheung AH, et al. Tuberculin skin test reaction and body mass index in old age home residents in Hong Kong. J Am Geriatr Soc 2007; 55(10):1592–7.
30. Tuberculosis and Chest Service. Annual report of tuberculosis and chest service 2007. Hong Kong (China): Department of Health; 2009.
31. Leung CC, Lam TH, Chan WM, et al. Lower risk of tuberculosis in obesity. Arch Intern Med 2007;167(12):1297–304.
32. Leung CC, Lam TH, Chan WM, et al. Diabetic control and risk of tuberculosis: a cohort study. Am J Epidemiol 2008;167(12):1486–94.
33. Dye C, Scheele S, Dolin P, et al. Consensus statement. Global burden of tuberculosis: estimated incidence, prevalence, and mortality by country. WHO Global Surveillance and Monitoring Project. JAMA 1999;282(7):677–86.
34. Chan-Yeung M, Tam CM, Wong H, et al. Molecular and conventional epidemiology of tuberculosis in Hong Kong: a population-based prospective study. J Clin Microbiol 2003;41(6):2706–8.
35. Abebe F, Holm-Hansen C, Wiker HG, et al. Progress in serodiagnosis of *Mycobacterium tuberculosis* infection. Scand J Immunol 2007;66:176–91.

36. World Health Organization. Laboratory -based evaluation of 19 commercially available rapid diagnostic tests for tuberculosis (Diagnostic Evaluation Series No. 2). Geneva (Switzerland): World Health Organization; 2008.
37. Leung CC, Yew WW, Chang KC, et al. Risk of active tuberculosis among school-children in Hong Kong. Arch Pediatr Adolesc Med 2006;160(3):247–51.
38. Stead WW, To T. The significance of the tuberculin skin test in elderly persons. Ann Intern Med 1987;107:837–42.
39. Pai M, Zwerling A, Menzies D. Systematic review: T-cell-based assays for the diagnosis of latent tuberculosis infection: an update. Ann Intern Med 2008;149: 177–84.
40. Lalvani A, Pathan AA, Durkan H, et al. Enhanced contact tracing and spatial tracking of *Mycobacterium tuberculosis* infection by enumeration of antigen-specific T cells. Lancet 2001;23:2017–21.
41. Leung CC, Yam WC, Yew WW, et al. Comparison of T-Spot.TB and tuberculin skin test among silicotic patients. Eur Respir J 2008;31(2):266–72.
42. Kobashi Y, Mouri K, Miyashita N, et al. QuantiFERON TB-2G test for patients with active tuberculosis stratified by age groups. Scand J Infect Dis 2009;14:1–6.
43. Detjen AK, Keil T, Roll S, et al. Interferon-gamma release assays improve the diagnosis of tuberculosis and nontuberculous mycobacterial disease in children in a country with a low incidence of tuberculosis. Clin Infect Dis 2007; 45:322–8.
44. Kobashi Y, Mouri K, Yagi S, et al. Clinical utility of the QuantiFERON TB-2G test for elderly patients with active tuberculosis. Chest 2008;133(5):1196–202.
45. Dewan PK, Grinsdale J, Kawamura LM. Low sensitivity of a whole-blood inter-feron-gamma release assay for detection of active tuberculosis. Clin Infect Dis 2007;44:69–73.
46. Kang YA, Lee I IW, Hwang SS, et al. Usefulness of whole-blood interferon-gamma assay and interferon-gamma enzyme-linked immunospot assay in the diagnosis of active pulmonary tuberculosis. Chest 2007;132:959–65.
47. Leung CC, Chang KC. Role of interferon gamma release assays in tuberculosis. Respirology 2009;14(2):156–8.
48. A double-blind placebo-controlled clinical trial of three anti-tuberculosis chemo-prophylaxis regimens in patients with silicosis in Hong Kong. Hong Kong Chest Service/Tuberculosis Research Centre, Madras/British Medical Research Council. Am Rev Respir Dis 1992;145:36–41.
49. International Union Against Tuberculosis, Committee on Prophylaxis. Efficacy of various durations of isoniazid preventive therapy for tuberculosis. Bull World Health Organ 1982;60:555–64.
50. Kopanoff DE, Snider DE, Caras GJ. Isoniazid-related hepatitis: a US Public Health Service cooperative surveillance study. Am Rev Respir Dis 1978;117: 991–1001.
51. Snider DE, Carasn GJ, Koplan JP. Preventive therapy with isoniazid: cost-effectiveness of different durations of therapy. JAMA 1986;255:1579–83.
52. Centers for Disease Control and Prevention/American Thoracic Society. Update: adverse event data and revised American Thoracic Society/CDC recommendations against the use of rifampin and pyrazinamide for treatment of latent tuberculosis infection—United States, 2003. MMWR Morb Mortal Wkly Rep 2003;52: 735–9.
53. Nolan CM, Goldberg SV, Buskin SE. Hepatotoxicity associated with isoniazid preventive therapy: a 7-year survey from a public health tuberculosis clinic. JAMA 1999;281:1014–8.

54. Menzies D, Dion MJ, Rabinovitch B, et al. Treatment completion and costs of a randomized trial of rifampin for 4 months versus isoniazid for 9 months. Am J Respir Crit Care Med 2004;170:445–9.

55. Schechter M, Zajdenverg R, Falco G, et al. Weekly rifapentine/isoniazid or daily rifampin/pyrazinamide for latent tuberculosis in household contacts. Am J Respir Crit Care Med 2006;173:922–6.

56. Halsey NA, Coberly JS, Desormeaux J, et al. Randomised trial of isoniazid versus rifampicin and pyrazinamide for prevention of tuberculosis in HIV-1 infection. Lancet 1998;351:786–92.

57. Gordin F, Chaisson RE, Matts JP, et al. Rifampin and pyrazinamide vs isoniazid for prevention of tuberculosis in HIV-infected persons: an international randomized trial. JAMA 2000;283:1445–50.

58. Jasmer RM, Saukkonen JJ, Blumberg HM, et al. Short-course rifampin and pyrazinamide compared with isoniazid for latent tuberculosis infection: a multicenter clinical trial. Ann Intern Med 2002;137:640–7.

59. Leung CC, Law WS, Chang KC, et al. Initial experience of a randomized controlled trial on the treatment of latent tuberculosis infection among silicotic subjects in Hong Kong: two months of rifampin and pyrazinamide versus six months of isoniazid. Chest 2003;124:2112–8.

60. Ijaz K, Jereb JA, Lambert LA, et al. Severe or fatal liver injury in 50 patients in the United States taking rifampin and pyrazinamide for latent tuberculosis infection. Clin Infect Dis 2006;42:346–55.

61. Yew WW, Leung CC. Antituberculosis drugs and hepatotoxicity. Respirology 2006;11(6):699–707.

62. Blumberg HM, Leonard MK Jr, Jasmer RM. Update on the treatment of tuberculosis and latent tuberculosis infection. JAMA 2005;293:2776–84.

63. Cegielski JP, McMurray DN. The relationship between malnutrition and tuberculosis: evidence from studies in humans and experimental animals. Int J Tuberc Lung Dis 2004;8:286–98.

64. Africa's Health in 2010 project/Academy for Educational Development. Nutrition and tuberculosis: a review of the literature and considerations for TB control programs. Washington, DC: United States Agency for International Development; 2008.

65. Chocano-Bedoya P, Ronnenberg AG. Vitamin D and tuberculosis. Nutr Rev 2009; 67(5):289–93.

66. Yamshchikov AV, Desai NS, Blumberg HM, et al. Vitamin D for treatment and prevention of infectious diseases: a systematic review of randomized controlled trials. Endocr Pract 2009;15(5):438–49.

67. Jensen PA, Lambert LA, Iademarco MF, et al. CDC Guidelines for preventing the transmission of *Mycobacterium tuberculosis* in health-care settings, 2005. MMWR Recomm Rep 2005;54:1–141, V.

68. Schluger NW. Tuberculosis and non-tuberculous Mycobacterial infections in older adults. Clin Chest Med 2007;28(4):773–83.

69. Yang Z, Kong Y, Wilson F, et al. Identification of risk factors for extrapulmonary tuberculosis. Clin Infect Dis 2004;38(2):199–205.

70. Morris CDW. Pulmonary tuberculosis in the elderly: a different disease? Thorax 1990;45:912–3.

71. Fullerton JM, Dyer L. Unsuspected tuberculosis in the aged. Lond. Tubercle 1965;46:193–8.

72. Iseman MD. Tuberculosis in the elderly; treating the "white plague". Geriatrics 1988;35:90–107.

Nontuberculous Mycobacterial Lung Diseases

Babafemi Taiwo, MBBS[a],*, Jeff Glassroth, MD[b]

KEYWORDS

- Nontuberculous mycobacteria • Lung disease • Macrolides
- *Mycobacterium tuberculosis*

Nontuberculous mycobacteria (NTM) are environmental mycobacteria that are distinct from *Mycobacterium leprae* and members of the *Mycobacterium tuberculosis* complex. Only relatively few of the more than 115 known NTM species have been implicated in lung disease (**Table 1**). The spectrum of NTM lung involvement ranges from isolation of mycobacteria that may be benignly colonizing an individual, to benign nodules (ie, granulomata), disease in ostensibly healthy immune competent persons, disease in immune compromised hosts who may be infected with unusual or rarely encountered NTM, and hypersensitivity syndrome.[1] Explanations for these varying presentations are imperfect, and studies of pathogenesis have yielded only few conclusive findings. Likewise, our approach to diagnosis and treatment continue to evolve.

EPIDEMIOLOGY

Precise data on the incidence and prevalence of NTM lung disease is limited by the fact that unlike tuberculosis, these infections are generally not reportable to public health authorities. However, between 1999 and 2000, sensitization to *Mycobacterium intracellulare* was found in 16.6% of 7384 noninstitutionalized civilians in the United States, representing a significant increase from the 11.2% found in a similar survey conducted between 1971 and 1972. This figure is consistent with increasing laboratory isolation of NTM. For example, approximately three-quarters of the mycobacterial isolates from 33 United States laboratories in 1992 were NTM,[2] up from one-third of 32,000 isolates between 1979 and 1980.[3] In Canada, the prevalence of NTM isolates (excluding *Mycobacterium gordonae*, a generally nonpathogenic species) increased at an annual rate of 8.4% between 1997 and 2003.[4] Similar trends have been described elsewhere in the world.

[a] Division of Infectious Diseases, Department of Medicine, Feinberg School of Medicine, Northwestern University, 645 North Michigan Avenue, Suite 900, Chicago, IL 60611, USA
[b] Division of Pulmonary and Critical Care, Department of Medicine, Feinberg School of Medicine, Northwestern University, 680 North Lake Shore Drive, Suite 1118, Chicago, IL 60611, USA
* Corresponding author.
E-mail address: b-taiwo@northwestern.edu

Infect Dis Clin N Am 24 (2010) 769–789
doi:10.1016/j.idc.2010.04.008
0891-5520/10/$ – see front matter © 2010 Elsevier Inc. All rights reserved.

id.theclinics.com

Table 1
NTM species more commonly implicated in human pulmonary disease

Species	Geographic Distribution of Reported Cases	Comments
MAC (*M intracellulare* and *M avium*)	Worldwide	Most common cause of NTM lung disease. Represents prototype of patterns of NTM lung disease
M kansasii	United States, Europe, South Africa	Clinical disease closely resembles TB. Associated with mining
M abscessus	Worldwide	Common cause of disease in CF patients. Difficult to eradicate with drugs alone
M xenopi	Europe, North America (United States and Canada)	Survives in hot water systems. Optimum growth temperature is 45°C. Pseudo-outbreaks from contaminated hospital water supplies
M chelonae	Probably worldwide	Usually seen in patients with underlying lung disease. Antibiotic susceptibility testing should guide therapy
M fortuitum	Probably worldwide	Associated with gastroesophageal disorders that predispose to aspiration such as achalasia. Treatment is needed only in a minority of cases where it is isolated. Antibiotic susceptibility testing should guide treatment selection

Species	Geographic distribution	Comments
M szulgai	Worldwide	Scotochromogenic at 37°C and photochromogenic at 25°C. Isolation represents true disease that requires treatment or close follow-up in virtually all cases. Usually favorable treatment outcomes
M malmoense	United Kingdom, Northern Europe. Rare cases from North America and Japan	Some strains require culture for 8–12 wk, thus may be underdiagnosed because many laboratories hold mycobacterial cultures for a shorter length of time
M simiae	Southwest United States	Can be easily mistaken for MTB because it produces niacin. Resistant to usual TB drugs, and has unpredictable antibiotic susceptibility
M scrofulaceum	Worldwide, South Africa. rarely in the United States	Classically a cause of scrofula (cervical lymphadenitis). Commonly isolated in South African miners
M smegmatis	United States, Europe	Associated with lipoid pneumonia
M celatum	United States, Asia, Europe	False-positive tests for MTB possible with DNA probe. DNA sequencing or HPLC is required for definitive diagnosis. Clinically indistinguishable from TB. Optimal therapy is unknown, although most patients have had some improvement with clarithromycin-based therapy

Rarer species include *M triplex, M hemophilum, M asiaticum*

Abbreviations: CF, cystic fibrosis; HPLC, high-performance liquid chromatography; MTB, *M tuberculosis*; TB, tuberculosis.

NTM are ubiquitous in environmental reservoirs, including domestic and natural water supplies, soil, food and animals.[5] Human infection is common but disease appears relatively rare given this ubiquity; infection is thought to occur mainly from water, soil, and aerosolized organisms from these sources. There is no persuasive evidence of human-to-human or animal-to-human transmission.

Partly because of their impermeable cell wall, NTM can survive environments with a wide range of acidity or alkalinity, and are intrinsically resistant to chlorine and biocides.[6] In addition, they can escape filtration.[7] *Mycobacterium avium*, *Mycobacterium chelonae*, *Mycobacterium phlei*, *Mycobacterium xenopi*, and *Mycobacterium scrofulaceum* are relatively viable at high temperature, with *M xenopi* being the most thermoresistant species.[8] Thus, water purification practices may inadvertently select NTM, and other modern practices such as a shift from bathing to showering and embrace of aquatic recreational activities may create new exposures. Common-source exposure can result in patient clusters of hypersensitivity phenomena following bathing in infected hot tubs[9] or occupational exposure to aerosolized NTM present in metal working fluid.[10]

Species of NTM Causing Lung Disease

The predominant NTM species responsible for lung disease depends on the geographic area and the patient population studied. Illustratively, in New York *M avium* complex (MAC), rapidly growing mycobacteria (RGM), *M xenopi*, and *Mycobacterium kansasii* were responsible for 80%, 9%, 6%, and 5% of cases, respectively.[11] In South Korea, analysis of NTM isolates from 195 patients with definite or probable NTM lung disease showed that the most common isolates were also MAC and *Mycobacterium abscessus*, but with very different frequencies (48% and 33%, respectively).[12] Those distributions contrast with data from South African miners, most of whom had a history of tuberculosis or silicosis. In that population, *M kansasii* accounted for 68% of isolates.[13] There have been fewer reported cases of NTM lung disease from developing countries, but more cases are likely to be identified as local diagnostic capabilities improve.

PATHOGENESIS
Virulence

The virulence of different NTM varies substantially. For example, *M kansasii* is often associated with lung disease whereas *M gordonae* rarely is. Of the 2 species described as MAC, *M intracellulare* may be relatively more pathogenic than *M avium*.[14] An MAC strain, designated 198, was recently reported to demonstrate hypervirulence in human macrophages in vitro, and produced clinical features of progressive lung disease.[15] Species differences in opsonization by complement have also been identified as a potential virulence factor.[16] RGM (*M abscessus*, *Mycobacterium fortuitum*, and *M chelonae*) are capable of biofilm formation in appropriate media,[17] but the impact of this property on the pulmonary pathogenicity, if any, is uncertain. Moreover, this would not explain why the majority of significant lung infections from RGM are due to *M abscessus*. Although mycobacterial virulence factors are likely important in lung disease, they remain largely uncharacterized.

Host Factors

Factors that may contribute to host susceptibility to NTM lung disease include defects in immune responses to the pathogen and dysfunctional local mechanical barriers due to pre-existing lung disease.

Cytokines and NTM lung disease

A recent review[18] describes the immune cascade that appears to be related to initial exposure to NTM lung disease. In brief, lipoarabinomannan from NTM cell wall binds to Toll-like receptor 2 (TLR-2) on macrophages, causing production of interleukin-12 (IL-12) and tumor necrosis factor (TNF). IL-12, in turn, binds to its receptor on lymphocytes and this interaction causes up-regulation of interferon-γ (IFN-γ). IFN-γ is a polyfunctional proinflammatory cytokine that binds to IFN-γ receptor (IFN-γR), and stimulates production of other proinflammatory cytokines including TNF-α, IL-12 (positive feedback), and free radicals. With other mediators, these cytokines orchestrate the immune cascade necessary for granuloma formation, host control, and eradication of intracellular pathogens including NTM,[19] and development of acquired (ie, specific) immunity.

Profound defects in the pathway for synthesis and response to IL-12 and IFN-γ exist in some patients with disseminated NTM.[20] Although anomalies of comparable severity have not been consistently demonstrated in those with disease limited to the lungs, measurable defects in these pathways exist in some patients.[21] In vitro, peripheral blood mononuclear (PBMCs) from 4 patients with NTM lung disease showed poor purified protein derivative (PPD)-induced IFN-γ production, and even lower cytokine production when stimulated by pathogenic NTM.[22] Similarly, defective secretion of IFN-γ was demonstrated in 5 patients with persistent NTM lung disease.[23] Other investigators have also found lower production of IFN-γ or IFN-γ receptor, TNF-α, and IL-12 in PBMCs of patients with MAC and *M abscessus* disease compared with healthy controls.[24]

Altered local host defense

The presence of preexisting lung disease such as bronchiectasis, chronic obstructive pulmonary disease (COPD), cystic fibrosis, pneumoconiosis, or prior tuberculosis in many patients with fibrocavitary NTM lung disease suggests that disruption of local defenses plays a central role in disease predisposition. Unlike *M tuberculosis*, which can adhere to normal mucosa, NTM tend to adhere to damaged respiratory mucosa through a fibronectin-mediated process.[25,26] Even in the absence of known preexisting lung disease, NTM can cause nodular disease with bronchiectasis and perhaps ultimately cavitation predominantly in older women,[27] although more subtle abnormalities have not been entirely excluded in such patients. Illustratively, women with nodular bronchiectatic disease tend to be taller and leaner, while scoliosis is present in up to 50%, pectus excavatum in 11% to 27%, and mitral valve prolapse in 9%.[20,28] Because this morphotype is strongly associated with NTM lung disease it has been speculated that it may signify underlying mucociliary, immune, or epithelial defects. Mutations in the cystic fibrosis transmembrane conductance regulator (CFTR) gene may also be more common in these patients than in the general population.[20]

Other systemic immune deficiency

Specific immune responses against NTM are CD4+ T lymphocyte dependent. Thus, advanced human immunodeficiency virus (HIV) infection and other causes of cellular immune deficiency are predisposing factors, whereas neutropenia and humoral immune defects seem much less important. Curiously, lung disease reportedly occurs in as few as 2.5% of AIDS patients in contrast to disseminated MAC, which is more common.[29] Iatrogenic immune suppression after solid organ or stem cell transplantation[30] and use of immune-modulatory agents such as TNF-α inhibitors[31] have become recognized predisposing conditions. NTM reside almost exclusively in macrophages, and it appears that some polymorphisms of the human solute carrier (SLC) 11A/natural resistance associated macrophage protein (NRAMP) 1 gene may influence development of MAC and perhaps other NTM lung disease.[32]

CLINICAL FEATURES

NTM lung disease usually presents with nonspecific pulmonary symptoms, especially cough or dyspnea. Chest pain and hemoptysis are less common. Fever, malaise, night sweats, and asthenia [33] tend to be seen with advanced/extensive disease. Symptoms related to comorbid conditions may be present as well. Given these protean presentations, precise characterization of a patient's illness requires comprehensive history and physical examination whereby attention is paid to subtle details, including occupational and recreational exposures, antecedent lung disease, and the patient's body habitus.

Immune Competent Hosts

In immune competent persons, the presentation is likely to be in 1 of 3 prototypical forms: fibrocavitary disease, nodular bronchiectatic disease, (with some overlap between the 2), or hypersensitivity pneumonitis syndrome. Those with underlying immune compromise tend to exhibit more florid, often atypical, syndromic manifestations and may be susceptible to uncommon and less pathogenic NTM. The 3 prototypes of disease were defined largely based on MAC-related disease, but other NTM species presumably have the ability to cause similar disease patterns and their frequency reflects their prevalence and virulence. Presentations such as solitary pulmonary nodule pose unique diagnostic challenges.[34]

Fibrocavitary disease

Fibrocavitary, "tuberculosis-like" disease (**Fig. 1**) is classically seen in middle-aged or older men with substantial smoking histories and underlying lung disease such as bronchiectasis, COPD, pneumoconiosis, prior tuberculosis, or sarcoidosis. There is

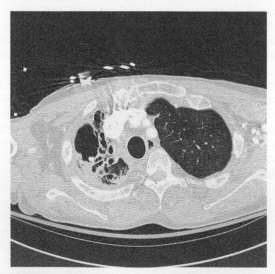

Fig. 1. Severe fibrocavitary disease with calcification at the right apex. Note also the extensive pleural thickening. (*Courtesy of* Dr Eric Hart, Feinberg School of Medicine, Northwestern University, Chicago.)

a predilection for apical and posterior segments of the upper lobe, although multiple lung segments may be involved. Cavitation typically includes thick walls, no air fluid level, and often is associated with pleural thickening that is more extensive than seen with *M tuberculosis*. Pleural effusion and substantial lymph node enlargement are less common than in tuberculosis.[35–38]

Nodular bronchiectasis

This pattern typically occurs without preexisting pulmonary disease, and is seen most commonly in older women nonsmokers; persistent cough is the cardinal symptom at presentation. In 1992, Reich and Johnson[39] hypothesized that affected patients habitually suppressed the impulse to cough, which led to pooled secretions that became secondarily infected by MAC with consequent nonspecific inflammation, especially in dependent pulmonary areas. These investigators termed involvement of the right middle lobe or lingula, which are anatomically pre-disposed to impaired clearance of secretions, Lady Windermere syndrome.[39,40] However, proof of the proposed association with habitual cough suppression is lacking. Pulsed field electrophoresis and seroagglutination studies showed substantial genetic diversity, over time, among the MAC strains found in patients with nodular bronchiectasis and no underlying lung disease, whereas only single strains were present in patients with the fibrocavitary phenotype. This finding may reflect a still uncharacterized predisposition of those with nodular bronchiec-tasis to NTM reinfection.[41] Nodular bronchiectasis can result in severe lung damage, although many patients experience a chronic less aggressive course.

Radiologic features include single or multiple nodules that are usually less than 5 mm in diameter with or without bronchiectasis. Computed tomography (CT) scans early in the disease process may reveal a nonspecific "tree-in-bud" pattern representing bronchiolar inflammation (**Fig. 2**). In contrast to the fibrocavitary proto-type, cavitation is uncommon early in this pattern of disease but may develop later in the course of the illness. The right middle lobe or lingula tend to be

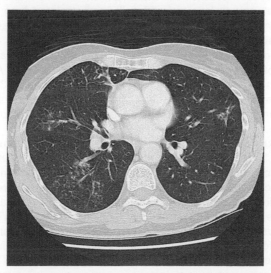

Fig. 2. Tree-in-bud opacities in the superior segment of the right lower lobe and ill-defined opacities in portions of the right middle lobe, right upper lobe, and lingula. (*Courtesy of* Dr Eric Hart, Feinberg School of Medicine, Northwestern University, Chicago.)

disproportionately affected, but not all studies have found a predilection for specific lobes.[27] The better sensitivity of CT scan for identifying characteristic abnormalities makes it the preferred imaging modality for this form of disease; suspicious CT findings may be the sentinel clue that leads the clinician to consider a diagnosis of NTM disease.[42]

Hypersensitivity syndrome

This pattern classically follows exposure to NTM-infected hot tubs, or medicinal pools, hence the name "hot tub lung."[9,10] However, other contaminated water sources have been implicated.[43] Symptoms typically include subacute or acute dyspnea and cough; fever may be prominent. It is likely that both direct infection and hypersensitivity to inflammatory products released by the offending NTM are involved in this syndrome. Symptom recrudescence on reexposure to the NTM source, as well as improvement of symptoms, radiologic appearance, and objective assessments of pulmonary function with removal of the offending NTM, support a hypersensitivity pathogenesis.[44] Use of systemic corticosteroids is sometimes needed, but it is unclear whether specific antimycobacterial therapy hastens recovery.[45] A role for direct infection is supported by the occasional recovery of NTM from lung tissue of affected patients, and formation of granulomata that are more exuberant than the loose, poorly circumscribed variety that is characteristic of most hypersensitivity pneumonias.[46]

There are no pathognomonic radiologic findings for this syndrome, but high-resolution CT (HRCT) scan usually demonstrates an alveolar-interstitial process with patchy or diffuse ground-glass infiltrates, interstitial nodules, and thickened interlobular septae.[47] Other patients may have ground-glass alveolar infiltrates or nonspecific alveolitis only. The distribution of CT findings matches areas of granulomatous inflammation, and a normal HRCT scan essentially excludes the diagnosis.

Immunocompromised Hosts

Disseminated MAC, the most common manifestation of NTM in AIDS patients, usually occurs at CD4 cell counts less than 50 cells/mm^3. Isolated lung disease is rare, whereas respiratory colonization without clinically apparent lung disease is relatively common with disseminated MAC.[48,49] Of the NTM, M kansasii has most often been associated with lung disease in the setting of HIV coinfection, perhaps reflecting the greater virulence of this species. HIV-infected gold miners in South Africa developed M kansasii lung disease at relatively high CD4 cell counts (median, 381 cells/mm^3).[50] Overall, HIV-infected persons and other cellular immunocompromised hosts have attenuated immune responses to NTM; therefore atypical clinical presentations are more common.

Escalation of existing symptoms or emergence of new symptoms or signs (such as recrudescent fever, lymph node enlargement, and worsening of radiologic abnormalities) is characteristic of immune reconstitution inflammatory syndrome (IRIS). In HIV-infected patients, IRIS can be provoked when antiretroviral therapy controls HIV replication, and increases CD4 cell counts, culminating in a robust immune response to circulating antigens, including those of NTM. The clinical features of IRIS usually appear within a few weeks to a few months of initiating HIV treatment. Effective treatment of HIV or the underlying lung disease may avert the need for specific treatment of potentially less virulent NTM such as M xenopi.[51]

Patients with other forms of acquired immune defects such as transplant recipients and those receiving TNF-α antagonists are at risk of severe NTM infections, sometimes caused by low-virulence NTM. For example, *Mycobacterium peregrinum*, a rarely encountered NTM, caused fatal pneumonia in a patient receiving infliximab for polymyositis and dermatomyositis.[52]

Cystic Fibrosis Patients

Fibrocavitary NTM lung disease occurs at a younger age in patients with cystic fibrosis (CF). In one study, respiratory NTM "colonization" in a cohort of CF patients (n = 385) increased with age, reaching a peak of 15% at 15 years. Of note, *M abscessus* was found in all age groups whereas MAC was present only in the older patients.[53] Allergic bronchopulmonary aspergillosis (ABPA) and use of systemic corticosteroids appear to be risk factors for NTM lung disease in this population.[54] Unlike other risk groups, screening for NTM at least yearly is recommended for CF patients.[55,56] Screening is also recommended for those who experience a decline in lung function, as well as before and during macrolide monotherapy for immune modulation. Macrolide immune modulation is not advisable in those with persistently positive NTM cultures. The presence of NTM pretransplant is a strong predictor of invasive lung disease posttransplant, but this should not automatically contraindicate transplantation because invasive cases may be treatable.[57]

DISEASE PATTERNS WITH NTM OTHER THAN MAC
Mycobacterium kansasii

M kansasii is the second most common cause of NTM lung disease in the United States. Subtype 1 is the most frequently implicated subtype in immune competent hosts, while most persons with disease due to subtype 2 are immune compromised.[58] The pulmonary disease caused by this NTM is clinically and radiologically more like reactivation tuberculosis than disease caused by other NTM. Accordingly, cavitary and upper lobe disease are typical, although nodular bronchiectasis without cavitation can occur as well. Isolation of *M kansasii* usually indicates disease that needs treatment.[59]

Rapidly Growing Mycobacteria

RGM are most commonly associated with skin and soft tissue infection, but they are also an important cause of lung disease. In the United States, approximately 80% of pulmonary diseases due to RGM are caused by *M abscessus*, the most common presentation being nodular bronchiectasis; cavitation occurs in fewer than 1 in 5 patients.[60] MAC is a coinfection in approximately 15% of patients with *M abscessus* lung disease.[60] *M abscessus* infection is particularly difficult to manage.[54,61] *M fortuitum* and *M chelonae* account for virtually all the remaining cases of RGM lung disease in the United States, although *Mycobacterium immunogenicum* has been the etiologic agent in some outbreaks of hypersensitivity illness.

Mycobacterium malmoense

Following initial reports from Sweden and a few other Northern European countries, this organism has been described in other geographic areas, including the United States and Japan.[62–64] *M malmoense* exhibits a strong association with underlying lung disease, and typically presents as fibrocavitary disease with symptoms and signs that are indistinguishable from tuberculosis. Radiographic findings are nonspecific, although cavities larger than 6 cm, air-fluid levels, and loss of lung volume may be more common with *M malmoense* than other mycobacteria.[65]

Mycobacterium xenopi

M xenopi is the most commonly isolated NTM in some geographic areas and, for example, it was the most common cause of NTM lung disease in a recent review of 24 cases from Croatia. Ninety percent of the patients in that series had a comorbidity, most frequently COPD. Approximately three-quarters of the patients had cavitary disease on chest radiograph.[66] Elderly and HIV-infected patients appear to be at increased risk.[67]

Other Notable NTM

M gordonae is very commonly isolated as a nonpathogenic contaminant, though rarely it has caused disease in immunocompromised hosts. *Mycobacterium terrae* complex and *Mycobacterium scrofulaceum* are also usually contaminants or the cause of extrapulmonary disease, respectively, although they have been the etiologic agents in lung disease.[49] *Mycobacterium szulgai* tends to affect persons with underlying lung disease,[68] and *Mycobacterium smegmatis* has been reported in the setting of lipoid pneumonia.[69]

DIAGNOSIS

NTM lung disease is likely underrecognized, partly because NTM are of lower pathogenicity than *M tuberculosis* and may be contaminants of clinical specimens. Hence, they are often erroneously described as "colonizers." In addition, diagnostic approaches geared to more acute conditions such as tuberculosis are not well suited to the more chronic conditions often caused by these organisms. However, our understanding of the potential of these organisms to invade tissue and cause bronchiolitis, bronchiectasis, and granulomatous inflammation is evolving,[70,71] and newer diagnostic methods are facilitating identification of NTM disease. Indeed, some have suggested that the term NTM "colonization" should be discarded and that patients from whom NTM are isolated should be categorized into those who require immediate treatment and those for whom treatment can be deferred.[71,72] The American Thoracic Society (ATS)/Infectious Diseases Society of America (IDSA)[56] Statement, summarized in **Table 2**, offers guidance for diagnosing NTM disease. Key elements in the diagnosis include: exclusion of other diseases, particularly tuberculosis and tumor;

Table 2
Recommendations of the ATS for diagnosis of pulmonary disease caused by NTM

Clinical criteria (all required)
- Pulmonary symptoms
- Imaging showing nodular or cavitary opacities on chest radiograph, or multifocal bronchiectasis with or without multiple small nodules on chest CT scan
- Exclusion of other diseases

Microbiologic criteria (only one required)
- Positive cultures from two separate expectorated sputum samples
- Positive culture from at least one bronchial wash or lavage
- Transbronchial or other lung biopsy with histopathologic changes (granulomatous inflammation or AFB) plus positive NTM culture, or histopathologic changes plus at least one positive NTM culture from sputum or bronchial washing

From Griffith DE, Aksamit T, Brown-Elliott BA, et al on behalf of the ATS Mycobacterial Diseases Subcommittee. An official ATS/IDSA statement: diagnosis, treatment, and prevention of nontuberculous mycobacterial diseases. Am J Respir Crit Care Med 2007;175:367–416; with permission from the American Thoracic Society.

microbiologic results; and radiologic evidence of disease consistent with NTM. The importance of repeated isolation of the same organism from respiratory secretions is emphasized but situations are acknowledged in which a single positive culture is sufficient for diagnosis if other clinical and radiologic findings, particularly chest CT, are consistent with NTM disease.

In most patients, radiologic findings, especially from chest CT (discussed earlier) provide valuable information that forms a rational basis for diagnosis and management decisions when interpreted in conjunction with baseline clinical and microbiologic data. Chest CT is the cornerstone imaging procedure in the diagnostic armamentarium because it provides better resolution of radiographic findings and therefore superior delineation of the disease severity (**Figs. 3** and **4**). CT may also provide prognostic information as, for example, when identifying those with extensive atelectasis, cavitation, and pleural thickening who are less likely to achieve sputum conversion after treatment.[73] Chest imaging also serves as a reference point for monitoring treatment response.

At least 3 expectorated or induced early morning sputum samples, ideally obtained over 3 separate days, should be evaluated to detect the presence of NTM. Bronchoscopy with bronchial washing or lavage is an alternative source of respiratory specimen when sputum is unavailable or nondiagnostic. Like other mycobacteria, NTM are acid-fast on smear microscopy. Commonly available staining techniques include fluorescence microscopy using a fluorochrome such as auramine or auramine-rhodamine, and carbol fuchsin (Ziehl-Neelsen [ZN] or Kinyoun) staining. The Kinyoun method is the least sensitive while fluorescence staining, the method recommended by ATS, has comparable sensitivity to the ZN technique but can be completed faster.[74] With the exception of M intracellulare and M avium, which are coclassified as MAC, all respiratory NTM should be fully speciated, a task that cannot be accomplished through smear microscopy.

Culture in solid media (eg, Lowenstein-Jensen agar or Middlebrook 7H10 and 7H11) and in broth media or in nonradiometric mycobacteria growth indicator tube, MGIT (Becton Dickinson Diagnostic Instrument Systems, Sparks, MD, USA), is recommended. Broth media are more sensitive and yield mycobacterial growth more rapidly

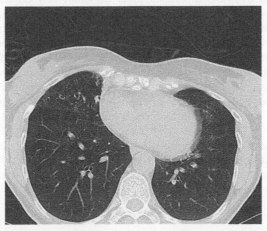

Fig. 3. Mild right middle lobe predominant disease with bronchial wall thickening, bronchiectasis, and a small amount of volume loss medially. (*Courtesy of* Dr Eric Hart, Feinberg School of Medicine, Northwestern University, Chicago.)

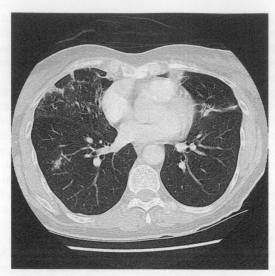

Fig 4. Moderately severe disease with more bronchial wall thickening and bronchiectasis, Also demonstrated are patchy right middle lobe consolidation, a small focus of consolidation in the right lower lobe, and minimal lingula volume loss. (*Courtesy of* Dr Eric Hart, Feinberg School of Medicine, Northwestern University, Chicago.)

(often within 2–3 weeks compared with 6–8 weeks). However, colony morphology, identification of infection with multiple species, and semiquantitative reporting are possible only with solid media. Although culture is a reliable method for isolating NTM, the results can take weeks for species other than RGM; evolving molecular identification methods now provide a more rapid adjunct for identifying certain common species.

In smear-positive patients, molecular techniques applied directly to the respiratory specimen have proven useful for rapid identification of those infected with *M tuberculosis*. Commercially available molecular tests generally rely on amplification using techniques like the polymerase chain reaction (PCR) of specific DNA or RNA sequences, with results available in as a few hours. These tests are highly specific but suffer from variable sensitivity. PCR-based techniques and gene probe can also be used to speciate several NTM isolates obtained from culture.[75] These techniques offer more rapid diagnosis than traditional methods that rely on testing biochemical properties and physical parameters such as growth rate, optimal growth temperature, and pigment production. The most widely used molecular test for culture isolates employs Acridium ester-labeled DNA probes that target released 16s rRNA to form DNA-rRNA hybrid (AccuProbe, Genprobe Inc, San Diego, CA, USA). AccuProbe is able to identify *M tuberculosis* complex, MAC, *M kansasii*, and *M gordonae*. Analysis of the mycolic acid in NTM cell wall using high-performance liquid chromatography (HPLC) can be used for species determination as well, but HPLC has lower specificity compared with the molecular techniques.[76]

TREATMENT

Treatment should be approached with the understanding that patients undergoing treatment for the first time have over twice the rate of culture response seen in previously treated patients.[77] Recommended initial treatment of NTM lung disease depends on the causative species, comorbidities, disease prototype, and severity of the condition (**Table 3**). Regimens for most NTM involve treatment for a period of 12 months following conversion to sputum culture negative status. In cases where sputum culture is initially negative (eg, diagnosed by bronchoscopy) a 12-month course of treatment would usually be pursued. As NTM tend to be slowly progressive, it may sometimes be prudent to defer treatment or attempt only to intermittently suppress symptoms rather than provide an extended course of poorly tolerated treatment that may have little likelihood of effecting cure in a particular patient. Treatment of hypersensitivity disease is addressed in an earlier section.

MAC

Macrolides form the cornerstone of MAC treatment. Although previously untreated "wild strains" are universally sensitive to macrolides, the ATS/IDSA recommend in vitro testing for clarithromycin susceptibility (results can be extrapolated to azithromycin).[56] The benefits of clarithromycin susceptibility testing are clearer in cases of retreatment or when the patient may be failing treatment. Routine susceptibility testing should not be performed for the other agents, as a correlation between in vitro susceptibility and response to treatment is unproven.[78,79] Because macrolide monotherapy can rapidly lead to resistance and treatment failure,[78] it is essential that additional agents be included in the regimen; a rifamycin and ethambutol are the preferred agents. The selected rifamycin can be rifampin or rifabutin with the understanding that as the more potent inducer of cytochrome P450, rifampin carries a greater risk of significant drug interactions. However, rifabutin tends to be less well tolerated.

An intermittent thrice-weekly regimen is recommended for most patients with nodular bronchiectatic disease but is less effective for cavitary disease, extensive bronchiectatic MAC, or patients with a history of previous treatment for MAC.[77] For those patients, daily therapy, possibly including a parenteral aminoglycoside (ie, streptomycin or amikacin) for the first 8 to 12 weeks, is recommended. Addition of an aminoglycoside is associated with more rapid sputum conversion to smear negative, although significant improvement in symptoms or radiographic appearance may lag behind or not occur.[80] Because these regimens may be poorly tolerated, many experts suggest gradual dose escalation over a period of 1 to 2 weeks. Ethambutol should not be excluded from the treatment regimen because of apparent in vitro resistance.[77] As with most NTM, treatment duration should include 12 months of negative sputum cultures.[56]

Sputum evaluation should be performed monthly while on therapy.[56] Conversion to smear negative tends to be associated with improvement or resolution of pulmonary nodules, but pleural thickening is less responsive. Factors predictive of decreased likelihood of sputum conversion include prior therapy, extensive bronchiectasis, atelectasis, cavities, and pleural thickening.[73] Strongly positive sputum acid-fast bacilli (AFB) stain pretherapy, low body mass index, persistently elevated C-reactive protein, and certain strains of MAC (eg, serovar 4) have also been associated with poor outcomes. Repeatedly positive cultures after completion of macrolide-based therapy in patients with nodular bronchiectasis usually represent reinfection with new strains rather than relapse.[81]

Resistance to macrolides is usually due to mutation in the 23S r-RNA gene at positions 2058 and 2059, and was recently reported to occur in only 4% of patients treated with a regimen of clarithromycin, ethambutol, and a rifamycin. In contrast, 76% (39/51) of patients receiving macrolide monotherapy or macrolide plus a fluoroquinolone

Table 3
Initial medical treatment of common NTM pulmonary disease

NTM Species	Recommended Susceptibility Testing	Potential Regimens
MAC	Clarithromycin (especially if retreatment); with or without aminoglycoside, rifabutin, ethambutol; possibly quinolone if macrolide resistant	Macrolide, rifampin, ethambutol (add aminoglycoside for extensive/cavitary disease) treatment 3 times weekly for limited disease. Treatment daily for extensive disease, repeat treatment or with coexisting COPD. For macrolide resistance use isoniazid, rifampin (possibly rifabutin), ethambutol, and amikacin/streptomycin (first 3–6 mo)
M kansasii	Rifampin for new (untreated) isolates; if rifampin resistant: macrolide, quinolones, isoniazid, ethambutol, rifabutin, amikacin, sulfamethoxazole	Daily rifampin, ethambutol, isoniazid (3 times weekly may be effective); if rifampin resistant, consider high-dose isoniazid, ethambutol plus 1–2 others (sulfa, amikacin/streptomycin, macrolide, quinolone), or macrolide/quinolone-based regimen
M szulgai	Isoniazid, rifampin, ethambutol, aminoglycoside, with/without quinolone and macrolide	Isoniazid, rifampin, ethambutol, with or without fourth drug; pyrazinamide may be effective
M malmoense	Ethambutol, isoniazid, rifampin, macrolide, quinolone, (correlation with outcome uncertain)	Isoniazid, rifampin, ethambutol, with/without macrolide and/or quinolone
M xenopi	Macrolide, rifampin, ethambutol, isoniazid, quinolone (correlation with outcome uncertain)	Isoniazid, rifampin, ethambutol, clarithromycin with/without streptomycin for first 3–6 mo; quinolones may be active
M abscessus	Macrolide, amikacin, cefoxitin, linezolid, imipenem, clofazimine, tigecycline; correlation with clinical response is poor	No clear curative medical regimen available; macrolide plus 1–2 parenteral drugs such as amikacin plus cefoxitin or imipenem may be useful for control of symptoms. Lung resection of limited disease or periodic treatment for symptom control. Amikacin plus cefoxitin (imipenem) when macrolide resistant
M chelonae	Tobramycin, amikacin, macrolide, quinolones, linezolid, imipenem, clofazimine, doxycycline	Clarithromycin plus one or more additional agents with in vitro susceptibility
M fortuitum	Macrolides (may be misleading), quinolones, doxycycline, minocycline, sulfa, amikacin, imipenem, cefoxitin	Two agents with in vitro susceptibility (macrolide with inducible resistance; use with caution)

Abbreviations: macrolide, clarithromycin/azithromycin; quinolone, moxifloxacin preferred.
Adapted from Glassroth J. Pulmonary disease due to nontuberculous mycobacteria. Chest 2008;133:243–51; with permission from the American College of Chest Physicians.

developed resistance.[82] Macrolide resistance is difficult to manage, often requiring intravenous aminoglycoside and surgical resection.[82]

Treatment of confirmed pulmonary MAC is similar in HIV-infected and HIV-negative persons, although optimization of antiretroviral therapy is an important additional element in HIV-infected patients, and drug interactions tend to be more problematic.

Mycobacterium kansasii

Rifampin is an essential drug for *M kansasii* treatment, and susceptibility testing is recommended for all new isolates.[56] Additional agents in a "standard" regimen for rifampin-susceptible isolates include isoniazid and ethambutol, all given daily. A rifampin, ethambutol, and macrolide regimen given thrice weekly has also been used successfully, though experience is limited.[83] Treatment duration should include 12 months of negative sputum cultures.[56] In a comparison of 12-month versus 18-month therapy, only one relapse occurred, which was in the 12-month arm.[84] Recently, Santin and colleagues[85] reported a relapse rate of 6.6% among patients treated with 12 months of rifampin, ethambutol, and isoniazid plus streptomycin in the first 3 months. Of note, there were no relapses in patients who were younger than 40 years and had no debilitating comorbidities. Susceptibility testing for other agents should be performed when there is documented rifamycin resistance.[56] Moxifloxacin and linezolid are active against *M kansasii* in vitro,[86] but the clinical value of these agents is unclear at this time.

Mycobacterium abscessus

Usual antituberculosis drugs are not active against *M abscessus*. Thus, treatment should be based on susceptibility testing. Short courses (2–4 months) of a combination macrolide plus parenteral agents such as amikacin plus cefoxitin or imipenem can slow disease progression and moderate symptoms, but rarely achieve cure.[87] Surgical resection of diseased lung, if possible, is usually necessary for cure. Intermittent cycles of treatment to control symptoms may be useful in patients who are not surgical candidates. Moxifloxacin and linezolid have in vitro activity against *M abscessus*; however, there is limited clinical experience with these agents.[88] A recent preliminary report suggests a role for clarithromycin based regimens.[89] By contrast, *M fortuitum* and *M chelonae* are curable medically using combinations of these same drugs as guided by in vitro susceptibility testing.

Mycobacterium xenopi

The optimal regimen and treatment duration for *M xenopi* lung disease are uncertain. A potential regimen is clarithromycin, rifampin, isoniazid, and ethambutol.[56] Quinolones, especially moxifloxacin, may be effective but experience is limited. Comorbidities significantly influence outcomes of *M xenopi* lung disease.[90] In a retrospective study of 31 patients with NTM lung disease, including 15 with *M xenopi*, there was no difference in survival between untreated and treated patients, even in the subset that was treated based on susceptibility results or treatment guidelines. The 5-year mortality was 71%, but only 30% of the deaths were primarily attributed to the mycobacterial disease.[91] This statistic illustrates the challenge of treatment decisions in patients with this species of NTM; the presence of persistent symptoms or evidence of radiographic progression are particularly important in the treatment selection process.

Surgical Therapy

Adjunctive surgical management should be considered for selected patients such as those with *M abscessus* infection, clarithromycin-resistant MAC, or inadequate response to antibiotic therapy alone. Surgery is best reserved for localized disease in patients who are otherwise also surgical candidates. Surgery is typically performed after a period of antibiotic therapy and while antibiotics are continued. Although associated with high complication rates, surgery can be highly effective in properly selected patients and at centers experienced in this type of surgery. For example, all 53 patients who underwent pneumonectomy at a center with experienced surgeons achieved clearance of sputum NTM; one patient had recurrent disease and died 4 years after the procedure, and another patient died within a year due to respiratory failure.[92]

SUMMARY

Human exposure to NTM is unavoidable and increasing, and in some cases results in lung disease. While the rapidity of laboratory identification of some NTM has been enhanced by advances in molecular techniques, further research into the pathogenesis, clinical course, and epidemiology of these organisms is needed to refine the criteria for therapeutic intervention, to expand the list of effective drugs, and to increase the odds of achieving a cure.

REFERENCES

1. Glassroth J. Pulmonary disease due to nontuberculous mycobacteria. Chest 2008;133:243–51.
2. Ostroff S, Hutwagner L, Collin S. Mycobacterial species and drug resistance patterns reported by state laboratories-1992. 93rd American Society for Microbiology. General Meeting, May 16, 1993, Atlanta (GA); abstract U-9:170
3. Good RC, Snider DE. Isolation of nontuberculous mycobacteria in the United States, 1980. J Infect Dis 1982;146:829–33.
4. Marras TK, Chedore P, Ying AM, et al. Isolation prevalence of pulmonary nontuberculous mycobacteria in Ontario, 1997-2003. Thorax 2007;62:661–6.
5. Falkinham JO 3rd. Nontuberculous mycobacteria in the environment. Clin Chest med 2002;23(3):529–51.
6. Taylor RH, Falkinham JO 3rd, Norton CD, et al. Chlorine, chloramine, chlorine dioxide, and ozone susceptibility of Mycobacterium avium. Appl Environ Microbiol 2000;66:1702–5.
7. Hilborn ED, Covert TC, Yakrus MA, et al. Persistence of nontuberculous mycobacteria in a drinking water system after addition of filtration treatment. Appl Environ Microbiol 2006;72(9):5864–9.
8. Schulze-Robbecke R, Buchholtz K. Heat susceptibility of aquatic mycobacteria. Appl Environ Microbiol 1992;58(6):1869–73.
9. Khoor A, Leslie KO, Tazelaar HD, et al. Diffuse pulmonary disease caused by nontuberculous mycobacteria in immune competent people (hot tub lung). Am J Clin Pathol 2001;115:755–62.
10. Centers for Disease Control and Prevention (CDC). Respiratory illness in workers exposed to metal working fluid contaminated with nontuberculous mycobacteria. Ohio, 2001. MMWR Morb Wkly Rep 2002;51(16):349–52.
11. Bodle EE, Cunningham JA, Della-Latta P, et al. Epidemiology of nontuberculous mycobacteria in patients without HIV infection, New York City. Emerg Infect Dis 2008;14(3):390–6.
12. Koh WJ, Kwon OJ, Jeon K, et al. Clinical significance of nontuberculous mycobacteria isolated from respiratory specimens in Korea. Chest 2006;129:341–8.

13. Corbett EL, Hay M, Churchyard GJ, et al. *Mycobacterium kansasii* and *M. scrofulaceum* isolates from HIV-negative South African gold miners: incidence, clinical significance and radiology. Int J Tuberc Lung Dis 1999;3(6):501–7.

14. Han XY, Tarrand JJ, Infante R, et al. Clinical significance and epidemiologic analyses of *Mycobacterium avium* and *Mycobacterium intracellulare* among patients without AIDS. J Clin Microbiol 2005;43(9):4407–12.

15. Tateishi Y, Hirayama Y, Ozeki Y, et al. Virulence of *Mycobacterium avium* complex strains isolated from immunocompetent patients. Microb Pathol 2009;46(1):6–12.

16. Schorey JS, Carroll MC, Brown EJ. A macrophage invasion mechanism for pathogenic mycobacteria. Science 1997;277:1091–3.

17. Esteban J, Martin-de-Hijas N, Kinnari TJ, et al. Biofilm development by potentially pathogenic non-pigmented rapidly growing bacteria. BMC Microbiol 2008;8:184.

18. Sexton P, Harrison AC. Susceptibility to nontuberculous mycobacterial lung disease. Eur Respir J 2008;31:1322–33.

19. Vankayalapati R, Wizel B, Samten B, et al. Cytokine profiles in immunocompetent persons infected with *Mycobacterium avium* complex. J Infect Dis 2001;183(3): 478–84.

20. Dorman SE, Holland SM. Interferon-gamma and interleukin-12 pathway defects in human disease. Cytokine Growth Factor Rev 2000;11:321–33.

21. Kim RD, Greenberg DE, Ehrmantraut ME, et al. Pulmonary nontuberculous mycobacterial disease: prospective study of a distinct preexisting syndrome. Am J Respir Crit Care Med 2008;178:1066–74.

22. Greinert U, Schlaak M, Rusch-Gerdes S, et al. Low in vitro production of interferon gamma and tumor necrosis factor-alpha in HIV seronegative patients with pulmonary disease caused by nontuberculous bacteria. J Clin Immunol 2000;20:445–52.

23. Safdar A, White DA, Stover D, et al. Profound interferon gamma deficiency in patients with chronic pulmonary nontuberculosis mycobacteriosis. Am J Med 2002;113:756–9.

24. Kwon YS, Kim EJ, Lee S, et al. Decreased cytokine production in patients with nontuberculous mycobacterial lung disease. Lung 2007;185:337–41.

25. Middleton AM, Chadwick MV, Nicholson AG, et al. Inhibition of adherence of *Mycobacterium avium* complex and *Mycobacterium tuberculosis* to fibronectin on the respiratory mucosa. Respir Med 2004;98:1203–6.

26. Middleton AM, Chadwick MV, Nicholson AG, et al. The role of *Mycobacterium avium* complex fibronectin attachment protein in adherence to the human respiratory mucosa. Mol Microbiol 2000;38:381–91.

27. Huang JH, Kao PN, Adi V, et al. *Mycobacterium avium*-intracellulare pulmonary infection in HIV-negative patients without preexisting lung disease: diagnostic and management limitations. Chest 1999;115(4):1033–40.

28. Iseman MD, Buschman DL, Ackerson LM. Pectus excavatum and scoliosis: thoracic anomalies associated with pulmonary disease caused by *Mycobacterium avium* complex. Am Rev Respir Dis 1991;144:914–6.

29. Kalayjian RC, Toossi Z, Tomashefski JF Jr, et al. Pulmonary disease due to infection by *Mycobacterium avium* complex in patients with AIDS. Clin Infect Dis 1995; 20(5):1186–94.

30. Doucette K, Fishman JA. Nontuberculous mycobacterial infection in hematopoietic stem cell and solid organ transplant recipients. Clin Infect Dis 2004;38(10): 1428–39.

31. Salvana EM, Cooper GS, Salata RA. Mycobacterium other than tuberculosis (MOTT) infection: an emerging disease in infliximab-treated patients. J Infect 2007;55(6):484–7.

32. Tanaka G, Shojima J, Matsushita I, et al. Pulmonary *Mycobacterium avium* complex infection: association with NRAMP1 polymorphism. Eur Respir J 2007; 30:90–6.

33. Dailloux M, Abalain ML, Laurain C, et al. Respiratory infections associated with nontuberculous mycobacteria in non-HIV patients. Eur Respir J 2006;28(6): 1211–5.

34. Kobashi Y, Fukuda M, Yoshida K, et al. Four cases of pulmonary *Mycobacterium avium intracellulare* complex presenting as a solitary pulmonary nodule and a review of the other cases in Japan. Respirology 2006;11:317–21.

35. Woodring JH, Vandiviere HM, Melvin IG, et al. Roentgenographic features of pulmonary disease caused by atypical mycobacteria. South Med J 1987; 80(12):1488–97.

36. Reich JM, Johnson RE. *Mycobacterium avium* complex pulmonary disease. Incidence, presentation, and response to therapy in a community setting. Am Rev Respir Dis 1991;143:1381–5.

37. Christensen EE, Dietz GW, Ahn CH, et al. Initial roetgenographic manifestations of pulmonary *Mycobacterium tuberculosis*. *M kansasii* and *M intracellularis* infections. Chest 1981;80(2):132–6.

38. Albelda SM, Kern JA, Marinelli DL, et al. Expanding spectrum of pulmonary disease caused by nontuberculous mycobacteria. Radiology 1985;157:289–96.

39. Reich JM, Johnson RE. *Mycobacterium avium* complex pulmonary disease presenting as an isolated lingula or middle lobe pattern. The Lady Windermere syndrome. Chest 1992;101(6):1605–9.

40. Bradham RR, Sealy WC, Young WG Jr, et al. Chronic middle lobe infection. Factors responsible for its development. Ann Thorac Surg 1966;2:612–6.

41. Wallace RJ, Zhang Y, Brown BA, et al. Polyclonal *Mycobacterium avium* complex infections in patients with nodular bronchiectasis. Am J Respir Crit Care Med 1998;158(4):1235–44.

42. Tanaka E, Amitani R, Niimi A, et al. Yield of computed tomography and bronchoscopy for the diagnosis of *Mycobacterium avium* complex pulmonary disease. Am J Respir Crit Care Med 1997;155(6):2041–6.

43. Marras TK, Wallace RJ Jr, Koth LL, et al. Hypersensitivity pneumonitis reaction to *Mycobacterium avium* in household water. Chest 2005;127:664–71.

44. Embil J, Warren P, Yakrus M, et al. Pulmonary illness associated with exposure to *Mycobacterium avium* complex in hot tub water. Hypersensitivity pneumonitis or infection? Chest 1997;111:813–6.

45. Marchetti N, Criner K, Criner GJ. Characterization of functional, radiologic and lung function recovery post treatment of hot tub lung. A case report and review of the literature. Lung 2004;182:271–7.

46. Agarwal R, Nath A. Hot-tub lung: hypersensitivity to *Mycobacterium avium* but not hypersensitivity pneumonitis. Respir Med 2006;100(8):1478.

47. Pham RV, Vydareny KH, Gal AA. High-resolution computed tomography appearance of pulmonary *Mycobacterium avium* complex infection after exposure to hot tub: case of hot-tub lung. J Thorac Imaging 2003;18:48–52.

48. Benson CA, Ellner JJ. *Mycobacterium avium* complex and AIDS: advances in theory and practice. Clin Infect Dis 1993;17:7–20.

49. Salama C, Policar M, Venkataraman M. Isolated pulmonary *Mycobacterium avium* complex infection in patients with human immunodeficiency virus infection: case reports and literature review. Clin Infect Dis 2003;37:e35–40.

50. Corbett EL, Blumberg L, Churchyard GJ, et al. Nontuberculous mycobacteria: defining disease in a prospective cohort of South African miners. Am J Respir Crit Care Med 1999;160:15–21.

51. Kerbiriou L, Ustianowski A, Johnson MA, et al. Human immunodeficiency virus type 1-related pulmonary *Mycobacterium xenopi* infection: a need to treat? Clin Infect Dis 2003;37:1250–4.

52. Marie I, Heliot P, Roussel F, et al. Fatal *Mycobacterium peregrinum* pneumonia in refractory polymyositis treated with infliximab. Rheumatology (Oxford) 2005;44: 1201–2.

53. Pierre-Audigier C, Ferroni A, Sermet-Gaudeleus I, et al. Age-related prevalence and distribution of nontuberculous mycobacterial species among patients with cystic fibrosis. J Clin Microbiol 2005;3:3467–70.

54. Mussaffi H, Rivlin J, Shalit I, et al. Nontuberculous mycobacteria in cystic fibrosis associated with allergic bronchopulmonary aspergillosis and steroid therapy. Eur Respir J 2005;25:324–8.

55. Olivier KN. NTM in CF Study Group. The natural history of nontuberculous mycobacteria in patients with cystic fibrosis. Paediatr Respir Rev 2004;5(Suppl A): S213–6.

56. Griffith DE, Aksamit T, Brown-Elliott BA, et al. on behalf of the ATS Mycobacterial Diseases Subcommittee. An official ATS/IDSA statement: diagnosis, treatment, and prevention of nontuberculous mycobacterial diseases. Am J Respir Crit Care Med 2007;175:367–416.

57. Chalermskulrat W, Sood N, Neuringer P, et al. Non-tuberculous mycobacteria in end stage cystic fibrosis: implications for lung transplantation. Thorax 2006;61: 507–13.

58. Taillard C, Greub G, Weber R, et al. Clinical implications of *Mycobacterium kansasii* species heterogeneity: Swiss National Survey. J Clin Microbiol 2003;41(3): 1240–4.

59. Lillo M, Orengo S, Cernoch P, et al. Pulmonary and disseminated infection due to *Mycobacterium kansasii*: a decade of experience. Rev Infect Dis 1990;12(5): 760–7.

60. Griffith DE, Girard WM, Wallace RJ Jr. Clinical features of pulmonary disease caused by rapidly growing mycobacteria. An analysis of 154 patients. Am Rev Respir Dis 1993;147:1271.

61. Cullen AR, Cannon CL, Mark EJ, et al. *Mycobacterium abscessus* infection in cystic fibrosis. Colonization or infection? Am J Respir Crit Care Med 2000; 161(2 Pt 1):641–5.

62. Ohno H, Matsuo N, Suyama N, et al. The first surgical case of pulmonary *Mycobacterium malmoense* infection in Japan. Intern Med 2008;47(24):2187–90.

63. Henriques B, Hoffner SE, Petrini B, et al. Infection with *Mycobacterium malmoense* in Sweden: report of 221 cases. Clin Infect Dis 1994;18(4):596–600.

64. Buchholz UT, McNeil MM, Keyes LE, et al. Mycobacterium malmoense infections in the United States, January 1993 through June 1995. Clin Infect Dis 1998;27(3): 551–8.

65. Evans AJ, Crisp AJ, Colville A, et al. Pulmonary infections caused by *Mycobacterium malmoense* and *Mycobacterium tuberculosis*: comparison of radiographic features. AJR Am J Roentgenol 1993;161:733–7.

66. Murasic A, Katalinic-Jankovic V, Popovic-Grie S, et al. *Mycobacterium xenopi* pulmonary disease—epidemiology and clinical features in non-immunocompromised patients. J Infect 2009;589:108–12.

67. Jiva TM, Jacoby HM, Weymouth LA, et al. *Mycobacterium xenopi*: innocent bystander or emerging pathogen? Clin Infect Dis 1997;24:226–32.
68. Tortoli E, Besozzi G, Lacchini C, et al. Pulmonary infection due to *Mycobacterium szulgai*, case report and review of the literature. Eur Respir J 1998;11:975–7.
69. Ergan B, Coplu L, Alp A, et al. *Mycobacterium smegmatis* pneumonia. Respirology 2004;9:283–5.
70. Fujita J, Ohtsuki Y, Suemitsu I, et al. Pathological and radiological changes in resected lung specimens in *Mycobacterium avium intracellulare* complex pulmonary disease. Eur Respir J 1999;13:535–40.
71. Rossman MD. Colonization with *Mycobacterium avium* complex—an outdated concept. Eur Respir J 1999;13(3):479.
72. Olivier KN, Yankaskas JR, Knowles MR, et al. Non-tuberculous mycobacterial pulmonary disease in cystic fibrosis. Semin Respir Infect 1996;11:272–84.
73. Kuroishi S, Nakamura Y, Hayakawa H, et al. *Mycobacterium avium* complex disease: prognostic implications of high-resolution computed tomography findings. Eur Respir J 2008;32(1):147–52.
74. Somoskovi A, Hotaling JE, Fitzgerald M, et al. Lessons from a proficiency testing event for acid-fast microscopy. Chest 2001;120(1):250–7.
75. Neonakis IK, Gitti Z, Krambovitis E, et al. Molecular diagnostic tools in mycobacteriology. J Microbiol Methods 2008;75:1–11.
76. Daley P, Petrich A, May K, et al. Comparison of in-house and commercial 16S rRNA sequencing with high-performance liquid chromatography and genotype AS and CM for identification of nontuberculous mycobacteria. Diagn Mcrobiol Infect Dis 2008;61(3):284–93.
77. Lam PK, Griffith DE, Aksamit TR. Factors related to response to intermittent treatment of *Mycobacterium avium* complex lung disease. Am J Respir Crit Care Med 2006;173:1283–9.
78. Wallace RJ, Brown BA, Griffith DE, et al. Initial clarithromycin monotherapy for *Mycobacterium avium-intracellulare* complex lung disease. Am J Respir Crit Care Med 1994;149(5):1335–41.
79. Kobashi Y, Yoshida K, Miyashita N, et al. Relationship between clinical efficacy of treatment of pulmonary *Mycobacterium avium* complex disease and drug-sensitivity testing of *Mycobacterium avium* complex isolates. J Infect Chemother 2006;12:195–202.
80. Kobashi Y, Matsushima T, Ok M. A double blind randomized study of aminoglycoside infusion with combined therapy for pulmonary *Mycobacterium avium* complex disease. Respir Med 2007;101:130–8.
81. Wallace RJ Jr, Zhang Y, Brown-Elliott BA, et al. Repeat positive cultures in *Mycobacterium intracellulare* lung disease after macrolide therapy represent new infections in patients with nodular bronchiectasis. J Infect Dis 2002;186(2):266–73.
82. Griffith DE, Brown-Elliott BA, Langsjoen B, et al. Clinical and molecular analysis of macrolide resistance in *Mycobacterium avium* complex lung disease. Am J Respir Crit Care Med 2006;174:928–34.
83. Griffith DE, Brown-Elliott BA, Wallace RJ Jr. Thrice-weekly clarithromycin-containing regimen for treatment of *Mycobacterium kansasii* lung disease: results of a preliminary study. Clin Infect Dis 2003;37(9):1178–82.
84. Sauret J, Hernandez-Flix S, Castro E, et al. Treatment of pulmonary disease caused by *Mycobacterium kansasii*: results of 18 vs 12 months' chemotherapy. Tuber Lung Dis 1995;76(2):104–8.

85. Santin M, Dorca J, Alcaide F, et al. Long-term relapses after 12-month treatment for *Mycobacterium kansasii* lung disease. Eur Respir J 2009;33:148–52.
86. Alcaide F, Calatayud L, Santin M, et al. Comparative in vitro activities of linezolid, telithromycin, clarithromycin, levofloxacin, moxifloxacin and four conventional antimycobacterial drugs against *Mycobacterium kansasii*. Antimicrobial Agents Chemother 2004;48(12):4562–5.
87. Daley CL, Griffith DE. Pulmonary disease caused by rapidly growing mycobacteria. Clin Chest Med 2002;23(3):623–32.
88. Rodriguez Diaz JC, Lopez M, Ruiz M, et al. In vitro activity of new fluoroquinolones and linezolid against non-tuberculous mycobacteria. Int J Antimicrob Agents 2003;21(6):585–8.
89. Jeon K, Kwon OJ, Lee NY; et al. Antibiotic treatment of Mycobacterium abscessus lung disease: a retrospective analysis of 65 patients. Am J Respir Crit Care med 2009;180(9):896–902.
90. Jenkins PA, Campbell IA, Research Committee of The British Thoracic Society. Pulmonary disease caused by *Mycobacterium xenopi* in HIV-negative patients: five-year follow-up of patients receiving standardized treatment. Respir Med 2003;97:439–44.
91. Andrejak C, Lescure FX, Douadi, et al. Non-tuberculous mycobacteria pulmonary infection: management and follow-up of 31 infected patients. J Infect 2007;55(1): 34–40.
92. Shiraishi Y, Nakajima Y, Katsuragi N, et al. Pneumonectomy for nontuberculous mycobacterial infections. Ann Thorac Surg 2004;78:399–403.

Emerging Advances in Rapid Diagnostics of Respiratory Infections

David R. Murdoch, MD, MSc, DTM&H, FRACP, FRCPA[a,b,*],
Lance C. Jennings, PhD, FRCPath[a,b], Niranjan Bhat, MD[c],
Trevor P. Anderson, MSc[b]

KEYWORDS

- Respiratory infection • Pneumonia • Polymerase chain reaction
- Diagnostics • Antigen detection

Diagnostic laboratories play a central role in the recognition of new and emerging infections. The identification of the severe acute respiratory syndrome (SARS) coronavirus in 2003 highlighted how modern diagnostic tools and collaboration between clinicians, public health professionals, and laboratorians can lead to the rapid characterization of a new respiratory pathogen.[1] Similarly, the development and rapid dissemination of a polymerase chain reaction (PCR) method to detect the novel H1N1 influenza A strain by the US Centers for Disease Control and Prevention in 2009, relied on the most recent diagnostic technology and played an important role in the response to the latest influenza pandemic.[2] These events remind us of how much recent developments in diagnostics have improved our ability to identify respiratory

---

D.R.M. and N.B. performed part of this work under the Pneumonia Etiology Research for Child Health (PERCH) program at the Johns Hopkins Bloomberg School of Public Health funded by a grant from The Bill & Melinda Gates Foundation. N.B. is supported by grant 1KL2RR025006-01 from the National Center for Research Resources (NCRR), a component of the National Institutes of Health (NIH), and NIH Roadmap for Medical Research. Its contents are solely the responsibility of the authors and do not necessarily represent the official view of NCRR or NIH. Information on NCRR is available at http://www.ncrr.nih.gov/. Information on Reengineering the Clinical Research Enterprise can be obtained from http://nihroadmap. nih.gov/clinicalresearch/overview-translational.asp.

[a] Department of Pathology, University of Otago Christchurch, PO Box 4345, Christchurch 8140, New Zealand
[b] Microbiology Unit, Canterbury Health Laboratories, PO Box 151, Christchurch 8140, New Zealand
[c] Division of Infectious Diseases, Department of Pediatrics, Johns Hopkins School of Medicine, 600 North Wolfe Street, Baltimore, MD 21287, USA
* Corresponding author. Department of Pathology, University of Otago Christchurch, PO Box 4345, Christchurch 8140, New Zealand.
E-mail address: david.murdoch@cdhb.govt.nz

Infect Dis Clin N Am 24 (2010) 791–807
doi:10.1016/j.idc.2010.04.006

viruses. For nonviral respiratory pathogens, developments in laboratory technology have been less profound in general, but have still led to modest improvements in the diagnostic capability.

For the diagnostic microbiology laboratory, the routine evaluation of patients with suspected respiratory infections continues to rely on methods that have been used for a long time: microscopy and culture of respiratory tract specimens, blood cultures, detection of antigens in urine and upper respiratory specimens, and serology. Recent advances in pneumonia diagnostics have mostly occurred in the areas of antigen and nucleic acid detection. Despite these technological advances, there remain several major challenges that hinder the search for the causes of respiratory infections, particularly for pneumonia.[3] These challenges include difficulty collecting lower respiratory tract specimens, problems distinguishing colonization from infection, poor clinical (diagnostic) sensitivity of assays, and often inadequate evaluation of new diagnostics.

This review focuses on recent advances in laboratory diagnostics that enable rapid identification of respiratory pathogens.

ANTIGEN DETECTION

Assays to detect microbial antigens in body fluids have been used for the diagnosis of respiratory infections for many years, using various formats such as immunofluorescence, enzyme-linked immunosorbent assay (ELISA), latex agglutination, coagulation, and chromatographic immunoassay. These methods are the diagnostic tools most easily applied as near-patient tests, but development is reliant on the identification of suitable antigens that are present in detectable quantities in clinical specimens. To date, commercial assays have been developed only for a limited range of pathogens. The most widely available assays have focused on the detection of selected bacterial pathogens in urine and the detection of viruses in respiratory specimens.

Among bacterial respiratory pathogens, assays for *Streptococcus pneumoniae* and *Legionella pneumophila* are the most developed. A newer generation immunochromatographic test that detects the C-polysaccharide cell wall antigen in urine (NOW) has been an important advance in the diagnosis of pneumococcal disease.[4] This test has a sensitivity of 70% to 80% and a specificity of greater than 90% compared with conventional diagnostic methods for detection of pneumococcal pneumonia in adults. Unfortunately, the NOW test cannot be used reliably in children as it also detects pneumococcal carriage.[5] Alternative pneumococcal antigens for diagnostic purposes, such as pneumolysin, have shown promising results, although none has been demonstrated to perform better than existing commercial C-polysaccharide antigen assays.[6–8] The combination of a pneumolysin-specific antigen detection ELISA together with the NOW test may result in a better diagnostic yield because of the higher specificity of the pneumolysin detection ELISA.[7]

Detection of soluble *Legionella* antigen in urine is an established and valuable tool for the diagnosis of Legionnaires' disease, although current commercial assays can only reliably detect infection caused by *Legionella pneumophila* serogroup 1.[9] Some assays have been intended to detect other legionellae,[10] although the performance is not as good as for *L pneumophila* serogroup 1.

Detection of respiratory viral antigens in respiratory secretions has become an important diagnostic tool.[11–13] Antigen detection using immunofluorescent techniques were pioneered in the 1970s, and commercial reagents are now widely used for the detection of influenza viruses, respiratory syncytial virus (RSV), parainfluenza viruses, adenoviruses, and human metapneumovirus. These assays require technical expertise and have the advantage of allowing direct evaluation of specimen quality. More recently, commercial rapid diagnostic tests (RDTs) have become widely used for the detection of influenza or RSV directly in respiratory specimens. These diagnostic test kits, produced as dipsticks, cassettes, or cards, contain internal controls, and a positive result is signaled by a color change. Results are produced by these tests within 5 to 40 minutes.

The sensitivity of rapid tests for the detection of seasonal influenza in clinical specimens ranges from 10% to 96%,[14,15] and varies with virus type or subtype, timing of specimen collection, specimen type, patient age, and the test comparator.[16,17] With the emergence of the pandemic influenza A (H1N1) 2009 virus, RDTs have been widely used for patient triaging, although there are limited data available on their clinical accuracy.[18,19] The sensitivity of these assays for detecting this new strain is 10% to 69% compared with real-time PCR.[20–22] Specificity of RDTs for seasonal influenza is 90% to 100% according to the available data for H1N1 2009.[22] Commercial RSV RDTs have sensitivities of 71% to 95% and specificities of 80% to 100% compared with culture.[23–25] Poorer performance has been observed in adults,[26] which may be related to the decreased viral titer in adults compared with children.

To correctly interpret results of RDTs, the prevalence of influenza or RSV disease in a community must be considered.[15] During peak disease activity, positive predictive values are highest, but false-negative results more likely. The opposite is true during times of low disease activity.[17] When the disease prevalence is low or unknown, RDT results become difficult to interpret and of limited use.[17]

NUCLEIC ACID AMPLIFICATION TESTS

The use of nucleic acid amplification tests (NAATs) has transformed our understanding of respiratory infections, demonstrating the relevance of new agents such as human metapneumovirus, and providing new insights into previously recognized ones such as rhinoviruses. The progressive commercialization and clinical application of these methods is placing them at the forefront of respiratory diagnostics.

NAATs possess several advantages over more traditional techniques for the detection of respiratory pathogens.[27] These tests have improved sensitivity for detecting organisms that are fastidious, no longer viable, or present in small amounts. NAATs can provide rapid genetic information regarding sequence evolution, geographic variation, or the presence of virulence factors or antibiotic resistance. Their rapid turnaround times allow them a more prominent role in patient management, and the ability of NAATs to test for multiple pathogens simultaneously has aided in the diagnosis of nonspecific respiratory syndromes, such as in outbreak settings. Within the laboratory, NAATs offer enhanced opportunities for automation, and have a lower safety risk than culture for the detection of highly virulent pathogens.

Among the NAATs, the PCR is the most common and thoroughly evaluated method.[28,29] The PCR formats most relevant for respiratory diagnostics can be classified into conventional, real-time, and multiplex platforms, with various amplicon detection methods such as gel analysis, ELISA, DNA hybridization, or the use of fluorescent dyes or chemical tags. Real-time PCR has several features that place it at an advantage. First, the two steps of amplification and detection are combined in one reaction, increasing the speed and efficiency of testing and reducing the risks of operator error and cross-contamination. Real-time PCR also allows for the possibility of quantifying the amount of starting nucleic acid material.

Multiplex PCR systems, in which multiple PCR targets are sought after simultaneously in one reaction, have gained wider acceptance, particularly among commercial assays. These systems have the advantage of increasing the number of pathogens tested for, without increasing the required amount of operator time or specimen material. Multiplex assays have broadened the scope of respiratory surveillance studies, and have also led to the increasing recognition of dual or triple infections in the same individual.[30] As noted in **Table 1**, these assays can be differentiated by either their amplification or detection steps. In the amplification step, all multiplex platforms must balance the competing optimal PCR conditions for each individual target, and must overcome problems of competition and inhibition among the various primers and probes. Each platform uses a unique method to address these issues, such as nested primer combinations,[30,31] complex primer structures,[32,33] and nontraditional nucleotides.[34–36]

These assays are even more varied in their detection stages, where the common task is to differentially detect and report distinct populations of amplified targets. Several platforms involve solid-phase arrays, such as polystyrene microbead suspensions that use fluorescent dyes to differentiate targets,[34,37,38] or the microchip formats that identify targets by binding to a specific physical location.[39–41] The former has been developed into platforms detecting 17 to 20 targets, whereas the latter can identify between a few dozen to thousands of targets. The increased breadth of targets afforded by microarrays, however, comes at the expense of decreased sensitivity.[42] Multiplex PCR products can also be distinguished by their size, using resolution techniques such as agarose gel electrophoresis to differentiate by weight, and capillary-based auto-sequencers that identify targets by length and sequence.[32,33] Mass spectrometry can also be used for identification, either by the attachment of high molecular weight tags to primers[43–46] or by the analysis of specific nucleotide base ratios that can be resolved by molecular weight.[47]

Regardless of the platform, all PCR assays require good primer design taking into consideration gene target, gene number, mobility of genes between species, stability of gene, and the presence of mutations. Bacteria have large genomes with many genes for a fully functional organism, including their own genes for replication and enzyme product. Owing to the large genome size there are many targets available for specific detection of a bacterial species. Housekeeping genes, those genes that are essential for the survival of the organism, are desirable gene targets because they have conserved regions and hypervariable regions (eg, the 16S rRNA gene). Genes found in multicopies will also increase the sensitivity of PCR assays. The choices of viral pathogen gene targets are limited because of the limited size of the viral genome. Genes that are highly conserved are desirable targets for PCR because they allow the detection of many strains. Other genes that process areas of nucleotide hypervariability caused by genetic mutation should be avoided because changes over primer and probe sites can cause poor PCR efficiency and the potential for false-negative results. **Table 2** lists some of the more common respiratory pathogen target genes.

The published literature on NAATs can be difficult to interpret, because study designs vary and rarely involve head-to-head comparisons among the different assays. Calculation of clinical sensitivity and specificity is complicated because NAATs often are more sensitive than the reference culture-based standards. Comparisons of study results are also problematic because of the use of different specimen types that may have differential yields for pathogens.[48] Finally, several NAAT platforms require investment in specialized equipment, the cost of which can only be recovered through high-volume testing. Therefore, few NAAT assays for respiratory diagnosis are licensed for clinical use, and their daily use in clinical practice remains uncommon. To promote widespread adoption in the future, developers of NAAT diagnostics will need to standardize evaluation methods, particularly in comparison with reference techniques, reduce complexity and cost, and better demonstrate their utility in the clinical environment.

NAATs for Specific Respiratory Pathogens

Although NAATs have been developed for all important respiratory pathogens, the clinical application of these tests varies. Perhaps the area that NAATs have had the greatest impact is for the diagnosis of infections caused by respiratory viruses.[29,49,50] For most, if not all, respiratory viruses, detection of viral nucleic acid is the most sensitive diagnostic approach, and current "gold standards" (namely, culture and direct immunofluorescence) will be eventually replaced by NAATs.[50] PCR has become the diagnostic test of choice for some respiratory viral infections (eg, for influenza during the current influenza H1N1 pandemic), and is a useful epidemiologic tool for characterizing the role of viruses in various disease states.[51] NAATs can provide results rapidly and are able to detect many viral pathogens that are unable to be readily detected by culture. Perhaps more so than for other respiratory pathogens, considerable effort has been directed toward the development of multiplex assays to enable the simultaneous detection of multiple viral pathogens. Given the increasingly large number of respiratory viruses, this can be a challenging task.

The need for improved diagnostic tools for pneumococcal disease has lead to the evaluation of several NAATs. For pneumonia, PCR has a sensitivity for detecting S pneumoniae in blood samples ranging from 29% to 100%,[27] with a tendency for higher sensitivity in children than adults. The finding of positive pneumococcal PCR results from asymptomatic control subjects complicates interpretation.[52–54] When testing sputum samples from adults with pneumonia, PCR positivity has ranged from 68% to 100%,[27] although it is unclear how often this reflects upper respiratory tract colonization rather than infection.[55] Further refinement of PCR assays, including the use of multiple targets, has increased the specificity,[56] with lytA assays potentially offering advantages over other assays.[57,58] Quantification of S pneumoniae DNA load may provide additional diagnostic and prognostic information. Quantitative PCR may help distinguish colonization from infection, with a higher bacterial burden in pneumococcal disease than in a carrier state.[59] High pneumococcal DNA loads in blood have been recently shown to be associated with severe disease in various settings.[60–62]

NAATs have improved the ability of diagnostic laboratories to detect respiratory pathogens that are difficult to culture, such as Mycoplasma pneumoniae, Legionella species, and Chlamydophila pneumoniae. An extensive evaluation of 13 antibody detection assays using PCR as the comparator standard concluded that few commercial serologic assays for detection of M pneumoniae performed with sufficient sensitivity and specificity, and highlighted the increasing importance of NAATs.[63] Indeed PCR is considered by many to be the method of choice for detection of M pneumoniae infection.[64] Both upper and lower respiratory tract samples are suitable for testing for M pneumoniae by PCR, although throat swabs and nasopharyngeal samples may be preferred because of high sensitivity, high specificity, and convenience. In practice, PCR has been successfully used to rapidly diagnose mycoplasma pneumonia during outbreaks, and was particularly useful in children, immunocompromised patients, and in early-stage disease.[65,66]

Legionnaires' disease can be difficult to diagnose, and NAATs have proven a useful adjunct to culture and antigen detection.[9] PCR has repeatedly been shown to have sensitivity equal to or greater than culture when testing lower respiratory specimens.[67–73] Legionella DNA can also be detected in nonrespiratory specimens, such as urine, serum, and peripheral leukocytes,[9] although testing these specimen types is not well established.

Table 1
Comparison of nucleic acid amplification platforms

Platform	Targets Included	Assays Available	Analytical Performance	Clinical Performance	Development Timeframe	Flexibility	Turnaround Time	Specimen Requirements	Quantitation	Licensing Status
Real-time PCR (rtPCR)	Variable; maximum of 4–5 targets per assay, can run parallel reactions, limited by sample volume	Various in-house protocols	Likely highest sensitivity, eg, 1 pfu/mL, 10 copies/reaction	Good; singleplex rtPCR is often the gold standard molecular diagnostic	Depends on the originating laboratory	Multiplex must be optimized for each additional target, limited to 5 total targets	Half-day	None	Yes	Some approved for in vitro diagnosis (IVD), others research use only (RUO)
Microbead array	17–20 viral or bacterial targets in each assay	Qiagen (Resplex I [bacterial] and II [viral]), Luminex, and Eragen Biosciences	Varies by kit and pathogen; limits of detection reported at 60 copies/reaction, or 0.1–100 $TCID_{50}$/mL	Sensitivity 72%–100% compared with culture plus rtPCR; varies by target, reduced by dual infections	All are commercially available	Multiplex must be optimized for each additional target; up to 30 can be detected at once; commercial kits may be slow to modify	6–8 h	No	No	IVD (Luminex); RUO (Qiagen, Eragen)
Mass spectrometry	All main respiratory viruses and bacteria	MassTag, IBIS	MassTag: 500–1000 copies/reaction, 1 $TCID_{50}$/mL; IBIS: 50 copies/well (basically singleplex)	Not rigorously evaluated	Unknown	Requires optimization of multiplex; detection methods unrestricted	Half to 1 day	No	No	RUO

Commercial multiplex	All main respiratory viruses and bacteria	Seegene (Seeplex)	10–100 copies/reaction	96%–100% concordance with DFA and sequencing	Commercially available	Multiplex apparently tolerant of additional targets; detection method determined separately	6–8 h	No sputum	No	IVD in Europe and Canada, RUO in USA
Microarray	Several thousand viruses, bacteria, fungi, and parasites	Greenechip, Virochip, Autogenomics	10–10,000 copies/reaction	No data	Unknown	Not generally customizable	No data	No data	No	RUO
16S rRNA	All bacteria and mycobacteria	Viruses	Can detect low abundance organisms	For bacteremia, 87% sensitivity, 86% specificity vs blood culture	Assay for respective pathogens is in development	Not applicable	PCR 3–4 h, analysis time 3–4 h	ND	No	RUO
Ultrahigh throughput screening	All microbes	None	Limit of detection 5500 copies/mL	No data	No data	Not applicable	ND	ND; likely none	No	RUO

Abbreviations: DFA, direct fluorescence assay; ND, not determined; TCID$_{50}$, tissue culture infective dose needed to produce 50% change.

Table 2
Common gene targets for nucleic acid amplification tests

Organism	Genome	Size (nt)	Target	Function
Streptococcus pneumoniae	dsDNA	~2,040,000	*ply* *lytA* *psaA* *16S rRNA*	Detection
Haemophilus influenzae	dsDNA	~1,830,138	*16S rRNA* *BexA*	Detection
Moraxella catarrhalis	dsDNA	~1,940,000	*16S rRNA*	Detection
Legionella	dsDNA	~3,576,470	*16S rRNA* *mip*	Detection
Mycoplasma pneumoniae	dsDNA	~816,394	*16S rRNA* P1 adhesion gene CARDS toxin	Detection
Chlamydophila pneumoniae	dsDNA	~1,225,935	*omp-2* gene	Detection
Bordetella pertussis	dsDNA	~4,086,189	*IS481* adenylate cyclase toxin (ACT) gene	Detection
Mycobacterium tuberculosis	dsDNA	~4,411,532	*IS6110* *16S rRNA*	Detection
Pneumocystis jiroveci	dsDNA	~8,400,000	*18S rRNA*, mitochondrial (mt) rRNA *5S rRNA*	Detection
Adenovirus	dsDNA	~36,000	Hexon gene Fiber gene	Detection and genotyping
Enterovirus	ssRNA (+)	~7500	5'UTR VP1,2	Detection Genotyping

Rhinovirus	ssRNA (+)	~7500	5'UTR VP1,2	Detection Genotyping
Coronavirus 229E, OC43, SARS, NL63, HKU-1	ssRNA (+)	~30,000	Polymerase gene Nucleocapsid gene ORF1	Detection
Influenza A	ssRNA (−)	~12,000	Matrix protein gene	Detection
Influenza B	ssRNA (−)	~12,000	Hemagglutinin gene	Detection
Parainfluenza virus 1, 2, 3, and 4	ssRNA (−)	~15,600	Hemagglutinin gene	Detection
RSV	ssRNA (−)	~10,000	Fusion protein (F) Nucleoprotein (N)	Detection
hMPV	ssRNA (−)	~14,000	Fusion protein Nucleoprotein Large polymerase (L) protein gene	Detection
Bocavirus	ssDNA	~5,500	Viral protein (VP1) Nonstructural protein (NP1)	Detection

Abbreviations: ORF, open reading frame; UTR, untranslated region.

PCR has been extensively evaluated for the rapid diagnosis of *C pneumoniae* infection using various assays.[74] A standardized approach to *C pneumoniae* diagnostic testing was published in 2001 by the US Centers for Disease Control and Prevention and the Canadian Laboratory Center for Disease Control.[75] However, there are still few evaluations that have extensively used clinical samples, and the great variety in the methods used makes it difficult to make firm conclusions about performance. To further complicate matters, significant interlaboratory discordance of detection rates have been recorded for some assays.[76,77]

The diagnostic yield from PCR is consistently greater than for culture when testing nasopharyngeal samples for *Bordetella pertussis*.[27] PCR remains positive for a longer period after the onset of symptoms and thus is useful for individuals who present late in their illness.[78] In the investigation of a pertussis outbreak, the combination of PCR and culture for samples obtained 2 weeks or less after illness onset and PCR alone for samples obtained more than 2 weeks after illness onset proved to be the most diagnostically useful.[79]

PCR has greater sensitivity than cytologic methods for the detection of *Pneumocystis jiroveci*, although it has been difficult to interpret the common finding of PCR-positive samples that are negative by standard methods.[27] The latter may reflect *P jiroveci* colonization of uncertain clinical significance. The performance of PCR has been shown to vary with different assays,[80] although the results correlate well with clinical evidence of pneumocystis pneumonia.[81]

The need for improved diagnostic methods for tuberculosis has focused attention on the potential role of NAATs. Advances in this area have been relatively slow, with NAATs for mycobacteria failing to provide greater sensitivity than culture-based methods. The relatively high false-negative rate with NAATs for *Mycobacterium tuberculosis* probably reflects a combination of the paucibacillary nature of samples, presence of inhibitors in samples, and suboptimal DNA extraction methods. The situation is changing, with new developments in rapid diagnosis and antibiotic susceptibility testing.[82] For direct detection of *M tuberculosis* in respiratory samples, all commercial assays have high specificity (>98%), but variable sensitivities: 90% to 100% for smear-positive samples and 33% to 100% for smear-negative samples.[27] Consequently, it is recommended that use of these tests is restricted to only smear-positive samples. Evaluations of PCR for the diagnosis of tuberculosis in high-prevalence populations have been promising.[83–86] Alternative strategies under development to diagnose tuberculosis by molecular tools include detection of mycobacterial DNA in urine[87,88] and direct detection in respiratory specimens by microarray.[89]

New Pathogen Discovery

The NAATs discussed herein target known pathogens. When NAATs fail to identify an agent, additional tools are needed to pursue an etiologic diagnosis as might be indicated in an outbreak setting. These additional methods include microarrays and high-throughput sequencing.[42,90,91] Proteomics also has a potential for being developed as a tool for pathogen discovery.[92]

BREATH ANALYSIS

Breath analysis is an exciting new area with enormous diagnostic potential.[93–95] Alveolar breath contains many biomarkers derived from the blood by passive diffusion across the alveolar membrane,[93] and also contains direct markers of lung injury.[96–98] Breath testing is noninvasive, easily repeatable, and requires minimal specimen workup. Various testing methodologies and sample types have been used in breath research, usually involving the measurement of exhaled permanent gases, detection of volatile organic compounds, or analysis of exhaled breath condensate.

The use of breath analysis for the investigation of respiratory infections has not yet been extensively evaluated. Electronic nose devices detect volatile molecules as they interact with chemical sensor assays.[99–101] Based on the reactivity of multiple sensors to the volatile molecules, an electronic signature is generated. Testing of exhaled breath by a portable electronic nose has been used to diagnose pneumonia in mechanically ventilated patients.[102–104] The clinical impact of this device needs further evaluation, but it could be used as a trigger for further diagnostic studies in pneumonia such as bronchoscopy.

Microorganisms produce volatile metabolites that may be used as biomarkers.[105] Detection of these biomarkers in breath samples by gas chromatography/mass spectroscopy or similar methods may provide an etiologic diagnosis of respiratory tract infection. Ideally, specific biomarkers need to be identified, and it may be difficult to discover unique markers for each pathogen produced in sufficient quantities to enable detection. Potential biomarkers have been reported for some respiratory pathogens, such as *Aspergillus fumigatus*[106,107] and *M tuberculosis*,[108,109] but it is still uncertain whether they will prove to be useful as clinical diagnostic tools.

FUTURE PROSPECTS

Diagnostic tests for respiratory infections will continue to evolve and become more user-friendly. Antigen-detection assays in immunochromatographic or similar formats are rapid, simple to perform, and are most easily developed as near-patient tests. These methods are among the most attractive diagnostic tools, but further development is reliant on the discovery of suitable antigens that can be reliably detected in readily obtained specimens. NAATs have now been developed to a stage where multiplex assays that detect the common respiratory pathogens are commercially available, although not all have been rigorously evaluated in clinical settings. Further improvements in design and performance are expected, and an emphasis should be placed on clarifying the clinical usefulness of NAATs, developing standardized methods, producing even more user-friendly platforms, and exploring the role of quantitative assays. New approaches for respiratory pathogen detection are desperately needed. Breath analysis is an exciting new area with enormous potential, and it will be interesting to follow progress in this area over the next few years.

REFERENCES

1. Peiris JSM, Yuen KY, Osterhaus A, et al. Current concepts: the severe acute respiratory syndrome. N Engl J Med 2003;349:2431–41.
2. WHO Collaborating Center. CDC protocol of real-time RT-PCR for influenza A (H1N1), 2009. Available at: http://www.who.int/csr/resources/publications/swineflu/CDCRealtimeRTPCR_SwineH1Assay-2009_20090430.pdf. Accessed May 22, 2010.
3. Murdoch DR, O'Brien KL, Scott JAG, et al. Breathing new life into pneumonia diagnostics. J Clin Microbiol 2009;47:3405–8.
4. Werno AM, Murdoch DR. Laboratory diagnosis of invasive pneumococcal disease. Clin Infect Dis 2008;46:926–32.
5. Dowell SF, Garman RL, Liu G, et al. Evaluation of Binax NOW, an assay for the detection of pneumococcal antigen in urine samples, performed among pediatric patients. Clin Infect Dis 2001;32:824–5.

6. Cima-Cabal MD, Méndez FJ, Vázquez F, et al. Immunodetection of pneumolysin in human urine by ELISA. J Microbiol Methods 2003;54:47–55.

7. García-Suárez MDM, Cima-Cabal MD, Villaverde R, et al. Performance of a pneumolysin ELISA assay for the diagnosis of pneumococcal infections. J Clin Microbiol 2007;45:3549–54.

8. Rajalakshmi B, Kanungo R, Srinivasan S, et al. Pneumolysin in urine: a rapid antigen detection method to diagnose pneumococcal pneumonia in children. Ind J Med Microbiol 2002;20:183–6.

9. Murdoch DR. Diagnosis of Legionella infection. Clin Infect Dis 2003;36:64–9.

10. Harrison T, Uldum S, Alexiou-Daniel S, et al. A multicenter evaluation of the Biotest legionella urinary antigen EIA. Clin Microbiol Infect 1998;4:359–65.

11. Abanses JC, Dowd MD, Simon SD, et al. Impact of rapid influenza testing at triage on management of febrile infants and young children. Pediatr Emerg Care 2006;22:145–9.

12. Jafri HS, Ramilo O, Makari D, et al. Diagnostic virology practices for respiratory syncytial virus and influenza virus among children in the hospital setting: a national survey. Pediatr Infect Dis J 2007;26:956–8.

13. Jennings LC, Skopnik H, Burckhardt I, et al. Effect of rapid influenza testing on the clinical management of paediatric influenza. Influenza Other Respi Viruses 2009;3:91–8.

14. Hurt AC, Alexander R, Hibbert J, et al. Performance of six influenza rapid tests in detecting human influenza in clinical specimens. J Clin Virol 2007;39:132–5.

15. Uyeki TM. Influenza diagnosis and treatment in children: a review of studies on clinically useful tests and antiviral treatment for influenza. Pediatr Infect Dis J 2003;22:164–77.

16. Smit M, Beynon KA, Murdoch DR, et al. Comparison of the NOW Influenza A & B, NOW Flu A, NOW Flu B, and Directigen Flu A+B assays, and immunofluorescence with viral culture for the detection of influenza A and B viruses. Diagn Microbiol Infect Dis 2007;57:67–70.

17. World Health Organization. WHO recommendations on the use of rapid testing for influenza diagnosis. WHO, 2005; Available at: http://www.who.int/csr/disease/avian_influenza/guidelines/rapid_testing/en/index.html. Accessed May 22, 2010.

18. Chan KH, Lai ST, Poon LL, et al. Analytical sensitivity of rapid influenza antigen detection tests for swine-origin influenza virus (H1N1). J Clin Virol 2009;45:205–7.

19. Hurt AC, Baas C, Deng YM, et al. Performance of influenza rapid point-of-care tests in the detection of swine lineage A(H1N1) influenza viruses. Influenza Other Respir Viruses 2009;3:171–6.

20. Centers for Disease Control and Prevention. Evaluation of rapid influenza diagnostic tests for detection of novel influenza A (H1N1) virus—United States, 2009. MMWR Morb Mortal Wkly Rep 2009;58:826–9.

21. Faix DJ, Sherman SS, Waterman SH. Rapid-test sensitivity for novel swine-origin influenza A (H1N1) virus in humans. N Engl J Med 2009;361:728–9.

22. Ginocchio CC, Zhang F, Manji R, et al. Evaluation of multiple test methods for the detection of the novel 2009 influenza A (H1N1) during the New York City outbreak. J Clin Virol 2009;45:191–5.

23. Borek AP, Clemens SH, Gaskins VK, et al. Respiratory syncytial virus detection by Remel Xpect, Binax Now RSV, direct immunofluorescent staining, and tissue culture. J Clin Microbiol 2006;44:1105–7.

24. Selvarangan R, Abel D, Hamilton M. Comparison of BD Directigen EZ RSV and Binax NOW RSV tests for rapid detection of respiratory syncytial virus from

nasopharyngeal aspirates in a pediatric population. Diagn Microbiol Infect Dis 2008;62:157–61.

25. Zheng X, Quianzon S, Mu Y, et al. Comparison of two new rapid antigen detection assays for respiratory syncytial virus with another assay and shell vial culture. J Clin Virol 2004;31:130–3.

26. Casiano-Colón AE, Hulbert BB, Mayer TK, et al. Lack of sensitivity of rapid antigen tests for the diagnosis of respiratory syncytial virus infection in adults. J Clin Virol 2003;28:169–74.

27. Murdoch DR. Molecular genetic methods in the diagnosis of lower respiratory tract infections. APMIS 2004;112:713–27.

28. Barken KB, Haagensen JAJ, Tolker-Nielsen T. Advances in nucleic acid-based diagnostics of bacterial infections. Clin Chim Acta 2007;384:1–11.

29. Ieven M. Currently used nucleic acid amplification tests for the detection of viruses and atypicals in acute respiratory infections. J Clin Virol 2007;40:259–76.

30. Brunstein JD, Cline CL, McKinney S, et al. Evidence from multiplex molecular assays for complex multipathogen interactions in acute respiratory infections. J Clin Microbiol 2008;46:97–102.

31. Li H, McCormac MA, Estes RW, et al. Simultaneous detection and high-throughput identification of a panel of RNA viruses causing respiratory tract infections. J Clin Microbiol 2007;45:2105–9.

32. Kim SR, Ki CS, Lee NY. Rapid detection and identification of 12 respiratory viruses using a dual priming oligonucleotide system-based multiplex PCR assay. J Virol Methods 2009;156:111–6.

33. Roh KH, Kim J, Nam MH, et al. Comparison of the Seeplex reverse transcription PCR assay with the R-mix viral culture and immunofluorescence techniques for detection of eight respiratory viruses. Ann Clin Lab Sci 2008;38:41–6.

34. Lee WM, Grindle K, Pappas T, et al. High-throughput, sensitive, and accurate multiplex PCR-microsphere flow cytometry system for large-scale comprehensive detection of respiratory viruses. J Clin Microbiol 2007;45:2626–34.

35. Marshall DJ, Reisdorf E, Harms G, et al. Evaluation of a multiplexed PCR assay for detection of respiratory viral pathogens in a public health laboratory setting. J Clin Microbiol 2007;45:3875–82.

36. Nolte FS, Marshall DJ, Rasberry C, et al. MultiCode-PLx system for multiplexed detection of seventeen respiratory viruses. J Clin Microbiol 2007;45:2779–86.

37. Mahony J, Chong S, Merante F, et al. Development of a respiratory virus panel test for detection of twenty human respiratory viruses by use of multiplex PCR and a fluid microbead-based assay. J Clin Microbiol 2007;45:2965–70.

38. Pabbaraju K, Tokaryk KL, Wong S, et al. Comparison of the Luminex xTAG respiratory viral panel with in-house nucleic acid amplification tests for diagnosis of respiratory virus infections. J Clin Microbiol 2008;46:3056–62.

39. Chiu CY, Urisman A, Greenhow TL, et al. Utility of DNA microarrays for detection of viruses in acute respiratory tract infections in children. J Pediatr 2008;153:76–83.

40. Quan P-L, Palacios G, Jabado OJ, et al. Detection of respiratory viruses and subtype identification of influenza A viruses by GreeneChipResp oligonucleotide microarray. J Clin Microbiol 2007;45:2359–64.

41. Raymond F, Carbonneau J, Boucher N, et al. Comparison of automated microarray detection with real-time PCR assays for detection of respiratory viruses in specimens obtained from children. J Clin Microbiol 2009;47:743–50.

42. Quan P-L, Briese T, Palacios G, et al. Rapid sequence-based diagnosis of viral infection. Antiviral Res 2008;79:1–5.

43. Briese T, Palacios G, Kokoris M, et al. Diagnostic system for rapid and sensitive differential detection of pathogens. Emerg Infect Dis 2005;11:310–3.
44. Dominguez SR, Briese T, Palacios G, et al. Multiplex MassTag-PCR for respiratory pathogens in pediatric nasopharyngeal washes negative by conventional diagnostic testing shows a high prevalence of viruses belonging to a newly recognized rhinovirus clade. J Clin Virol 2008;43:219–22.
45. Lamson D, Renwick N, Kapoor V, et al. MassTag polymerase-chain-reaction detection of respiratory pathogens, including a new rhinovirus genotype, that caused influenza-like illness in New York State during 2004-2005. J Infect Dis 2006;194:1398–402.
46. Renwick N, Schweiger B, Kapoor V, et al. A recently identified rhinovirus genotype is associated with severe respiratory-tract infection in children in Germany. J Infect Dis 2007;196:1754–60.
47. Ecker DJ, Sampath R, Massire C, et al. Ibis T5000: a universal biosensor approach for microbiology. Nature Rev Microbiol 2008;6:553–8.
48. Loens K, Van Heirstraeten L, Malhotra-Kumar S, et al. Optimal sampling sites and methods for detection of pathogens possibly causing community-acquired lower respiratory tract infections. J Clin Microbiol 2009;47:21–31.
49. Fox JD. Nucleic acid amplification tests for detection or respiratory viruses. J Clin Virol 2007;40(Suppl 1):S15–23.
50. Mahony JB. Detection of respiratory viruses by molecular methods. Clin Microbiol Rev 2008;21:716–47.
51. Jennings LC, Anderson TP, Beynon KA, et al. Incidence and characteristics of viral community-acquired pneumonia in adults. Thorax 2008;63:42–8.
52. Dagan R, Shriker O, Hazan I, et al. Prospective study to determine clinical relevance of detection of pneumococcal DNA in sera of children by PCR. J Clin Microbiol 1998;36:669–73.
53. Rudolph KM, Parkinson AJ, Black CM, et al. Evaluation of polymerase chain reaction for diagnosis of pneumococcal pneumonia. J Clin Microbiol 1993;31: 2661–6.
54. Salo P, Ortqvist A, Leinonen M. Diagnosis of bacteremic pneumococcal pneumonia by amplification of pneumolysin gene fragment in serum. J Infect Dis 1995;171:479–82.
55. Murdoch DR, Anderson TP, Beynon KA, et al. Evaluation of a PCR assay for detection of Streptococcus pneumoniae in respiratory and nonrespiratory samples from adults with community-acquired pneumonia. J Clin Microbiol 2003;41:63–6.
56. Sheppard CL, Harrison TG, Morris R, et al. Autolysin-targeting LightCycler assay including internal process control for detection of Streptococcus pneumoniae DNA in clinical samples. J Med Microbiol 2004;53:189–95.
57. Carvalho MGS, Tondella ML, McCaustland K, et al. Evaluation and improvement of real-time PCR assays targeting lytA, ply, and psaA genes for detection of pneumococcal DNA. J Clin Microbiol 2007;45:2460–6.
58. Smith MD, Sheppard CL, Hogan A, et al. Diagnosis of Streptococcus pneumoniae infections in adults with bacteremia and community-acquired pneumonia: clinical comparison of pneumococcal PCR and urinary antigen detection. J Clin Microbiol 2009;47:1046–9.
59. Kais M, Spindler C, Kalin M, et al. Quantitative detection of Streptococcus pneumoniae, Haemophilus influenzae, and Moraxella catarrhalis in lower respiratory tract samples by real-time PCR. Diagn Microbiol Infect Dis 2006;55: 169–78.

60. Carrol ED, Guiver M, Nkhoma S, et al. High pneumococcal DNA loads are associated with mortality in Malawian children with invasive pneumococcal disease. Pediatr Infect Dis J 2007;26:416–22.
61. Peters RPH, de Boer RF, Schuurman T, et al. *Streptococcus pneumoniae* DNA load in blood as marker of infection in patients with community-acquired pneumonia. J Clin Microbiol 2009;47:3308–12.
62. Rello J, Lisboa T, Lujan M, et al. Severity of pneumococcal pneumonia associated with genomic bacterial load. Chest 2009;136:832–40.
63. Beersma MFC, Dirven K, van Dam AP, et al. Evaluation of 12 commercial tests and the complement fixation test for *Mycoplasma pneumoniae*-specific immunoglobulin G (IgG) and IgM antibodies, with PCR use as the "gold standard". J Clin Microbiol 2005;43:2277–85.
64. Daxboeck F, Krause R, Wenisch C. Laboratory diagnosis of *Mycoplasma pneumoniae* infection. Clin Microbiol Infect 2003;9:263–73.
65. Kim NH, Lee JA, Eun BW, et al. Comparison of polymerase chain reaction and the indirect particle agglutination antibody test for the diagnosis of *Mycoplasma pneumoniae* pneumonia in children during two outbreaks. Pediatr Infect Dis J 2007;26:897–903.
66. Liu F-C, Chen P-Y, Huang F-L, et al. Rapid diagnosis of *Mycoplasma pneumoniae* infection in children by polymerase chain reaction. J Microbiol Immunol Infect 2007;40:507–12.
67. Cloud JL, Carroll KC, Pixton P, et al. Detection of *Legionella* species in respiratory specimens using PCR with sequencing confirmation. J Clin Microbiol 2000; 38:1709–12.
68. Jaulhac B, Nowicki M, Bornstein N, et al. Detection of *Legionella* spp. in bronchoalveolar lavage fluids by DNA amplification. J Clin Microbiol 1992;30:920–4.
69. Jonas D, Rosenbaum A, Weyrich S, et al. Enzyme-linked immunoassay for detection of PCR-amplified DNA of legionellae in bronchoalveolar fluid. J Clin Microbiol 1995;33:1247–52.
70. Kessler HH, Reinthaler FF, Pschaid A, et al. Rapid detection of *Legionella* species in bronchoalveolar lavage fluids with the EnviroAmp *Legionella* PCR amplification and detection kit. J Clin Microbiol 1993;31:3325–8.
71. Lisby G, Dessau R. Construction of a DNA amplification assay for detection of *Legionella* species in clinical samples. Eur J Clin Microbiol Infect Dis 1994;13: 225–31.
72. Matsiota-Bernard P, Pitsouni E, Legakis N, et al. Evaluation of commercial amplification kit for detection of *Legionella pneumophila* in clinical specimens. J Clin Microbiol 1994;32:1503–5.
73. Weir SC, Fischer SH, Stock F, et al. Detection of *Legionella* by PCR in respiratory specimens using a commercially available kit. Am J Clin Pathol 1998;110: 295–300.
74. Kumar S, Hammerschlag MR. Acute respiratory infection due to *Chlamydia pneumoniae*: current status of diagnostic methods. Clin Infect Dis 2007;44: 568–76.
75. Dowell SF, Peeling RW, Boman J, et al. Standardizing *Chlamydia pneumoniae* assays: recommendations from the Centers for Diseases Control and Prevention (USA) and the Laboratory Centre for Disease Control (Canada). Clin Infect Dis 2001;33:492–503.
76. Apfalter P, Assadian O, Blasi F, et al. Reliability of nested PCR for detection of *Chlamydia pneumoniae* DNA in atheromas: results from a multicenter study applying standardized protocols. J Clin Microbiol 2002;40:4428–34.

77. Apfalter P, Blasi F, Boman J, et al. Multicenter comparison trial of DNA extraction methods and PCR assays for detection of *Chlamydia pneumoniae* in endarterectomy specimens. J Clin Microbiol 2001;39:519–24.

78. Muller FM, Hoppe JE, Wirsing von Kohig CH. Laboratory diagnosis of pertussis: state of the art in 1997. J Clin Microbiol 1997;35:2435–43.

79. Sotir MJ, Cappozzo DL, Warshauer DM, et al. Evaluation of polymerase chain reaction and culture for diagnosis of pertussis in the control of a county-wide outbreak focused among adolescents and adults. Clin Infect Dis 2007;44:1216–9.

80. Robberts FJL, Liebowitz LD, Chalkley LJ. Polymerase chain reaction detection of *Pneumocystis jiroveci*: evaluation of 9 assays. Diagn Microbiol Infect Dis 2007;58:385–92.

81. Azoulay E, Bergeron A, Chevret S, et al. Polymerase chain reaction for diagnosing pneumocystis pneumonia in non-HIV immunocompromised patients with pulmonary infiltrates. Chest 2009;135:655–61.

82. Balasingham SV, Davidsen T, Szpinda I, et al. Molecular diagnostics in tuberculosis: basis and implications for therapy. Mol Diagn Ther 2009;13:137–51.

83. Kibiki GS, Mulder B, van der Ven AJ, et al. Laboratory diagnosis of pulmonary tuberculosis in TB and HIV endemic settings and the contribution of real time PCR for *M. tuberculosis* in bronchoalveolar lavage fluid. Trop Med Int Health 2007;12:1210–7.

84. Kivihya-Ndugga L, van Cleeff M, Juma E, et al. Comparison of PCR with the routine procedure for diagnosis of tuberculosis in a population with high prevalences of tuberculosis and human immunodeficiency virus. J Clin Microbiol 2004;42:1012–5.

85. Ani A, Okpe S, Akambi M, et al. Comparison of a DNA based PCR method with conventional methods for the detection of M. tuberculosis in Jos, Nigeria. J Infect Dev Ctries 2009;3:470–5.

86. Ben Kahla I, Ben Selma W, Marzouk M, et al. Evaluation of a simplified IS6110 PCR for the rapid diagnosis of *Mycobacterium tuberculosis* in an area with high tuberculosis incidence. Pathol Biol. DOI:10.1016/j.patbio.2009.04.001.

87. Green C, Huggett JF, Talbot E, et al. Rapid diagnosis of tuberculosis through the detection of mycobacterial DNA in urine by nucleic acid amplification methods. Lancet Infect Dis 2009;9:505–11.

88. Gopinath K, Singh S. Urine as an adjunct specimen for the diagnosis of active pulmonary tuberculosis. Int J Infect Dis 2009;13:374–9.

89. Chang HJ, Huang MY, Yeh CS, et al. Rapid diagnosis of tuberculosis directly from clinical specimens by gene chip. Clin Microbiol Infect. DOI:10.1111/j.1469-0691.2009.03045.x.

90. Lipkin WI, Gustavo P, Thomas B. Diagnostics and discovery in viral hemorrhagic fevers. Ann N Y Acad Sci 2009;1171(S1):E6–11.

91. Palacios G, Druce J, Du L, et al. A new arenavirus in a cluster of fatal transplant-associated diseases. N Engl J Med 2008;358:991–8.

92. Ye Y, Mar E-C, Tong S, et al. Application of proteomics methods for pathogen discovery. J Virol Methods 2010;163:87–95.

93. Cao W, Duan Y. Breath analysis: potential for clinical diagnosis and exposure assessment. Clin Chem 2006;52:800–11.

94. Corradi M, Mutti A. Exhaled breath analysis: from occupational to respiratory medicine. Acta Biomed 2005;76(Suppl 2):20–9.

95. Risby TH, Solga SF. Current status of clinical breath analysis. Appl Phys B 2006; 85:421–6.
96. Majewska E, Kasielski M, Luczynski R, et al. Elevated exhalation of hydrogen peroxide and thiobarbituric acid reactive substances in patients with community acquired pneumonia. Respir Med 2004;98:669–76.
97. Romero PV, Rodríguez B, Martínez S, et al. Analysis of oxidative stress in exhaled breath condensate from patients with severe pulmonary infections. Arch Bronconeumol 2006;42:113–9.
98. Sack U, Scheibe R, Wötzel M, et al. Multiplex analysis of cytokines in exhaled breath condensate. Cytometry A 2006;69:169–72.
99. Nagle HT, Schiffman SS, Gutierrez-Osuna R. The how and why of electronic noses. IEEE Spectrum 1998;35:22–34.
100. Pearce TC. Computational parallels between the biological olfactory pathway and its analogue 'The Electronic Nose': Part I. Biological olfaction. Biosystems 1997;41:43–67.
101. Thaler ER, Hanson CW. Medical applications of electronic nose technology. Expert Rev Med Devices 2005;2:559–66.
102. Hanson CW, Thaler ER. Electronic nose prediction of a clinical pneumonia score: biosensors and microbes. Anesthesiology 2005;102:63–8.
103. Hockstein NG, Thaler ER, Lin Y, et al. Correlation of pneumonia score with electronic nose signature: a prospective study. Ann Otol Rhinol Laryngol 2005;114: 504–8.
104. Hockstein NG, Thaler ER, Torigian D, et al. Diagnosis of pneumonia with an electronic nose: correlation of vapor signature with chest computed tomography scan findings. Laryngoscope 2004;114:1701–5.
105. Allardyce RA, Langford VS, Hill AL, et al. Detection of volatile metabolites produced by bacterial growth in blood culture media by selected ion flow tube mass spectrometry (SIFT-MS). J Microbiol Meth 2006;65:361–5.
106. Syhre M, Scotter JM, Chambers ST. Investigation into the production of 2-pentylfuran by *Aspergillus fumigatus* and other respiratory pathogens *in vitro* and human breath samples. Med Mycol 2008;46:209–15.
107. Chambers ST, Syhre M, Murdoch DR, et al. Detection of 2-pentylfuran in the breath of patients with *Aspergillus fumigatus*. Med Mycol 2009;47:468–76.
108. Syhre M, Chambers ST. The scent of *Mycobacterium tuberculosis*. Tuberculosis 2008;88:317–23.
109. Syhre M, Manning L, Phuanukoonnon S, et al. The scent of *Mycobacterium tuberculosis*—Part II: breath. Tuberculosis 2009;89:263–6.

Antiviral Drug Resistance: Mechanisms and Clinical Implications

Lynne Strasfeld, MD*, Sunwen Chou, MD

KEYWORDS

- Drug resistance • Transplant • Cytomegalovirus
- Herpes simplex virus • Varicella zoster virus
- Hepatitis B virus

In the setting of intensive immunosuppression for the management of rejection in solid organ transplant (SOT) recipients, or graft-versus-host disease (GVHD) in hematopoietic stem cell transplant (HSCT) recipients, antiviral therapy is commonly used and drug-resistant viruses are increasingly encountered. Prolonged antiviral drug exposure and ongoing viral replication due to immunosuppression are key factors in the development of antiviral drug resistance, which may manifest as persistent or increasing viremia or disease despite therapy. Consequences of drug resistance range from toxicity inherent in use of second-line antivirals, to severe disease and even death from progressive viral infection when no effective alternative treatments are available. In this article, the authors review the mechanisms, implications, and management of resistance to antiviral drugs used to treat several viral infections that play a significant role in the clinical course of transplant recipients and oncology patients: cytomegalovirus (CMV), herpes simplex virus (HSV), varicella zoster virus (VZV), and hepatitis B virus (HBV).

HERPESVIRUSES

Antiviral Agents and Mechanism of Action

All of the currently licensed drugs for systemic treatment of herpesvirus infections share the same target, viral DNA polymerase. The most commonly used drugs are the nucleoside analogues acyclovir and ganciclovir. Acyclovir, its more bioavailable prodrug valacyclovir, and famciclovir (the prodrug of penciclovir) are used for HSV

Dr Chou was supported by NIH grant AI39938.

Division of Infectious Diseases, Oregon Health & Science University, 3181 SW Sam Jackson Park Road, mail code L457, Portland, OR 97239, USA

* Corresponding author.

E-mail address: strasfel@ohsu.edu

Infect Dis Clin N Am 24 (2010) 809–833

doi:10.1016/j.idc.2010.07.001

0891-5520/10/$ – see front matter © 2010 Elsevier Inc. All rights reserved.

id.theclinics.com

and VZV infections but have weak anti-CMV activity. Ganciclovir and its valine ester prodrug valganciclovir have in vitro activity against HSV, VZV, and CMV, and are Food and Drug Administration (FDA)-approved for CMV infection, for which antiviral potency outweighs the increased toxicity as compared with acyclovir.

Acyclovir is monophosphorylated by thymidine kinase (TK) expressed by HSV (UL23) or VZV (ORF36) and then converted by cellular kinases to the active form, acyclovir triphosphate. Acyclovir triphosphate inhibits HSV and VZV replication by competitive inhibition of viral DNA polymerase and by chain termination of viral DNA strands.[1,2] Selectivity is related to preferential activation of acyclovir by viral TK and to the greater sensitivity of viral compared with cellular DNA polymerase to acyclovir triphosphate. Penciclovir, the active metabolite of famciclovir, has a similar mechanism of activation and action. Ganciclovir is monophosphorylated by the CMV UL97 kinase, or HSV or VZV TK, with subsequent antiviral action analogous to acyclovir. Unlike acyclovir, ganciclovir is not an obligate chain terminator, but rather causes a slowing and subsequent cessation of viral DNA chain elongation.[3]

Foscarnet, a pyrophosphate analogue, and cidofovir, a nucleotide analogue, do not depend on prior activation by viral enzymes. Foscarnet binds selectively to viral DNA polymerase at the pyrophosphate-binding site, blocking cleavage of the pyrophosphate moiety from deoxynucleotide triphosphates, in turn halting DNA chain elongation. Cidofovir is phosphorylated by cellular enzymes, and once activated acts as a potent inhibitor of the viral DNA polymerase. Foscarnet and cidofovir are typically used as second- and third-line herpesvirus drugs, respectively, when there is either suspected or documented resistance to initial therapy or dose-limiting toxicities of first-line drugs.

Use of these antiviral drugs may be affected by dose-limiting toxicities. Although acyclovir is usually considered relatively nontoxic, high doses are associated with nephrotoxicity[4] and encephalopathy.[5,6] High-dose valacyclovir has been associated with thrombotic microangiopathy in immunocompromised hosts.[7] Ganciclovir and valganciclovir frequently cause myelosuppression, especially neutropenia.[8,9] Foscarnet is associated with significant nephrotoxicity and electrolyte abnormalities.[10,11] Cidofovir is associated with nephrotoxicity and neutropenia when administered intravenously,[12] and with application site irritation when administered topically.[13]

In Vitro Evaluation of Antiviral Susceptibility

In vitro drug susceptibility testing of herpesviruses is by phenotypic and/or genotypic assays. Phenotypic assays measure drug susceptibility by culturing a calibrated viral inoculum under serial drug dilutions, thereby arriving at the drug concentration required to inhibit viral growth by 50% or 90% from the level observed without drug, referred to as the IC_{50} or IC_{90}, respectively. The IC_{50} is the value usually reported because it is more reproducible than the IC_{90} value. The IC_{50} threshold for susceptible strains is assay dependent, with the cutoff for sensitivity typically set at 3 to 5 times the mean IC_{50} for susceptible strains. In the classic plaque reduction assay (PRA), viral growth is measured as the number of visible plaques formed in cell culture monolayers after a fixed incubation period. The PRA is poorly standardized as to what constitutes a viral plaque, is labor-intensive, and is affected by a variety of culture conditions such as the type, density, and growth phase of cells, the viral inoculum, and the drug concentration range. Efforts were made to standardize a PRA technique for CMV susceptibility testing,[14] though in practice a great deal of variability remains, and the assay is clinically impractical because of the slow growth of CMV and the increasing use of molecular diagnostic assays that do not yield a live isolate for phenotypic testing. On the other hand, phenotypic testing for the more rapidly growing HSV is a preferred approach to resistance testing for this virus. To improve assay efficiency and reduce subjectivity, plaque counting can be replaced by viral quantitation methods that depend on assay of viral antigen or nucleic acid, or a reporter gene that is activated by viral infection. A reporter-based yield reduction system has been used for rapid phenotypic testing of HSV clinical isolates and laboratory strains.[15]

Genotypic assays depend on knowledge of the viral mutations causing resistance to specific antiviral drugs and the level of resistance and cross-resistance conferred by single and multiple mutations. These assays work best when a limited number of characteristic mutations are regularly encountered in connection with resistance to a specific drug, and are well supported by an accessible information database necessary for accurate interpretation. Genotypic tests have a faster turnaround time than phenotype assays and use a common technology of polymerase chain reaction (PCR) amplification of viral sequences followed by analysis for diagnostic mutations. A viral culture isolate is not needed, and viral DNA can be amplified directly from blood, fluid, or tissue specimens. Limitations of genotypic assays include difficulties with interpretation of viral sequence changes not found in the current information database, and the effective levels of resistance that result from combinations of mutations. There are also technical issues relating to DNA amplification and the sensitivity of detection of viral mutations when present as a minor subpopulation mixed with wild-type virus.

Genotype-phenotype correlations are confirmed by recombinant phenotyping, also known as marker transfer, whereby individual mutations suspected of causing drug resistance are transferred to baseline viral strains and their effect on drug susceptibility is established by phenotypic assays. A large volume of this work has been done for CMV because of the dominant role of genotypic resistance testing for this virus. Recombinant phenotyping has also been done to determine the significance of various TK and DNA polymerase gene mutations for HSV and VZV drug resistance,[16,17] but given the number and variety of TK resistance mutations, resistance testing of HSV and VZV isolates is more reliant on phenotypic approaches.

HERPES SIMPLEX VIRUS
Epidemiology of Antiviral Resistance

Acyclovir, valacyclovir, and famciclovir are drugs of choice for mucocutaneous HSV infections and for preventive treatment, while intravenous acyclovir is used for serious invasive disease such as encephalitis. The first clinical cases of acyclovir-resistant HSV were reported in 1982, shortly after initial use of systemically administered acyclovir.[18,19] Despite the subsequent widespread use of acyclovir, clinically evident drug resistance remains largely confined to the immunocompromised population, and the frequency of isolation of acyclovir-resistant HSV has remained stable over time.[20] Drug-resistant HSV disease is rare in immunocompetent hosts (<1% in various reports), and typically is cleared without adverse clinical outcome.[20–24] In immunocompromised hosts the prevalence ranges from 3.5% to 14%, with the most the most immunosuppressed subset having the highest risk for resistance.[20–25] Prolonged use of acyclovir is an important risk factor for resistant HSV, but drug-resistant HSV has been isolated in the absence of a known history of acyclovir exposure.[26]

Mechanisms of Resistance

Resistance of HSV to acyclovir is related to viral TK or DNA polymerase mutations.[27] As viral TK is not essential for HSV replication, more than 90% of acyclovir resistance in clinical isolates is associated with TK mutations.[28] TK mutations may result in either a loss of TK activity (TK deleted or deficient virus) or, less commonly, an alteration in TK substrate specificity (TK altered virus).[28] Mutations in the TK gene are often due to addition or deletion of nucleotides in homopolymer runs of guanines and cytosines, resulting in frameshifting and loss of TK function.[29,30] The specific TK mutations resulting from penciclovir exposure differ from those selected by acyclovir; cross-resistance is expected with TK deficient mutants, though certain acyclovir-resistant TK altered mutants appear to retain in vitro sensitivity to penciclovir.[31] In addition, resistance to ganciclovir is presumed in the case of TK-deficient mutants.[32] Drug-resistant TK mutants retain susceptibility to drugs that are not dependent on virally mediated phosphorylation, including foscarnet and cidofovir, unless a viral DNA polymerase mutation is also present. Given the essential role of viral DNA polymerase in viral replication, mutations in this gene occur less frequently and have been observed to cluster in functional domains II and III. The cross-resistance patterns of these mutations vary and are evaluated by recombinant phenotyping.[3,33]

Clinical Implications and Management of Resistant Virus

The clinical implications of antiviral-resistant HSV are related to the direct effects of viral infection as well as the toxicities of second-line agents. Unchecked viral replication can lead to progressive and sometimes fatal invasive HSV disease.[32,34,35] Recurrent, chronic, and extensive mucocutaneous HSV ulcerations have been observed in immunocompromised individuals with drug-resistant virus.[36] Drug-resistant HSV has been associated with decreased neurovirulence in murine models when compared with wild-type virus,[37,38] with TK null mutants having the greatest reduction in virulence.[39] Though previously thought to lack the ability to establish and reactivate from latency, it is now appreciated that TK null mutants may be able to do so by way of reversion, due to ribosomal frameshifting or replication errors that create subpopulations of TK altered virus.[40,41] Human data for decreased pathogenicity of drug-resistant HSV are lacking.

In clinical practice, management of suspected or proven acyclovir-resistant HSV is generally with foscarnet, or less often with cidofovir. Management is often done empirically based on the frequency of TK mutations, but cross-resistance may result from DNA polymerase mutations, and emergence of both foscarnet and cidofovir resistance while on therapy has been reported.[36,42] Vidarabine, a purine analogue phosphorylated by cellular kinases with selectivity for HSV DNA polymerase, has in vitro activity against HSV,[43] but clinical experience has been disappointing for acyclovir-resistant HSV in the human immunodeficiency virus (HIV)-infected population.[44] Topical imiquimod, an immunomodulatory agent, or topical cidofovir have been used successfully to treat some cases of drug-resistant mucocutaneous HSV infection.[45,46] Topical treatments avoid the potential nephrotoxicity of systemically administered foscarnet or cidofovir. Management of drug-resistant HSV should include efforts to improve the immune status of the patient, when possible, by decreasing immunosuppressive therapy.

VARICELLA ZOSTER VIRUS
Epidemiology of Antiviral Resistance

The same antiviral drugs are used for VZV as for HSV. Given that acyclovir has less potent activity against VZV than HSV, intravenous administration, frequent and high oral doses, or the more bioavailable oral prodrugs (valacyclovir or famciclovir) are needed to ensure therapeutic antiviral blood levels.[47] Acyclovir-resistant VZV clinical isolates have been reported uncommonly and mostly in the HIV population,[48–51] with a few cases in oncology and transplant recipients.[52,53] Unlike HSV, there are no large surveillance studies of antiviral drug-resistant VZV, and available information exists as case reports and series. Of note, there are 2 cases in the pediatric oncology literature of chronic disseminated varicella disease attributable to the VZV vaccine strain Oka with in vitro documentation of acyclovir resistance.[54,55]

Mechanisms of Resistance

Like HSV, VZV also expresses a TK, and VZV drug resistance is for the most part attributable to TK mutations,[3] which often result in a premature stop codon that makes the virus TK deficient and appear to cluster at particular VZV TK gene loci.[3,53] Limited data from laboratory strains suggest that acyclovir-resistance mutations in the VZV DNA polymerase gene may partially overlap mutations conferring resistance to foscarnet.[3] Not much is known of penciclovir-resistant clinical isolates. Although acyclovir and penciclovir may select in vitro for different patterns of cross-resistance to other antivirals, cross-resistance between the 2 drugs is expected.[56]

Clinical Implications and Management of Resistant Virus

Similar to HSV, the clinical implications of drug-resistant VZV relate to the direct effects of viral replication and to the toxicities of alternative antiviral agents. Cases of visceral dissemination and death due to progressive VZV infection unresponsive to antiviral treatment were reported in HIV-infected subjects.[51] A chronic verrucous form of VZV is associated with drug-resistant virus in immunocompromised hosts.[52,55,57,58] Some VZV DNA polymerase mutants selected under foscarnet in cell culture have a slow-growth phenotype,[59] perhaps suggesting attenuated virulence, although this has not been clinically validated.

Management of suspected or proven acyclovir-resistant VZV is generally with foscarnet, as described mostly in HIV-infected individuals[51,60] and some oncology patients.[52,54,55] Emergence of foscarnet resistance was detected in a few patients being treated with the drug for acyclovir-resistant VZV,[60,61] and attributed to a viral DNA polymerase mutation.[61] Although the literature on cidofovir treatment for drug-resistant VZV is very limited,[62] cidofovir is expected to retain activity against acyclovir-resistant TK mutants.[63] Vidarabine shows in vitro activity against VZV DNA polymerase mutants,[64] though clinical experience is limited.[65] Susceptibility testing of VZV isolates should be performed when drug resistance is suspected on clinical grounds, and any immunosuppressive therapy should be minimized.

CYTOMEGALOVIRUS
Epidemiology of Antiviral Resistance

CMV is a well-recognized opportunistic pathogen in those with AIDS, in SOT and HSCT recipients, and occasionally in nontransplant oncology patients, particularly following major T-cell suppressive regimens.[66] Ganciclovir and valganciclovir are currently the principal drugs used for prevention and treatment of CMV infection, and are widely used in transplant populations. Shortly following the introduction of ganciclovir in the late 1980s, cases of ganciclovir resistance in immunocompromised hosts began to appear in the literature.[67] Much of our knowledge about CMV drug resistance comes from studies of CMV retinitis in the AIDS population in the 1990s.[68,69] More recently, studies have highlighted the problem in the SOT population.[70–78] The overall incidence of ganciclovir resistance among SOT recipients is 0% to 13%, and varies according to the type of organ transplant, the immunosuppressive regimen and antiviral prophylaxis used, and the specific criteria for determining resistance.[79] CMV seronegative recipients of organs from seropositive donors (D+/R− subset), those with prolonged ganciclovir exposure and potent immunosuppression, and lung transplant recipients are at higher risk for developing antiviral drug resistance. In the HSCT setting, the development of ganciclovir resistance is reported to be uncommon and generally limited to case reports and small case series,[80–85] with the exception of the pediatric population for which there have been reports of rapid emergence of resistance[86–88]; this may relate to less ganciclovir exposure in the HSCT population, where a preemptive as opposed to a prophylactic approach to CMV disease prevention is favored. Emergence of resistance to foscarnet and cidofovir has also been reported in the SOT and HSCT population.[76,80,81,86,89–91]

Mechanism of Resistance

The literature on CMV drug resistance mutations is extensive,[92–99] especially for ganciclovir. More than 90% of resistant CMV isolates obtained following ganciclovir exposure contain one or more characteristic mutations in the viral UL97 kinase gene,[98] which apparently decrease the phosphorylation of ganciclovir without impairing the important functions of this kinase in viral replication.[98,100,101] Unlike the case with HSV TK mutations, CMV UL97 drug resistance mutations cluster tightly at codons 460, 520, and 590-607 (**Fig. 1**). Mutations M460V/I, H520Q, C592G, A594V, L595S, and C603W are among the most frequently encountered in ganciclovir-resistant isolates.[98] These mutations individually confer moderate ganciclovir resistance, with an IC_{50} ratio of 5 to 10, except for C592G, which confers low-level ganciclovir resistance with an IC_{50} ratio of about 2.5.[98] These IC_{50} ratios are based on recombinant phenotyping data,[99] which are also available for many other less common UL97 mutations. The accumulated genotype-phenotype correlations are the basis for the CMV genotypic resistance testing that is available in various commercial and academic laboratories.

CMV UL54 DNA polymerase mutations can confer resistance to any or all of the current anti-CMV drugs. Many ganciclovir resistance mutations are located in the exonuclease domains (**Fig. 2**) and typically confer cross-resistance to cidofovir.[92,94] Mutations in and between catalytic regions II (eg, codons 700 and 715), III (eg, codons 802 and 809), VI (eg, codon 781), and at some nonconserved loci (eg, codon 756) confer foscarnet resistance, as well as low-grade ganciclovir or cidofovir cross-resistance in the case of mutations at region III.[3,92,95] Uncommonly, single UL54 mutations can confer simultaneous resistance to ganciclovir, cidofovir, and foscarnet.[89,94,97] The serial emergence of multiple mutations in patients on prolonged CMV antiviral therapy

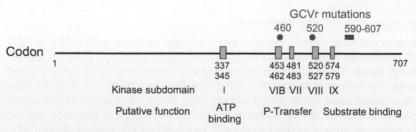

Fig. 1. Map of CMV UL97 gene functional domains and resistance mutations. Ganciclovir resistance (GCVr) mutations are clustered at codons 460, 520, and 590-607. In the latter region mutations A594V, L595S, C592G, and C603W are some of the most common, but a variety of point and in-frame deletion mutations are known to confer varying degrees of GCV resistance. Not all sequence changes at codons 590 to 607 confer ganciclovir resistance. ATP, adenosine triphosphate.

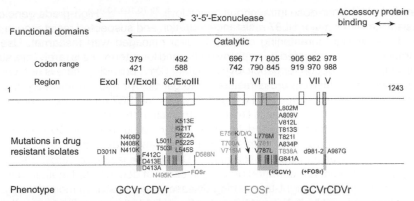

Fig. 2. Map of CMV DNA polymerase functional domains, resistance mutations, and associated phenotypes. All listed mutations have been found in clinical isolates and validated by recombinant phenotyping. Shaded regions indicate where resistance mutations are clustered, with associated phenotypes indicated below. GCVr, ganciclovir resistance; CDVr, cidofovir resistance; FOSr, foscarnet resistance. *Updated from* Chou S, Lurain NS, Thompson KD, et al. Viral DNA polymerase mutations associated with drug resistance in human cytomegalovirus. J Infect Dis 2003;188:32–9; with permission.

is well documented.[93,102] A UL97 mutation conferring ganciclovir typically appears first, followed by the addition of one or more UL54 polymerase mutations after prolonged therapy. The eventual phenotype of these isolates is often high-level resistance to ganciclovir, with additional resistance to foscarnet and/or cidofovir.

Clinical Implications and Management of Resistant Virus

As with untreated CMV infection, the clinical consequences of infection with drug-resistant CMV range from asymptomatic to severe. While asymptomatic infection with drug-resistant virus has been noted, especially in clinical antiviral trials for disease prevention,[103] and persistent viremia without overt disease also occurs, drug-resistant CMV has been reported more commonly in connection with severe disease,[75,77,80,83,84] probably because the host factors that predispose to serious CMV disease are the same as those that favor the emergence of drug resistance. There is insufficient evidence to assess the relative clinical virulence of wild-type and drug-resistant CMV strains, even though several drug-resistant CMV DNA polymerase mutants have been reported to have a slow-growth phenotype in vitro.[3,80,86,96]

CMV drug resistance should be suspected in the setting of high or rising viral load and/or progressive CMV disease despite appropriate induction doses of antiviral therapy for at least 2 weeks, and with a history of cumulative antiviral drug exposure of at least 6 weeks, except in some pediatric settings as noted earlier. When resistance is suspected, laboratory testing for resistance should be pursued and immunosuppressive therapy should be minimized. There are no controlled studies to guide the treatment of drug-resistant CMV infection. The degree of drug resistance, the antiviral drug(s) and dose used, the competence of host immune response, and the site and extent of CMV disease all play a role in determining outcome.

In the absence of immediate, life- or sight-threatening CMV disease, selection of antiviral therapy should be guided by genotypic analysis of UL97 and UL54 genes. The degree of phenotypic resistance known to be associated with a particular gene mutation(s) has significant implications for choice of therapy. Low-grade ganciclovir resistance in the case of non–life- or sight-threatening disease can potentially be addressed with higher-dose intravenous ganciclovir.[78,79,104,105] High-grade ganciclovir resistance with a major UL97 resistance mutation and suspected resistance in the case of life- or sight-threatening disease is best managed with foscarnet. Use of foscarnet is often complicated by nephrotoxicity, and long-term use is rarely tolerated. Cidofovir is another option for ganciclovir-resistant CMV, providing there is not a polymerase mutation conferring cross-resistance to ganciclovir and cidofovir. Significant nephrotoxicity has been associated with cidofovir use in HSCT recipients[106]; however, the experience in SOT recipients is limited. Combination therapy with ganciclovir and foscarnet has been recommended for treatment of drug-resistant CMV infection, based on limited in vitro data[107] and a small case series advocating reduced-dose ganciclovir and escalating-dose foscarnet.[108] Despite the lack of controlled studies, combination treatment is a common practice in cases of documented multidrug resistance or cases of life- or sight-threatening disease unresponsive to monotherapy.

Given the significant limitations of the currently available therapies for drug-resistant CMV infection, alternative agents, both investigational compounds and drugs currently licensed for other indications, have been studied. Maribavir, a benzimidazole riboside, is a potent inhibitor of the CMV UL97 kinase, an enzyme important in various aspects of CMV replication. Because maribavir inhibits UL97-mediated ganciclovir phosphorylation, it antagonizes the antiviral action of ganciclovir, but may have an additive anti-CMV effect when combined with foscarnet or cidofovir.[109] No cross-resistance has been observed between maribavir and other current anti-CMV drugs.[110] Maribavir-resistant laboratory CMV strains have been isolated in vitro[111,112] and have been found to contain mutations in the UL97 and/or UL27 genes, which confer high- and low-grade resistance, respectively.[111–113] Maribavir was successfully tested in phase 1 and 2 trials, which suggested low toxicity and in vivo antiviral activity.[114] However, two phase 3 trials as a CMV prophylactic agent in HSCT and liver transplant recipients did not meet expectations of antiviral efficacy at the dosing regimens chosen. Higher doses of maribavir could still be useful in treating drug-resistant CMV, although clinical experience to date is limited to several transplant recipients, some of whom may have benefited, albeit maribavir-resistant virus was isolated in one case.[115]

Other experimental anti-CMV therapies are considerably less clinically developed than maribavir. Inhibitors of viral DNA cleavage and processing include tomeglovir (BAY-384766), and a benzimidazole D-riboside, GW-275175X, both of which underwent preliminary clinical studies to demonstrate tolerability, but neither of which has proceeded to more advanced clinical trials.[116] In vitro resistance to tomeglovir maps to the CMV UL89, UL56, and UL104 genes,[117] supporting the novel mechanism of action and expected lack of cross-resistance to current drugs. A lipid ester oral prodrug of cidofovir (hexadecyloxypropyl-CDV, or CMX001) has been shown to have in vitro and in vivo activity against CMV, with excellent oral bioavailability and minimal nephrotoxicity in preclinical studies.[118–120] CMX001 may offer a better alternative to the intravenous cidofovir formulation currently available. Cyclopropavir, a purine nucleoside analogue, has been shown to have potent in vitro and in vivo activity against CMV[121,122] but has not undergone clinical trials. While cyclopropavir appears to have a mechanism of action similar to ganciclovir, one study reported that some ganciclovir-resistant isolates exhibited only slightly reduced susceptibility to cyclopropavir[122]; more data are needed on the extent of cross-resistance between the 2 drugs.

Several drugs licensed for other indications and with no defined viral target appear to have anti-CMV activity, although clinical experience is limited to case reports, small case series, and retrospective cohort studies, with no controlled treatment data available. Their role in the treatment of drug-resistant CMV is unclear at this time but would likely be adjunctive to other antivirals. Several retrospective studies in SOT recipients,[123–129] as well as a few studies in HSCT recipients,[130,131] have demonstrated a lower incidence of CMV infection in patients who have received immunosuppressive regimens that included a target of rapamycin inhibitor, either sirolimus or everolimus. Leflunomide, an immunosuppressive drug with an indication for the treatment of rheumatoid arthritis, has been demonstrated to inhibit CMV replication in vitro and in a rat model.[132] Clinical data on the use of leflunomide for treatment of CMV infection in transplant recipients is mixed. When used as adjunctive therapy, a few successes have been reported in the treatment of drug-resistant CMV[81,133]; however, leflunomide is associated with significant hematologic and hepatic toxicity, and treatment failures have been reported as well.[134] Lastly, the antimalarial drug artesunate has been shown to have inhibitory activity against CMV in vitro and in vivo.[135,136] Artesunate appears to have additive effects with ganciclovir, foscarnet, and cidofovir.[135] There is one report of successful use in an HSCT recipient with foscarnet- and ganciclovir-resistant CMV infection.[137]

HEPATITIS B VIRUS
Antiviral Agents and Mechanism of Action

There are currently 7 FDA-approved agents for the treatment of hepatitis B. Three are nucleoside analogues (lamivudine, entecavir, and telbivudine) and 2 are nucleotide analogues (adefovir and tenofovir). Alpha-interferon, approved in 1992 for this indication, and more recently pegylated interferon, remains an important treatment option. Lastly, passive immunization with hepatitis B immune globulin (HBIG) is used after liver transplantation, in combination with a nucleoside or nucleotide analogue for the prevention of HBV recurrence.[138,139]

All of the nucleoside and nucleotide analogues selectively target HBV DNA polymerase, which includes reverse transcriptase activity. Drugs in this class are phosphorylated by cellular enzymes to active form and then incorporated into growing DNA, resulting in premature chain termination, amongst other inhibitory functions related to viral replication. While drug-related side effects are generally minimal with this class, adefovir is associated with nephrotoxicity in up to 12% of liver transplant recipients,[140,141] and caution is advised in patients receiving concomitant nephrotoxins. Although these antiviral compounds are effective to varying degrees in providing long-term suppression, they do not eradicate HBV, which persists in hepatocytes in the form of covalently closed circular DNA (cccDNA).[142] In vitro studies have demonstrated that antiviral therapy has little or no effect on cccDNA.[143] Therefore, treatment of chronic HBV infection is typically prolonged and issues of antiviral drug resistance become important.

Historically, sequential and combination therapy was used to treat chronic HBV infection, with changes made in response to the frequent emergence of antiviral drug resistance. More recently, because of higher potency and lower rates of resistance, entecavir and tenofovir have largely supplanted lamivudine and adefovir as preferred first-line agents for antiviral naïve individuals.[144] For the significant number of patients who have been successfully treated with lamivudine and adefovir, with undetectable serum HBV DNA, there is no recommendation to change therapy.

In Vitro Evaluation of Antiviral Susceptibility

Genotypic resistance testing involves the detection of characteristic HBV polymerase gene mutations, which can be performed at varying levels of sensitivity using broadly applicable methods, such as standard sequencing of PCR products, restriction fragment length polymorphism, reverse hybridization, and single genome sequencing.[145] Conventional dideoxy sequencing is insensitive at detecting minor subpopulations of mutant virus that comprise less than 20% of the circulating virus population. The more sensitive assays can detect HBV DNA mutants that represent 5% to 10% of the entire HBV quasispecies, potentially allowing for earlier identification of genotypic resistance. With the advent of newer sequencing technologies, such as "ultra-deep" pyrosequencing, mutants comprising less than 1% of the viral pool can be identified and characterized.[146] The clinical utility and value of these more sensitive techniques remains to be determined. Genotypic testing is standard clinical practice as it is rapid and practical, but subject to the usual limitation that it cannot interpret novel or previously uncharacterized mutations and cannot directly assess such properties as the replication fitness of drug-resistant mutants.

Standardized phenotypic testing for HBV drug susceptibility has been limited by the absence of a cell culture system that allows fully permissive infection. A human hepatoma cell line maintained with dimethyl sulfoxide and hydrocortisone to promote cell differentiation and phenotypic stability[147] has been developed as a means of comparing the relative antiviral susceptibility and growth fitness of HBV mutants.[148] Cell culture systems may involve transient transfection of HBV clones or construction of cell lines that permanently express drug-resistant mutants.[149] Alternatively, biochemical assays of expressed HBV polymerase have been used to assess inhibition by drug, independent of cell culture. Although current HBV recombinant phenotyping approaches may not accurately model viral replication in vivo, they are necessary for validating the interpretation of genotypic resistance testing data.

Epidemiology of Antiviral Resistance

Given the high viral replication rate and the error-prone nature of HBV reverse transcriptase, emergence of drug resistance is expected.[150] Drug resistance has been associated with a variety of patient and viral factors. Host factors that contribute to an increased risk for drug resistance include older age, high body mass index (weight in kilograms divided by height in meters squared), medication noncompliance, immunosuppression, high pretreatment HBV DNA levels, baseline hepatic enzyme elevations, and abundant replication space (large number of uninfected hepatocytes, as in a newly transplanted liver).[151–156] The viral mutation frequency, the magnitude and rate of virus replication, and the overall replication fitness of the mutant are critical viral determinants in risk for drug resistance.[157]

Apart from host and virus factors, the potency and genetic barrier to resistance of the antiviral drug is of critical importance in determining risk for drug resistance.[150] The genetic barrier reflects the number and type of mutations that must be accumulated in order for the virus to develop significant drug resistance while maintaining adequate growth. Lamivudine is an intermediate potency drug with a low genetic barrier to resistance, resulting in high resistance rates. Adefovir is a low potency drug with an intermediate genetic barrier to resistance, and therefore an intermediate rate of resistance. Telbivudine is a high-potency drug, though with a low genetic barrier to resistance, and so resistance rates are intermediate. Lastly, entecavir and tenofovir are considered high-potency antivirals, with a high genetic barrier to resistance, and therefore low rates of resistance. Among antiviral-naïve patients, drug resistance has been reported in up to 70% of patients treated with 5 years of lamivudine therapy, 29% after 5 years of adefovir, 20% after 2 years of telbivudine, and 1% after 5 years of entecavir.[152,158–162] Resistance rates are significantly higher in patients with prior exposure to lamivudine, with rates of up to 18% at 1 year following switch to adefovir monotherapy and 51% at 5 years following switch to entecavir.[150,163]

Mechanism of Resistance

The HBV polymerase gene is the target for nucleoside and nucleotide analogues. The enzyme has 4 functional domains (terminal protein, spacer, Pol/rt [polymerase/reverse transcriptase], and RNaseH), with 7 catalytic subdomains (A–G) in the Pol/rt region (**Fig. 3**).[150] Antiviral drug-resistant strains have signature mutations in the reverse transcriptase domains of the viral polymerase gene, with most substitutions occurring in domains B, C, and D. Resistance mutations alter the interaction between HBV polymerase and drug.[164] Molecular modeling studies of the interaction of wild-type and mutant HBV polymerase with natural thymidine triphosphate substrate and with anti-HBV agents highlight the important conformational changes in mutants that confer drug resistance.[165] While the interaction of each nucleoside or nucleotide analogue with HBV polymerase appears to be mechanistically unique with regard to binding affinity and shifting after ligand attachment, all drug-resistant mutants seem to exhibit either altered binding of substrate or downstream structural changes that interfere with the inhibitory effect of drug on viral polymerase. After emergence of primary resistance mutations, compensatory mutations that restore replication capacity may arise, as well as secondary resistance mutations that increase drug resistance when they accumulate on the same viral genome.

High-level lamivudine resistance is most often caused by mutations M204I/V, which are in the YMDD (tyrosine-methionine-aspartate-aspartate) motif in the C domain of the polymerase gene,[166] and infrequently by A181V/T mutations.[167] M204V is almost always accompanied by compensatory mutations L180M and/or V173L, resulting in restored fitness of the mutant.[166,168] The M204I mutation confers high-level cross-resistance to telbivudine, but M204I/V mutations do not appear to reduce susceptibility to adefovir and tenofovir.[162,169] The signature mutation associated with

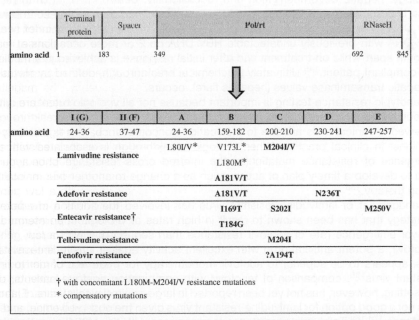

	Terminal protein	Spacer	Pol/rt				RNaseH
amino acid	1	183	349			692	845

	I (G)	II (F)	A	B	C	D	E
amino acid	24-36	37-47	24-36	159-182	200-210	230-241	247-257
Lamivudine resistance			L80I/V*	V173L* L180M* A181V/T	M204I/V		
Adefovir resistance				A181V/T		N236T	
Entecavir resistance†				I169T T184G	S202I		M250V
Telbivudine resistance					M204I		
Tenofovir resistance				?A194T			

† with concomitant L180M-M204I/V resistance mutations
* compensatory mutations

Fig. 3. Map of HBV polymerase gene functional domains (terminal protein, spacer, Pol/rt, RNaseH), catalytic subdomains (A–G), and resistance mutations. Pol/rt, polymerase/reverse transcriptase.

telbivudine resistance is M204I, either alone or in association with the secondary mutations L80I/V or L180M.[162]

N236T and A181V/T are adefovir-resistance mutations.[159,170] Although the resistance conferred by these mutations is less than that associated with M204I/V and lamivudine resistance, virological breakthrough is seen.[169–171] The N236T mutation reduces viral replicative capacity in vitro and confers cross-resistance to tenofovir but not to lamivudine or telbivudine.[172]

Resistance to entecavir appears to occur though a 2-hit mechanism, whereby classic lamivudine-resistant mutants (L180M, M204I/V) are selected in patients on lamivudine or, less frequently, in patients on primary therapy with entecavir.[173] During continued entecavir treatment, additional mutations at I169T and M250V or T184G and S202I are selected, conferring resistance to entecavir.[174–176]

Resistance to tenofovir currently appears to be unusual,[177] although more experience with this drug for treatment of chronic HBV is needed. There is a report of virologic breakthrough on tenofovir in 2 HBV/HIV coinfected patients with prior lamivudine exposure (L180M-M204V mutations) and an A194T mutation.[178] However, A194T was not shown to confer resistance to tenofovir in vitro,[179] suggesting that it may instead be a viral sequence polymorphism or a lamivudine compensatory mutation.[180]

Clinical Implications and Management of Resistant Virus

With the availability of safe and effective oral HBV antiviral agents in the late 1990s and the switch from HBIG monotherapy to combination therapy (HBIG plus antivirals) in HBV-infected liver transplant recipients, HBV recurrence rates have decreased significantly.[181–183] Antiviral drug resistance remains an important factor in HBV reinfection after liver transplantation. Clinical consequences of the emergence of drug-resistant HBV range from asymptomatic viremia to serum transaminase flares, worsening liver histology, hepatic decompensation and, occasionally, death.[152,171,184] Drug resistance is associated with virologic breakthrough,[185] defined as an increase in serum HBV DNA by at least 1.0 $\log_{10}$ (10-fold) above nadir, or the reappearance of serum HBV DNA with previously undetectable HBV DNA on 2 or more occasions at least 1 month apart while on treatment and after initial response is achieved in a medication-compliant patient.[145] Ultimately biochemical breakthrough, defined by elevation of hepatic transaminase values (hepatitis flare), occurs.

Genotypic resistance testing is important because not all virologic breakthrough is attributable to drug resistance. As many as 30% to 50% of viral breakthroughs observed in clinical trials are due to medication noncompliance,[145] a figure likely to be higher in clinical practice. When virologic breakthrough is associated with the emergence of resistance mutation(s), the inferred cross-resistance phenotype is used to develop a timely plan of action, such as a change to another drug or combination therapy.[186]

Management of lamivudine-resistant virus has involved the addition of adefovir, a strategy that has been shown to result in high rates of virologic suppression and a lower emergence rate of adefovir resistance than sequential monotherapy.[186,187] Tenofovir, a potent antiviral drug with excellent activity against lamivudine-resistant virus, appears to be superior to adefovir monotherapy for treatment of lamivudine-resistant virus[188]; comparison of tenofovir with combination adefovir-lamivudine in this setting, however, has not yet been reported in large-scale clinical studies. Entecavir is not a good option for lamivudine-resistant virus given the observed emergence of resistance.[176,189] Telbivudine resistance is associated with the M204I mutation, and although there are in vitro data demonstrating telbivudine activity against the M204V lamivudine-resistant mutant,[190] clinical data are not available at this time.

Telbuvidine should not be relied on for treatment of lamivudine-resistant virus, and management of telbivudine resistance should be similar to management of lamivudine resistance. Management of adefovir-resistant virus is dependent on the type of mutation(s) and the antiviral drug history of the patient. Lamivudine has proved to be effective in suppressing adefovir-resistant HBV with the N236 T mutation,[170,191] and it is presumed that telbivudine would also be effective based on in vitro data.[190] The durability of response in patients with previous lamivudine resistance, however, is unclear, with a report of reemergence of lamivudine resistance after reintroduction of drug.[192] There are in vitro data to suggest that entecavir may be a reasonable choice for N236T mutants,[193] with the caveat that the benefit may be short-lived in patients with prior lamivudine resistance. For patients with the N236T mutation, options include switching to or adding entecavir, adding lamivudine (or telbivudine), or switching to tenofovir. The activity of lamivudine (and likely telbivudine) against the A181 V adefovir-resistant mutants is decreased compared with wild-type HBV.[167] Whereas the A181T mutant has been shown in vitro to have decreased susceptibility to tenofovir,[167] in the clinical setting entecavir and tenofovir have been effective in suppressing replication of A181T adefovir-resistant mutants.[194,195] In the case of an A181T mutation, management options include switching to or adding entecavir, or switching to tenofovir; lamivudine should not be used in this scenario given the risk of cross-resistance.[167]

There are no large-scale clinical studies yet available to guide the treatment of entecavir-resistant HBV. From in vitro data and case reports it appears that adefovir and tenofovir are effective for entecavir-resistant HBV.[176,196,197] Based for the most part on expert opinion, a recommended approach for entecavir-resistant virus is to add tenofovir or adefovir.[145,150,194] Data on management of tenofovir-resistant HBV are not yet available, given the low rate of resistance observed with early use of this drug.

Emtricitabine, a potent nucleoside analogue that is currently FDA-approved for the treatment of HIV, is currently in late phase clinical trial for management of chronic HBV.[198] At the target treatment dose of 200 mg daily, resistance to emtricitabine was observed in 9% of treatment-naïve patients at 1 year and rose to 20% after 2 years.[198] Emtricitabine resistance is conferred by the M204I/V mutation with or without the accompanying L180M and V173L mutations, therefore implying cross-resistance to lamivudine and telbivudine.

THE FUTURE

As antiviral therapy becomes widely used in immunosuppressed patient populations, concerns about drug resistance will require a better understanding of the relevant virus-, host-, and drug-related factors. Knowledge of genetic mechanisms and associated viral mutations has allowed for development of genotypic techniques for the timely diagnosis of resistance. The accuracy of this testing will be improved by recombinant phenotyping data that validate the drug resistance properties associated with the many viral sequence changes detected in clinical specimens. An accessible and authoritative database of drug resistance mutations needs to be available for each virus to guide therapeutic decisions. More comprehensive information on the epidemiologic, host, and drug exposure factors that favor the emergence of resistant virus can be used to develop better strategies for prevention, early detection, and appropriate treatment change. Ideally, controlled trials are needed to compare sequential and combination use of alternative therapies, optimize dosing schedules, and evaluate adjunctive therapies that seek to improve host conditions for antiviral drug efficacy. There is an ongoing need for less toxic but potent new antiviral drugs that preferably target different aspects of viral replication to reduce the risk of cross-resistance.

REFERENCES

1. Elion GB, Furman PA, Fyfe JA, et al. The selectivity of action of an antiherpetic agent, 9-(2-hydroxyethoxymethyl) guanine. Proc Natl Acad Sci USA 1977;74(12):5716–20.
2. Elion GB. Acyclovir: discovery, mechanism of action, and selectivity. J Med Virol 1993;41(Suppl 1):2–6.
3. Gilbert C, Bestman-Smith J, Boivin G. Resistance of herpesviruses to antiviral drugs: clinical impacts and molecular mechanisms. Drug Resist Updat 2002; 5(2):88–114.
4. Wagstaff AJ, Faulds D, Goa KL. Aciclovir. A reappraisal of its antiviral activity, pharmacokinetic properties and therapeutic efficacy. Drugs 1994;47(1): 153–205.
5. Haefeli WE, Schoenenberger RA, Weiss P, et al. Acyclovir-induced neurotoxicity: concentration-side effect relationship in acyclovir overdose. Am J Med 1993;94(2):212–5.
6. Lowance D, Neumayer HH, Legendre CM, et al. Valacyclovir for the prevention of cytomegalovirus disease after renal transplantation. International Valacyclovir Cytomegalovirus Prophylaxis Transplantation Study Group. N Engl J Med 1999; 340(19):1462–70.
7. Ormrod D, Scott LJ, Perry CM. Valaciclovir: a review of its long term utility in the management of genital herpes simplex virus and cytomegalovirus infections. Drugs 2000;59(4):839–63.
8. Kalil AC, Freifeld AG, Lyden ER, et al. Valganciclovir for cytomegalovirus prevention in solid organ transplant patients: an evidence-based reassessment of safety and efficacy. PLoS One 2009;4(5):e5512.
9. Crumpacker CS. Ganciclovir. N Engl J Med 1996;335(10):721–9.
10. Wagstaff AJ, Bryson HM. Foscarnet. A reappraisal of its antiviral activity, pharmacokinetic properties and therapeutic use in immunocompromised patients with viral infections. Drugs 1994;48(2):199–226.
11. Deray G, Martinez F, Katlama C, et al. Foscarnet nephrotoxicity: mechanism, incidence and prevention. Am J Nephrol 1989;9(4):316–21.
12. Safrin S, Cherrington J, Jaffe HS. Clinical uses of cidofovir. Rev Med Virol 1997;7(3):145–56.
13. Lalezari J, Schacker T, Feinberg J, et al. A randomized, double-blind, placebo-controlled trial of cidofovir gel for the treatment of acyclovir-unresponsive mucocutaneous herpes simplex virus infection in patients with AIDS. J Infect Dis 1997;176(4):892–8.
14. Landry ML, Stanat S, Biron K, et al. A standardized plaque reduction assay for determination of drug susceptibilities of cytomegalovirus clinical isolates. Antimicrob Agents Chemother 2000;44(3):688–92.
15. Wang YC, Kao CL, Liu WT, et al. A cell line that secretes inducibly a reporter protein for monitoring herpes simplex virus infection and drug susceptibility. J Med Virol 2002;68(4):599–605.
16. Frobert E, Ooka T, Cortay JC, et al. Herpes simplex virus thymidine kinase mutations associated with resistance to acyclovir: a site-directed mutagenesis study. Antimicrob Agents Chemother 2005;49(3):1055–9.
17. Suzutani T, Saijo M, Nagamine M, et al. Rapid phenotypic characterization method for herpes simplex virus and varicella-zoster virus thymidine kinases to screen for acyclovir-resistant viral infection. J Clin Microbiol 2000;38(5): 1839–44.

18. Burns WH, Saral R, Santos GW, et al. Isolation and characterisation of resistant Herpes simplex virus after acyclovir therapy. Lancet 1982;1(8269):421–3.
19. Sibrack CD, Gutman LT, Wilfert CM, et al. Pathogenicity of acyclovir-resistant herpes simplex virus type 1 from an immunodeficient child. J Infect Dis 1982; 146(5):673–82.
20. Stranska R, Schuurman R, Nienhuis E, et al. Survey of acyclovir-resistant herpes simplex virus in The Netherlands: prevalence and characterization. J Clin Virol 2005;32(1):7–18.
21. Nugier F, Colin JN, Aymard M, et al. Occurrence and characterization of acyclovir-resistant herpes simplex virus isolates: report on a two-year sensitivity screening survey. J Med Virol 1992;36(1):1–12.
22. Englund JA, Zimmerman ME, Swierkosz EM, et al. Herpes simplex virus resistant to acyclovir. A study in a tertiary care center. Ann Intern Med 1990;112(6): 416–22.
23. Christophers J, Clayton J, Craske J, et al. Survey of resistance of herpes simplex virus to acyclovir in northwest England. Antimicrob Agents Chemother 1998;42(4):868–72.
24. Danve-Szatanek C, Aymard M, Thouvenot D, et al. Surveillance network for herpes simplex virus resistance to antiviral drugs: 3-year follow-up. J Clin Microbiol 2004;42(1):242–9.
25. Chakrabarti S, Pillay D, Ratcliffe D, et al. Resistance to antiviral drugs in herpes simplex virus infections among allogeneic stem cell transplant recipients: risk factors and prognostic significance. J Infect Dis 2000;181(6):2055–8.
26. Malvy D, Treilhaud M, Bouee S, et al. A retrospective, case-control study of acyclovir resistance in herpes simplex virus. Clin Infect Dis 2005;41(3): 320–6.
27. Coen DM, Schaffer PA. Two distinct loci confer resistance to acycloguanosine in herpes simplex virus type 1. Proc Natl Acad Sci U S A 1980;77(4):2265–9.
28. Morfin F, Thouvenot D. Herpes simplex virus resistance to antiviral drugs. J Clin Virol 2003;26(1):29–37.
29. Morfin F, Souillet G, Bilger K, et al. Genetic characterization of thymidine kinase from acyclovir-resistant and -susceptible herpes simplex virus type 1 isolated from bone marrow transplant recipients. J Infect Dis 2000;182(1):290–3.
30. Gaudreau A, Hill E, Balfour HH Jr, et al. Phenotypic and genotypic characterization of acyclovir-resistant herpes simplex viruses from immunocompromised patients. J Infect Dis 1998;178(2):297–303.
31. Bacon TH, Levin MJ, Leary JJ, et al. Herpes simplex virus resistance to acyclovir and penciclovir after two decades of antiviral therapy. Clin Microbiol Rev 2003; 16(1):114–28.
32. Ljungman P, Ellis MN, Hackman RC, et al. Acyclovir-resistant herpes simplex virus causing pneumonia after marrow transplantation. J Infect Dis 1990;162(1):244–8.
33. Bestman-Smith J, Boivin G. Drug resistance patterns of recombinant herpes simplex virus DNA polymerase mutants generated with a set of overlapping cosmids and plasmids. J Virol 2003;77(14):7820–9.
34. Longerich T, Eisenbach C, Penzel R, et al. Recurrent herpes simplex virus hepatitis after liver retransplantation despite acyclovir therapy. Liver Transpl 2005;11(10): 1289–94.
35. Frangoul H, Wills M, Crossno C, et al. Acyclovir-resistant herpes simplex virus pneumonia post-unrelated stem cell transplantation: a word of caution. Pediatr Transplant 2007;11(8):942–4.

36. Chen Y, Scieux C, Garrait V, et al. Resistant herpes simplex virus type 1 infection: an emerging concern after allogeneic stem cell transplantation. Clin Infect Dis 2000;31(4):927–35.
37. Coen DM, Kosz-Vnenchak M, Jacobson JG, et al. Thymidine kinase-negative herpes simplex virus mutants establish latency in mouse trigeminal ganglia but do not reactivate. Proc Natl Acad Sci U S A 1989;86(12):4736–40.
38. Andrei G, Fiten P, Froeyen M, et al. DNA polymerase mutations in drug-resistant herpes simplex virus mutants determine in vivo neurovirulence and drug-enzyme interactions. Antivir Ther 2007;12(5):719–32.
39. Coen DM. Acyclovir-resistant, pathogenic herpesviruses. Trends Microbiol 1994;2(12):481–5.
40. Griffiths A, Chen SH, Horsburgh BC, et al. Translational compensation of a frameshift mutation affecting herpes simplex virus thymidine kinase is sufficient to permit reactivation from latency. J Virol 2003;77(8):4703–9.
41. Griffiths A, Link MA, Furness CL, et al. Low-level expression and reversion both contribute to reactivation of herpes simplex virus drug-resistant mutants with mutations on homopolymeric sequences in thymidine kinase. J Virol 2006;80(13):6568–74.
42. Wyles DL, Patel A, Madinger N, et al. Development of herpes simplex virus disease in patients who are receiving cidofovir. Clin Infect Dis 2005;41(5):676–80.
43. De Clercq E. The antiviral spectrum of (E)-5-(2-bromovinyl)-2'-deoxyuridine. J Antimicrob Chemother 1984;14(Suppl A):85–95.
44. Safrin S, Crumpacker C, Chatis P, et al. A controlled trial comparing foscarnet with vidarabine for acyclovir-resistant mucocutaneous herpes simplex in the acquired immunodeficiency syndrome. The AIDS Clinical Trials Group. N Engl J Med 1991;325(8):551–5.
45. Martinez V, Molina JM, Scieux C, et al. Topical imiquimod for recurrent acyclovir-resistant HSV infection. Am J Med 2006;119(5):e9–11.
46. Sims CR, Thompson K, Chemaly RF, et al. Oral topical cidofovir: novel route of drug delivery in a severely immunosuppressed patient with refractory multidrug-resistant herpes simplex virus infection. Transpl Infect Dis 2007;9(3):256–9.
47. Biron KK, Elion GB. In vitro susceptibility of varicella-zoster virus to acyclovir. Antimicrob Agents Chemother 1980;18(3):443–7.
48. Boivin G, Edelman CK, Pedneault L, et al. Phenotypic and genotypic characterization of acyclovir-resistant varicella-zoster viruses isolated from persons with AIDS. J Infect Dis 1994;170(1):68–75.
49. Jacobson MA, Berger TG, Fikrig S, et al. Acyclovir-resistant varicella zoster virus infection after chronic oral acyclovir therapy in patients with the acquired immunodeficiency syndrome (AIDS). Ann Intern Med 1990;112(3):187–91.
50. Saint-Leger E, Caumes E, Breton G, et al. Clinical and virologic characterization of acyclovir-resistant varicella-zoster viruses isolated from 11 patients with acquired immunodeficiency syndrome. Clin Infect Dis 2001;33(12):2061–7.
51. Breton G, Fillet AM, Katlama C, et al. Acyclovir-resistant herpes zoster in human immunodeficiency virus-infected patients: results of foscarnet therapy. Clin Infect Dis 1998;27(6):1525–7.
52. Crassard N, Souillet AL, Morfin F, et al. Acyclovir-resistant varicella infection with atypical lesions in a non-HIV leukemic infant. Acta Paediatr 2000;89(12):1497–9.
53. Morfin F, Thouvenot D, De Turenne-Tessier M, et al. Phenotypic and genetic characterization of thymidine kinase from clinical strains of varicella-zoster virus resistant to acyclovir. Antimicrob Agents Chemother 1999;43(10):2412–6.

54. Levin MJ, Dahl KM, Weinberg A, et al. Development of resistance to acyclovir during chronic infection with the Oka vaccine strain of varicella-zoster virus, in an immunosuppressed child. J Infect Dis 2003;188(7):954–9.

55. Bryan CJ, Prichard MN, Daily S, et al. Acyclovir-resistant chronic verrucous vaccine strain varicella in a patient with neuroblastoma. Pediatr Infect Dis J 2008;27(10):946–8.

56. Andrei G, De Clercq E, Snoeck R. In vitro selection of drug-resistant varicella-zoster virus (VZV) mutants (OKA strain): differences between acyclovir and penciclovir? Antiviral Res 2004;61(3):181–7.

57. Pahwa S, Biron K, Lim W, et al. Continuous varicella-zoster infection associated with acyclovir resistance in a child with AIDS. JAMA 1988;260(19):2879–82.

58. Linnemann CC Jr, Biron KK, Hoppenjans WG, et al. Emergence of acyclovir-resistant varicella zoster virus in an AIDS patient on prolonged acyclovir therapy. AIDS 1990;4(6):577–9.

59. Visse B, Huraux JM, Fillet AM. Point mutations in the varicella-zoster virus DNA polymerase gene confers resistance to foscarnet and slow growth phenotype. J Med Virol 1999;59(1):84–90.

60. Safrin S, Berger TG, Gilson I, et al. Foscarnet therapy in five patients with AIDS and acyclovir-resistant varicella-zoster virus infection. Ann Intern Med 1991;115(1): 19–21.

61. Visse B, Dumont B, Huraux JM, et al. Single amino acid change in DNA polymerase is associated with foscarnet resistance in a varicella-zoster virus strain recovered from a patient with AIDS. J Infect Dis 1998;178(Suppl 1):S55–7.

62. Schliefer K, Gumbel HO, Rockstroh JK, et al. Management of progressive outer retinal necrosis with cidofovir in a human immunodeficiency virus-infected patient. Clin Infect Dis 1999;29(3):684–5.

63. Snoeck R, Andrei G, De Clercq E. Novel agents for the therapy of varicella-zoster virus infections. Expert Opin Investig Drugs 2000;9(8):1743–51.

64. Kamiyama T, Kurokawa M, Shiraki K. Characterization of the DNA polymerase gene of varicella-zoster viruses resistant to acyclovir. J Gen Virol 2001;82(Pt 11):2761–5.

65. Reusser P, Cordonnier C, Einsele H, et al. European survey of herpesvirus resistance to antiviral drugs in bone marrow transplant recipients. Infectious diseases working party of the European group for blood and marrow transplantation (EBMT). Bone Marrow Transplant 1996;17(5):813–7.

66. Laurenti L, Piccioni P, Cattani P, et al. Cytomegalovirus reactivation during alemtuzumab therapy for chronic lymphocytic leukemia: incidence and treatment with oral ganciclovir. Haematologica 2004;89(10):1248–52.

67. Erice A, Chou S, Biron KK, et al. Progressive disease due to ganciclovir-resistant cytomegalovirus in immunocompromised patients. N Engl J Med 1989;320(5): 289–93.

68. Jabs DA, Enger C, Dunn JP, et al. Cytomegalovirus retinitis and viral resistance: ganciclovir resistance. CMV Retinitis and Viral Resistance Study Group. J Infect Dis 1998;177(3):770–3.

69. Jabs DA, Enger C, Forman M, et al. Incidence of foscarnet resistance and cidofovir resistance in patients treated for cytomegalovirus retinitis. The Cytomegalovirus Retinitis and Viral Resistance Study Group. Antimicrob Agents Chemother 1998;42(9):2240–4.

70. Reddy AJ, Zaas AK, Hanson KE, et al. A single-center experience with ganciclovir-resistant cytomegalovirus in lung transplant recipients: treatment and outcome. J Heart Lung Transplant 2007;26(12):1286–92.

71. Li F, Kenyon KW, Kirby KA, et al. Incidence and clinical features of ganciclovir-resistant cytomegalovirus disease in heart transplant recipients. Clin Infect Dis 2007;45(4):439–47.

72. Limaye AP, Raghu G, Koelle DM, et al. High incidence of ganciclovir-resistant cytomegalovirus infection among lung transplant recipients receiving preemptive therapy. J Infect Dis 2002;185(1):20–7.

73. Limaye AP, Corey L, Koelle DM, et al. Emergence of ganciclovir-resistant cytomegalovirus disease among recipients of solid-organ transplants. Lancet 2000; 356(9230):645–9.

74. Bhorade SM, Lurain NS, Jordan A, et al. Emergence of ganciclovir-resistant cytomegalovirus in lung transplant recipients. J Heart Lung Transplant 2002; 21(12):1274–82.

75. Eid AJ, Arthurs SK, Deziel PJ, et al. Emergence of drug-resistant cytomegalovirus in the era of valganciclovir prophylaxis: therapeutic implications and outcomes. Clin Transplant 2008;22(2):162–70.

76. Lurain NS, Bhorade SM, Pursell KJ, et al. Analysis and characterization of antiviral drug-resistant cytomegalovirus isolates from solid organ transplant recipients. J Infect Dis 2002;186(6):760–8.

77. Isada CM, Yen-Lieberman B, Lurain NS, et al. Clinical characteristics of 13 solid organ transplant recipients with ganciclovir-resistant cytomegalovirus infection. Transpl Infect Dis 2002;4(4):189–94.

78. Kruger RM, Shannon WD, Arens MQ, et al. The impact of ganciclovir-resistant cytomegalovirus infection after lung transplantation. Transplantation 1999;68(9): 1272–9.

79. Limaye AP. Ganciclovir-resistant cytomegalovirus in organ transplant recipients. Clin Infect Dis 2002;35(7):866–72.

80. Marfori JE, Exner MM, Marousek GI, et al. Development of new cytomegalovirus UL97 and DNA polymerase mutations conferring drug resistance after valganciclovir therapy in allogeneic stem cell recipients. J Clin Virol 2007;38(2):120–5.

81. Avery RK, Bolwell BJ, Yen-Lieberman B, et al. Use of leflunomide in an allogeneic bone marrow transplant recipient with refractory cytomegalovirus infection. Bone Marrow Transplant 2004;34(12):1071–5.

82. Erice A, Borrell N, Li W, et al. Ganciclovir susceptibilities and analysis of UL97 region in cytomegalovirus (CMV) isolates from bone marrow recipients with CMV disease after antiviral prophylaxis. J Infect Dis 1998;178(2):531–4.

83. Hamprecht K, Eckle T, Prix L, et al. Ganciclovir-resistant cytomegalovirus disease after allogeneic stem cell transplantation: pitfalls of phenotypic diagnosis by in vitro selection of an UL97 mutant strain. J Infect Dis 2003;187(1): 139–43.

84. Julin JE, van Burik JH, Krivit W, et al. Ganciclovir-resistant cytomegalovirus encephalitis in a bone marrow transplant recipient. Transpl Infect Dis 2002;4(4): 201–6.

85. Seo SK, Regan A, Cihlar T, et al. Cytomegalovirus ventriculoencephalitis in a bone marrow transplant recipient receiving antiviral maintenance: clinical and molecular evidence of drug resistance. Clin Infect Dis 2001;33(9):e105–8.

86. Springer KL, Chou S, Li S, et al. How evolution of mutations conferring drug resistance affects viral dynamics and clinical outcomes of cytomegalovirus-infected hematopoietic cell transplant recipients. J Clin Microbiol 2005;43(1): 208–13.

87. Eckle T, Lang P, Prix L, et al. Rapid development of ganciclovir-resistant cytomegalovirus infection in children after allogeneic stem cell transplantation in

the early phase of immune cell recovery. Bone Marrow Transplant 2002;30(7): 433–9.

88. Prix L, Hamprecht K, Holzhuter B, et al. Comprehensive restriction analysis of the UL97 region allows early detection of ganciclovir-resistant human cytomegalovirus in an immunocompromised child. J Infect Dis 1999;180(2):491–5.

89. Scott GM, Weinberg A, Rawlinson WD, et al. Multidrug resistance conferred by novel DNA polymerase mutations in human cytomegalovirus isolates. Antimicrob Agents Chemother 2007;51(1):89–94.

90. Rodriguez J, Casper K, Smallwood G, et al. Resistance to combined ganciclovir and foscarnet therapy in a liver transplant recipient with possible dual-strain cytomegalovirus coinfection. Liver Transpl 2007;13(10):1396–400.

91. Oshima K, Kanda Y, Kako S, et al. Case report: persistent cytomegalovirus (CMV) infection after haploidentical hematopoietic stem cell transplantation using in vivo alemtuzumab: emergence of resistant CMV due to mutations in the UL97 and UL54 genes. J Med Virol 2008;80(10):1769–75.

92. Chou S, Lurain NS, Thompson KD, et al. Viral DNA polymerase mutations associated with drug resistance in human cytomegalovirus. J Infect Dis 2003;188(1):32–9.

93. Chou S, Marousek G, Guentzel S, et al. Evolution of mutations conferring multidrug resistance during prophylaxis and therapy for cytomegalovirus disease. J Infect Dis 1997;176(3):786–9.

94. Chou S, Marousek G, Li S, et al. Contrasting drug resistance phenotypes resulting from cytomegalovirus DNA polymerase mutations at the same exonuclease locus. J Clin Virol 2008;43(1):107–9.

95. Chou S, Marousek G, Parenti DM, et al. Mutation in region III of the DNA polymerase gene conferring foscarnet resistance in cytomegalovirus isolates from 3 subjects receiving prolonged antiviral therapy. J Infect Dis 1998;178(2):526–30.

96. Chou S, Marousek GI, Van Wechel LC, et al. Growth and drug resistance phenotypes resulting from cytomegalovirus DNA polymerase region III mutations observed in clinical specimens. Antimicrob Agents Chemother 2007;51(11): 4160–2.

97. Chou S, Miner RC, Drew WL. A deletion mutation in region V of the cytomegalovirus DNA polymerase sequence confers multidrug resistance. J Infect Dis 2000;182(6):1765–8.

98. Chou S, Waldemer RH, Senters AE, et al. Cytomegalovirus UL97 phosphotransferase mutations that affect susceptibility to ganciclovir. J Infect Dis 2002;185(2): 162–9.

99. Chou S, Van Wechel LC, Lichy HM, et al. Phenotyping of cytomegalovirus drug resistance mutations by using recombinant viruses incorporating a reporter gene. Antimicrob Agents Chemother 2005;49(7):2710–5.

100. Prichard MN, Gao N, Jairath S, et al. A recombinant human cytomegalovirus with a large deletion in UL97 has a severe replication deficiency. J Virol 1999; 73(7):5663–70.

101. Wolf DG, Courcelle CT, Prichard MN, et al. Distinct and separate roles for herpesvirus-conserved UL97 kinase in cytomegalovirus DNA synthesis and encapsidation. Proc Natl Acad Sci U S A 2001;98(4):1895–900.

102. Smith IL, Cherrington JM, Jiles RE, et al. High-level resistance of cytomegalovirus to ganciclovir is associated with alterations in both the UL97 and DNA polymerase genes. J Infect Dis 1997;176(1):69–77.

103. Boivin G, Goyette N, Gilbert C, et al. Clinical impact of ganciclovir-resistant cytomegalovirus infections in solid organ transplant patients. Transpl Infect Dis 2005;7(3–4):166–70.

104. Cytomegalovirus. Am J Transplant 2004;4(Suppl 10):51–8.
105. West P, Schmiedeskamp M, Neeley H, et al. Use of high-dose ganciclovir for a resistant cytomegalovirus infection due to UL97 mutation. Transpl Infect Dis 2008;10(2):129–32.
106. Ljungman P, Deliliers GL, Platzbecker U, et al. Cidofovir for cytomegalovirus infection and disease in allogeneic stem cell transplant recipients. The infectious diseases working party of the European group for blood and marrow transplantation. Blood 2001;97(2):388–92.
107. Drew WL. Is combination antiviral therapy for CMV superior to monotherapy? J Clin Virol 2006;35(4):485–8.
108. Mylonakis E, Kallas WM, Fishman JA. Combination antiviral therapy for ganciclovir-resistant cytomegalovirus infection in solid-organ transplant recipients. Clin Infect Dis 2002;34(10):1337–41.
109. Chou S, Marousek GI. Maribavir antagonizes the antiviral action of ganciclovir on human cytomegalovirus. Antimicrob Agents Chemother 2006;50(10):3470–2.
110. Drew WL, Miner RC, Marousek GI, et al. Maribavir sensitivity of cytomegalovirus isolates resistant to ganciclovir, cidofovir or foscarnet. J Clin Virol 2006;37(2):124–7.
111. Chou S, Wechel LC, Marousek GI. Cytomegalovirus UL97 kinase mutations that confer maribavir resistance. J Infect Dis 2007;196(1):91–4.
112. Chou S, Marousek GI, Senters AE, et al. Mutations in the human cytomegalovirus UL27 gene that confer resistance to maribavir. J Virol 2004;78(13):7124–30.
113. Chou S, Marousek GI. Accelerated evolution of maribavir resistance in a cytomegalovirus exonuclease domain II mutant. J Virol 2008;82(1):246–53.
114. Winston DJ, Young JA, Pullarkat V, et al. Maribavir prophylaxis for prevention of cytomegalovirus infection in allogeneic stem cell transplant recipients: a multicenter, randomized, double-blind, placebo-controlled, dose-ranging study. Blood 2008;111(11):5403–10.
115. Avery RK, Marty FM, Strasfeld L, et al. Oral maribavir (MBV) for treatment of resistant or refractory cytomegalovirus (CMV) infection in transplant recipients [abstract V-1256]. In: Programs and abstracts of the 49th Interscience Conference on Antimicrobial Agents and Chemotherapy (ICAAC). San Francisco, September 12–15, 2009.
116. Lischka P, Zimmermann H. Antiviral strategies to combat cytomegalovirus infections in transplant recipients. Curr Opin Pharmacol 2008;8(5):541–8.
117. Buerger I, Reefschlaeger J, Bender W, et al. A novel nonnucleoside inhibitor specifically targets cytomegalovirus DNA maturation via the UL89 and UL56 gene products. J Virol 2001;75(19):9077–86.
118. Ciesla SL, Trahan J, Wan WB, et al. Esterification of cidofovir with alkoxyalkanols increases oral bioavailability and diminishes drug accumulation in kidney. Antiviral Res 2003;59(3):163–71.
119. Quenelle DC, Collins DJ, Pettway LR, et al. Effect of oral treatment with (S)-HPMPA, HDP-(S)-HPMPA or ODE-(S)-HPMPA on replication of murine cytomegalovirus (MCMV) or human cytomegalovirus (HCMV) in animal models. Antiviral Res 2008;79(2):133–5.
120. Quenelle DC, Collins DJ, Wan WB, et al. Oral treatment of cowpox and vaccinia virus infections in mice with ether lipid esters of cidofovir. Antimicrob Agents Chemother 2004;48(2):404–12.
121. Kern ER, Bidanset DJ, Hartline CB, et al. Oral activity of a methylenecyclopropane analog, cyclopropavir, in animal models for cytomegalovirus infections. Antimicrob Agents Chemother 2004;48(12):4745–53.

122. Kern ER, Kushner NL, Hartline CB, et al. In vitro activity and mechanism of action of methylenecyclopropane analogs of nucleosides against herpesvirus replication. Antimicrob Agents Chemother 2005;49(3):1039–45.
123. Webster AC, Lee VW, Chapman JR, et al. Target of rapamycin inhibitors (TOR-I; sirolimus and everolimus) for primary immunosuppression in kidney transplant recipients. Cochrane Database Syst Rev 2006;(2):CD004290.
124. Hill JA, Hummel M, Starling RC, et al. A lower incidence of cytomegalovirus infection in de novo heart transplant recipients randomized to everolimus. Transplantation 2007;84(11):1436–42.
125. Kobashigawa JA, Miller LW, Russell SD, et al. Tacrolimus with mycophenolate mofetil (MMF) or sirolimus vs. cyclosporine with MMF in cardiac transplant patients: 1-year report. Am J Transplant 2006;6(6):1377–86.
126. Buchler M, Caillard S, Barbier S, et al. Sirolimus versus cyclosporine in kidney recipients receiving thymoglobulin, mycophenolate mofetil and a 6-month course of steroids. Am J Transplant 2007;7(11):2522–31.
127. Haririan A, Morawski K, West MS, et al. Sirolimus exposure during the early post-transplant period reduces the risk of CMV infection relative to tacrolimus in renal allograft recipients. Clin Transplant 2007;21(4):466–71.
128. Demopoulos L, Polinsky M, Steele G, et al. Reduced risk of cytomegalovirus infection in solid organ transplant recipients treated with sirolimus: a pooled analysis of clinical trials. Transplant Proc 2008;40(5):1407–10.
129. San Juan R, Aguado JM, Lumbreras C, et al. Impact of current transplantation management on the development of cytomegalovirus disease after renal transplantation. Clin Infect Dis 2008;47(7):875–82.
130. Cutler C, Kim HT, Hochberg E, et al. Sirolimus and tacrolimus without methotrexate as graft-versus-host disease prophylaxis after matched related donor peripheral blood stem cell transplantation. Biol Blood Marrow Transplant 2004;10(5):328–36.
131. Marty FM, Bryar J, Browne SK, et al. Sirolimus-based graft-versus-host disease prophylaxis protects against cytomegalovirus reactivation after allogeneic hematopoietic stem cell transplantation: a cohort analysis. Blood 2007;110(2):490–500.
132. Waldman WJ, Knight DA, Blinder L, et al. Inhibition of cytomegalovirus in vitro and in vivo by the experimental immunosuppressive agent leflunomide. Intervirology 1999;42(5–6):412–8.
133. Levi ME, Mandava N, Chan LK, et al. Treatment of multidrug-resistant cytomegalovirus retinitis with systemically administered leflunomide. Transpl Infect Dis 2006;8(1):38–43.
134. Battiwalla M, Paplham P, Almyroudis NG, et al. Leflunomide failure to control recurrent cytomegalovirus infection in the setting of renal failure after allogeneic stem cell transplantation. Transpl Infect Dis 2007;9(1):28–32.
135. Kaptein SJ, Efferth T, Leis M, et al. The anti-malaria drug artesunate inhibits replication of cytomegalovirus in vitro and in vivo. Antiviral Res 2006;69(2):60–9.
136. Efferth T, Romero MR, Wolf DG, et al. The antiviral activities of artemisinin and artesunate. Clin Infect Dis 2008;47(6):804–11.
137. Shapira MY, Resnick IB, Chou S, et al. Artesunate as a potent antiviral agent in a patient with late drug-resistant cytomegalovirus infection after hematopoietic stem cell transplantation. Clin Infect Dis 2008;46(9):1455–7.
138. Tung BY, Kowdley KV. Hepatitis B and liver transplantation. Clin Infect Dis 2005;41(10):1461–6.

139. Marzano A, Salizzoni M, Debernardi-Venon W, et al. Prevention of hepatitis B virus recurrence after liver transplantation in cirrhotic patients treated with lamivudine and passive immunoprophylaxis. J Hepatol 2001;34(6): 903–10.

140. Schiff ER, Lai CL, Hadziyannis S, et al. Adefovir dipivoxil therapy for lamivudine-resistant hepatitis B in pre- and post-liver transplantation patients. Hepatology 2003;38(6):1419–27.

141. Schiff E, Lai CL, Hadziyannis S, et al. Adefovir dipivoxil for wait-listed and post-liver transplantation patients with lamivudine-resistant hepatitis B: final long-term results. Liver Transpl 2007;13(3):349–60.

142. Wong DK, Yuen MF, Yuan H, et al. Quantitation of covalently closed circular hepatitis B virus DNA in chronic hepatitis B patients. Hepatology 2004;40(3): 727–37.

143. Moraleda G, Saputelli J, Aldrich CE, et al. Lack of effect of antiviral therapy in nondividing hepatocyte cultures on the closed circular DNA of woodchuck hepatitis virus. J Virol 1997;71(12):9392–9.

144. Keeffe EB, Dieterich DT, Han SH, et al. A treatment algorithm for the management of chronic hepatitis B virus infection in the United States: 2008 update. Clin Gastroenterol Hepatol 2008;6(12):1315–41 [quiz: 286].

145. Lok AS. How to diagnose and treat hepatitis B virus antiviral drug resistance in the liver transplant setting. Liver Transpl 2008;14(Suppl 2):S8–14.

146. Margeridon-Thermet S, Shulman NS, Ahmed A, et al. Ultra-deep pyrosequencing of hepatitis B virus quasispecies from nucleoside and nucleotide reverse-transcriptase inhibitor (NRTI)-treated patients and NRTI-naïve patients. J Infect Dis 2009;199(9):1275–85.

147. Gripon P, Rumin S, Urban S, et al. Infection of a human hepatoma cell line by hepatitis B virus. Proc Natl Acad Sci U S A 2002;99(24):15655–60.

148. Villet S, Billioud G, Pichoud C, et al. In vitro characterization of viral fitness of therapy-resistant hepatitis B variants. Gastroenterology 2009;136(1): 168–76, e2.

149. Zoulim F. In vitro models for studying hepatitis B virus drug resistance. Semin Liver Dis 2006;26(2):171–80.

150. Yuen MF, Fung J, Wong DK, et al. Prevention and management of drug resistance for antihepatitis B treatment. Lancet Infect Dis 2009;9(4):256–64.

151. Fung SK, Chae HB, Fontana RJ, et al. Virologic response and resistance to adefovir in patients with chronic hepatitis B. J Hepatol 2006;44(2):283–90.

152. Lai CL, Dienstag J, Schiff E, et al. Prevalence and clinical correlates of YMDD variants during lamivudine therapy for patients with chronic hepatitis B. Clin Infect Dis 2003;36(6):687–96.

153. Benhamou Y, Bochet M, Thibault V, et al. Long-term incidence of hepatitis B virus resistance to lamivudine in human immunodeficiency virus-infected patients. Hepatology 1999;30(5):1302–6.

154. Litwin S, Toll E, Jilbert AR, et al. The competing roles of virus replication and hepatocyte death rates in the emergence of drug-resistant mutants: theoretical considerations. J Clin Virol 2005;34(Suppl 1):S96–107.

155. Chang ML, Chien RN, Yeh CT, et al. Virus and transaminase levels determine the emergence of drug resistance during long-term lamivudine therapy in chronic hepatitis B. J Hepatol 2005;43(1):72–7.

156. Zoulim F, Poynard T, Degos F, et al. A prospective study of the evolution of lamivudine resistance mutations in patients with chronic hepatitis B treated with lamivudine. J Viral Hepat 2006;13(4):278–88.

157. Locarnini S, Warner N. Major causes of antiviral drug resistance and implications for treatment of hepatitis B virus monoinfection and coinfection with HIV. Antivir Ther 2007;12(Suppl 3):H15–23.

158. Lok AS, Lai CL, Leung N, et al. Long-term safety of lamivudine treatment in patients with chronic hepatitis B. Gastroenterology 2003;125(6):1714–22.

159. Hadziyannis SJ, Tassopoulos NC, Heathcote EJ, et al. Long-term therapy with adefovir dipivoxil for HBeAg-negative chronic hepatitis B for up to 5 years. Gastroenterology 2006;131(6):1743–51.

160. Tenney DJ, Rose RE, Baldick CJ, et al. Long-term monitoring shows hepatitis B virus resistance to entecavir in nucleoside-naïve patients is rare through 5 years of therapy. Hepatology 2009;49(5):1503–14.

161. Nguyen MH, Keeffe EB. Chronic hepatitis B: early viral suppression and long-term outcomes of therapy with oral nucleos(t)ides. J Viral Hepat 2009;16(3): 149–55.

162. Liaw YF, Gane E, Leung N, et al. 2-Year GLOBE trial results: telbivudine Is superior to lamivudine in patients with chronic hepatitis B. Gastroenterology 2009; 136(2):486–95.

163. Lee YS, Suh DJ, Lim YS, et al. Increased risk of adefovir resistance in patients with lamivudine-resistant chronic hepatitis B after 48 weeks of adefovir dipivoxil monotherapy. Hepatology 2006;43(6):1385–91.

164. Das K, Xiong X, Yang H, et al. Molecular modeling and biochemical characterization reveal the mechanism of hepatitis B virus polymerase resistance to lamivudine (3TC) and emtricitabine (FTC). J Virol 2001;75(10):4771–9.

165. Sharon A, Chu CK. Understanding the molecular basis of HBV drug resistance by molecular modeling. Antiviral Res 2008;80(3):339–53.

166. Allen MI, Deslauriers M, Andrews CW, et al. Identification and characterization of mutations in hepatitis B virus resistant to lamivudine. Lamivudine Clinical Investigation Group. Hepatology 1998;27(6):1670–7.

167. Villet S, Pichoud C, Billioud G, et al. Impact of hepatitis B virus rtA181V/T mutants on hepatitis B treatment failure. J Hepatol 2008;48(5):747–55.

168. Delaney WE 4th, Yang H, Westland CE, et al. The hepatitis B virus polymerase mutation rtV173L is selected during lamivudine therapy and enhances viral replication in vitro. J Virol 2003;77(21):11833–41.

169. Yang H, Qi X, Sabogal A, et al. Cross-resistance testing of next-generation nucleoside and nucleotide analogues against lamivudine-resistant HBV. Antivir Ther 2005;10(5):625–33.

170. Angus P, Vaughan R, Xiong S, et al. Resistance to adefovir dipivoxil therapy associated with the selection of a novel mutation in the HBV polymerase. Gastroenterology 2003;125(2):292–7.

171. Fung SK, Andreone P, Han SH, et al. Adefovir-resistant hepatitis B can be associated with viral rebound and hepatic decompensation. J Hepatol 2005;43(6): 937–43.

172. Yang H, Westland C, Xiong S, et al. In vitro antiviral susceptibility of full-length clinical hepatitis B virus isolates cloned with a novel expression vector. Antiviral Res 2004;61(1):27–36.

173. Kobashi H, Fujioka S, Kawaguchi M, et al. Two cases of development of entecavir resistance during entecavir treatment for nucleoside-naïve chronic hepatitis B. Hepatol Int 2009;3(2):403–10.

174. Tenney DJ, Levine SM, Rose RE, et al. Clinical emergence of entecavir-resistant hepatitis B virus requires additional substitutions in virus already resistant to Lamivudine. Antimicrob Agents Chemother 2004;48(9):3498–507.

175. Langley DR, Walsh AW, Baldick CJ, et al. Inhibition of hepatitis B virus polymerase by entecavir. J Virol 2007;81(8):3992–4001.

176. Tenney DJ, Rose RE, Baldick CJ, et al. Two-year assessment of entecavir resistance in Lamivudine-refractory hepatitis B virus patients reveals different clinical outcomes depending on the resistance substitutions present. Antimicrob Agents Chemother 2007;51(3):902–11.

177. Marcellin P, Heathcote EJ, Buti M, et al. Tenofovir disoproxil fumarate versus adefovir dipivoxil for chronic hepatitis B. N Engl J Med 2008;359(23):2442–55.

178. Sheldon J, Camino N, Rodes B, et al. Selection of hepatitis B virus polymerase mutations in HIV-coinfected patients treated with tenofovir. Antivir Ther 2005;10(6):727–34.

179. Delaney WE, Ray AS, Yang H, et al. Intracellular metabolism and in vitro activity of tenofovir against hepatitis B virus. Antimicrob Agents Chemother 2006;50(7): 2471–7.

180. Fung S, Mazzulli T, Sherman M, et al. Presence of rtA194T at baseline does not reduce efficacy to tenofovir (TDF) in patients with lamivudine (LAM)-resistant chronic hepatitis B. In: Programs and abstracts of the 58th Annual Meeting of the American Association for the Study of Liver Disease (AASLD). San Francisco, October 31–November 4, 2008 [abstract: 880].

181. Markowitz JS, Martin P, Conrad AJ, et al. Prophylaxis against hepatitis B recurrence following liver transplantation using combination lamivudine and hepatitis B immune globulin. Hepatology 1998;28(2):585–9.

182. Gane EJ, Angus PW, Strasser S, et al. Lamivudine plus low-dose hepatitis B immunoglobulin to prevent recurrent hepatitis B following liver transplantation. Gastroenterology 2007;132(3):931–7.

183. Angus PW, Patterson SJ, Strasser SI, et al. A randomized study of adefovir dipivoxil in place of HBIG in combination with lamivudine as post-liver transplantation hepatitis B prophylaxis. Hepatology 2008;48(5):1460–6.

184. Bock CT, Tillmann HL, Torresi J, et al. Selection of hepatitis B virus polymerase mutants with enhanced replication by lamivudine treatment after liver transplantation. Gastroenterology 2002;122(2):264–73.

185. Fournier C, Zoulim F. Antiviral therapy of chronic hepatitis B: prevention of drug resistance. Clin Liver Dis 2007;11(4):869–92, ix.

186. Lampertico P, Vigano M, Manenti E, et al. Adefovir rapidly suppresses hepatitis B in HBeAg-negative patients developing genotypic resistance to lamivudine. Hepatology 2005;42(6):1414–9.

187. Fung J, Lai CL, Yuen JC, et al. Adefovir dipivoxil monotherapy and combination therapy with lamivudine for the treatment of chronic hepatitis B in an Asian population. Antivir Ther 2007;12(1):41–6.

188. van Bommel F, Wunsche T, Mauss S, et al. Comparison of adefovir and tenofovir in the treatment of lamivudine-resistant hepatitis B virus infection. Hepatology 2004;40(6):1421–5.

189. Sherman M, Yurdaydin C, Sollano J, et al. Entecavir for treatment of lamivudine-refractory, HBeAg-positive chronic hepatitis B. Gastroenterology 2006;130(7): 2039–49.

190. Seifer M, Patty A, Serra I, et al. Telbivudine, a nucleoside analog inhibitor of HBV polymerase, has a different in vitro cross-resistance profile than the nucleotide analog inhibitors adefovir and tenofovir. Antiviral Res 2009;81(2):147–55.

191. Villeneuve JP, Durantel D, Durantel S, et al. Selection of a hepatitis B virus strain resistant to adefovir in a liver transplantation patient. J Hepatol 2003;39(6): 1085–9.

192. Yim HJ, Hussain M, Liu Y, et al. Evolution of multi-drug resistant hepatitis B virus during sequential therapy. Hepatology 2006;44(3):703–12.
193. Brunelle MN, Jacquard AC, Pichoud C, et al. Susceptibility to antivirals of a human HBV strain with mutations conferring resistance to both lamivudine and adefovir. Hepatology 2005;41(6):1391–8.
194. Fung SK, Fontana RJ. Management of drug-resistant chronic hepatitis B. Clin Liver Dis 2006;10(2):275–302, viii.
195. Trojan J, Stuermer M, Teuber G, et al. Treatment of patients with lamivudine-resistant and adefovir dipivoxil-resistant chronic hepatitis B virus infection: is tenofovir the answer? Gut 2007;56(3):436–7 [author reply: 37].
196. Yatsuji H, Hiraga N, Mori N, et al. Successful treatment of an entecavir-resistant hepatitis B virus variant. J Med Virol 2007;79(12):1811–7.
197. Villet S, Ollivet A, Pichoud C, et al. Stepwise process for the development of entecavir resistance in a chronic hepatitis B virus infected patient. J Hepatol 2007; 46(3):531–8.
198. Gish RG, Trinh H, Leung N, et al. Safety and antiviral activity of emtricitabine (FTC) for the treatment of chronic hepatitis B infection: a two-year study. J Hepatol 2005;43(1):60–6.

Index

Note: Page numbers of article titles are in **boldface** type.

A

Aceintobacter spp., HAP due to, 645–646

Aging, of TB patient population, 751–754. See also *Tuberculosis (TB), in global aging population.*

Alveolar echinococcosis, pulmonary, cestodes and, 593

Amebiasis, pulmonary, 580–582

Ancylostomiasis, pulmonary, nematodes and, 585–586

Antibiotic(s), for influenza virus infections, 612

Antibody(ies), human monoclonal, for SARS, 626–627

Antigen detection, in respiratory infections, emerging advances in, 792–793

Antiviral drug resistance, **809–833.** See also specific disorders, e.g., *Herpesviruses, antiviral drug resistance in.*

    future directions in, 821

    in CMV, 813–817

    in HBV, 817–821

    in herpesviruses, 809–811

    in HSV, 811–812

    in VZV, 812–813

Ascariasis, pulmonary, nematodes and, 584–585

Aspergillus spp., in transplantation, 544 545

Avian influenza A (H5N1) virus, 605

    clinical presentation of, 608

B

Babesiosis, pulmonary, 583

Bacteria

    drug-resistant, respiratory infections due to, **639–653.** See also specific infections and *Respiratory infections.*

    nontuberculous, described, 769

Bacterial respiratory infections, emerging, in transplantation, 542–544

    Myobacterium abscessus, 543–544

    Nocardia spp., 542–544

    Rhodococcus equi, 544

Blastomycosis, 560, 563, 565–566

Breath analysis, in respiratory infections, emerging advances in, 800–801

Bronchiectasis, nodular, 775–776

C

CAP. See *Community-acquired pneumonia (CAP).*

Cestodes, pulmonary diseases due to, 589–593

Infect Dis Clin N Am 24 (2010) 835–844

doi:10.1016/S0891-5520(10)00051-6

0891-5520/10/$ – see front matter © 2010 Elsevier Inc. All rights reserved.

id.theclinics.com